Ovarian Carcinoma

Etiology, Diagnosis, and Treatment

Hugh R. K. Barber, M. D.

Director, Department of Obstetrics and Gynecology
Lenox Hill Hospital
New York, New York

Clinical Professor of Obstetrics and Gynecology
Cornell Medical College
New York, New York

Attending Surgeon Gynecological Service
Memorial Hospital
New York, New York

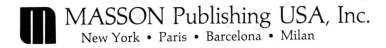 MASSON Publishing USA, Inc.
New York • Paris • Barcelona • Milan

Dedication

To my sister, Mary Cecelia Barber Nugent, and her late husband Joseph, my nieces Elizabeth Ann, Ellen, and Mary Hugh; to Bridget (Bridie) Flavin McGuire, her husband Patrick, and their children Ann Marie and Hugh John.

Acknowledgment

I am grateful to Margaret Ryon Uibel of the Department of Medical Photography, Lenox Hill Hospital, for the preparation of illustrations.

Foreword

The story of ovarian cancer is complex because many types of cancers develop from the ovary. While the individual types have distinctive clinical characteristics and pathologic features, they are often not identified adequately during treatment. This is due in part to the lack of a well-written monograph on ovarian cancer. Dr. Barber has mastered the conglomeration of facts known currently about ovarian cancer and presents them in a direct, very readable and learnable manner. While he has not unraveled the often conflicting literature which is snarled because many authors have composited their data and grouped various histologic types together when reporting clinical experiences in ovarian cancer, the references used by the author are ample and wisely chosen. However, he has not attempted to review the literature on each type of ovarian cancer in presenting this overall story. To do so is unnecessary and would have produced confusing and burdensome reading because much of the literature about cancer of the ovary is clinically useless. Fortunately, the author bypasses this jumble to present comprehensive information based on current data and knowledge, much of which is from his own experience.

This is a book of facts, useful for a range of physicians. Medical students will be pleased with the uncluttered presentation about the where, why, and how of detection, diagnosis, and management. For the clinicians, the recommendations for diagnostic procedures and guidelines for studying patients suspected of having ovarian cancer will be appreciated. The standard treatment methods outlined will be valuable information for any physician who treats women. The resident will find new understanding about facts he already knows for the author presents liberal background information. The gynecologic oncologist will find a well-organized base for building additional knowledge of this disease. The nongynecologic physician has a ready reference in this book.

The facts are organized in chapters arranged in conventional order dealing with the most basic aspects of the disease first and concluding with the more current data such as treatment methods. The chapters presenting epidemiology, pathology, clinical features, treatment by surgery, x-ray and chemotherapy are the longest; the shorter chapters deal with subjects about which there is less information such as the postmenopausal palpable ovary, tumor marker substances, treatment by radioisotopes, second look operations, etc. With this arrangement, the book provides a ready reference for the busy physician who may selectively read about topics of immediate concern. At the same time, information provided in this book is readable in its entirety.

There is little controversy discussed, and consequently the author teaches with clear, direct statements. The reader's comprehension is further assisted by statements in the opening of each chapter telling what to expect. In the first paragraph of each chapter, the contents are outlined briefly and sources of material quoted. Often the author's own publications are the source. At the end of each chapter the author summarizes briefly what the preceding material was about, emphasizing the important points.

Since Dr. Barber is an accomplished gynecologic oncologist, his professional career dedicated to this specialty, we can be confident that we are reading the best information currently available. We can feel secure that selection of material has been tempered with his extensive clinical experience in treating patients and his research in this disease. While the author's pessimism about reducing the annual mortality for ovarian cancer is realistic, there is still a great opportunity to improve management with our currently available tools. For example, little is being done to identify the high-risk patients through genetic surveillance; currently many patients believed to have early stage disease are not receiving postoperative x-ray therapy or chemotherapy promptly; there is confusion about which patient should have x-ray and which chemotherapy; thus, time is lost and patients' prescribed. Too often the surgeon does not accomplish maximum resection because of timidity or inadequate understanding. Correcting this situation is a high-priority goal among gynecologic oncologists, and this book will make a valuable contribution towards improving the treatment of this disease.

This book is long overdue. It will contribute significantly toward a better knowledge of this disease among all physicians who see women. Such knowledge is of great importance, for the symptoms of ovarian cancer may simulate those more typical of other abdominal organ systems. An awareness will speed the discovery at an earlier stage.

Felix Rutledge, M.D.
Head, Department of Gynecology
M.D. Anderson Hospital and Tumor Institute
Houston, Texas 77030

Preface

When the American Board of Obstetrics and Gynecology established the Division of Gynecologic Oncology, it recognized the increasing importance of special knowledge areas, techniques, and skills within the discipline of obstetrics and gynecology.

With the exception of ovarian cancer patients, most women having a gynecologic malignancy today can be cured with good treatment.

On the basis of the Third National Cancer Survey data about 1.4%, or 1 of every 70 newborn girls, will develop cancer of the ovary at sometime during their lives.

The definition of a cancer of the ovary is difficult because of the diversity of histogenetic types of cancer originating in the ovary. It has been and is considered a family of malignancies. The ovary is complex in its embryology, histology, steroidogenesis, and potential for malignancy. It is made up of germ cells, gonadal stromal cells, as well as mesothelial cells. Each has its own potential to form a tumor. The ovary is unique in that it not only gives rise to a great variety of malignancies, but is itself a favorite site for metastases from many other organs.

Ovarian cancer is *now* the leading cause of death from gynecologic cancers in the United States. It is anticipated that there will be 17,000 new cases in 1977 and 11,000 deaths from ovarian cancer. The results of therapy in 1976 were no better than in the previous two decades.

The management of patients with ovarian cancer presents a constant challenge to the clinician. This challenge is reflected not so much in the incidence of the disease (25% of gynecologic cancers), but rather in its high mortality rates (44% of all deaths from cancers of the genital tract). Thus, while 10 of every 1,000 women in the United States over age 40 will develop ovarian cancer, only 1 or 2 will be cured. The remainder will suffer repeated bouts of intestinal obstruction as the tumor spreads over the surface of the bowel; they will develop inanition, malnutrition, and literally vomit to death. This pathology, described as carcinomatosis ileus, is one of the few indications for the intermittent use of a nasogastric tube as definitive therapy to decompress the bowel. Those therapeutic nihilists who plead that patients should be left to "die with dignity" must face a dilemma when forced to apply their philosophy to the care of women with advanced ovarian cancer.

Because cancer of the ovary is such a frustrating problem for the clinician, I have attempted to assimilate in a concise form the prevailing opinions as an overview to ovarian cancer. I hope I have achieved this goal without being superficial.

Each chapter has a conclusion which not only covers pertinent material presented but includes ideas not covered in the chapter. A glossary and an index follow the last chapter. The glossary was included to define terms discussed in the text and to provide a ready reference for those pursuing the subject in more detail in other articles and textbooks.

The references at the end of each chapter are not meant to cover the entire field; they have been selected for their historical value or because they represent an original or significant contribution. In general, the references consist principally of recent articles, reviews, monographs, and books. The book has been developed from these sources.

I want to express my appreciation to Dr. Sheldon C. Sommers for the help he has given me in this undertaking. He has been particularly helpful in selecting material to illustrate histologic and nuclear grading as well as stromal reactions.

Dr. Margaret Long has kindly supplied illustrations and material from her large collection of photographs of ovarian tumors.

For taking time from a busy schedule which includes practice, research, teaching, lecturing, and administrative duties, I am most grateful to Dr. Felix Rutledge for reading the text and writing the foreword.

As always, I am very grateful to Marcia Miller for her help in writing this book. I have relied on her for her skilled typing, for locating and xeroxing articles, for making suggestions, and most important, for assisting me with her editorial expertise. These contributions lightened my burden and allowed me to concentrate on writing this book.

I am appreciative of the help and support of the entire Lenox Hill family—doctors, nurses, paramedics, librarians, administrators, and trustees. The house staff on obstetrics and gynecology at Lenox Hill Hospital has been most helpful with their suggestions and the stimulation that they supplied through their interest.

To Masson Publishing Company and to Alan Frankenfield, I want to express my appreciation for their suggestions and encouragement, and for the opportunity to bring this material to my colleagues.

Much of the work on which this book is based was supported by the John C. Kilroe Memorial Fund.

To my wife Mary Louise, family, and friends, I owe deep thanks for their patience and help in writing this book.

Friends, relatives, doctors, and nurses share my hope that this book will help those unfortunate women who develop ovarian cancer.

Contents

1

Introduction

The purpose of this book is to collect in a single volume pertinent material about ovarian malignancy which is either new or in which there has been a change in traditional concepts in terms of contemporary findings and knowledge. To accomplish this, it was necessary first to identify the problems associated with ovarian cancer, then to suggest solutions in light of the present phase of medical development. This chapter identifies problems related to ovarian cancer but does not discuss them in detail. The detailed discussion will be included in the appropriate chapters.

It is my hope that the information collected and presented here will satisfy the goals of this book as well as suggest new avenues of meeting the constant challenge presented by ovarian cancer. More than 10,800 women die from ovarian cancer each year, and the results in 1976 were no better than those of the previous two decades.

INCIDENCE

Cancers of the ovary account for roughly 5% of all cancers in women reported by the Third National Cancer Survey. Only cancers of the skin, breast, colon and rectum, uterus, and lung account for more new cases of female cancer than cancer of the ovary. Each year about 14 women per 100,000, 1.4%, are diagnosed with ovarian cancers. One of every 70 newborn girls will develop cancer of the ovary sometime during her life. It is estimated that in 1977 there will be 17,000 new cases of cancer of the ovary.

The age-specific incidence rates for ovarian cancer rise steadily up to age 80, then they drop off slightly in the older ages. It is obvious that the ovary gets too old to function, but never gets too old to form a cancer. By applying these rates to the estimated population for 1975, it is possible to determine the distribution of cases by age. The greatest number of cases is found in the age groups 50–54 and 55–59 years. The mean age was 62.3 while the median age was 59.0.

The trends by age through the years have shown that the age-adjusted rate for all ages has remained about the same throughout the period from 1940 to 1975. All age groups have generally shown the same trend as the all-ages rates, except age group 25–34, in which there has been a slight decrease through the years.

From 1940 to 1969, at least half of the patients whose ovary was the primary cancer site were found to have distant metastases. Data from the last period, 1965–1969, indicate that an additional 10% of the cases were considered to have distant disease, while the proportion of patients with regional involvement, which held steady at 17% from 1950 through 1964, dropped to 7%. A shift of this type may result from a change in diagnostic procedures. The percentage of patients with localized disease has hovered at about 28% for a long time.

There have been slight decreases in survival rates for all patients and for those with regional disease in the years 1965–1969. In contrast, survival rates for patients with distant metastases have been increasing; the 3-year rate increased from 9% in 1950–1959 to 16% in 1965–1969. This improvement may reflect a shift in stage classification.

MORTALITY

Deaths from cancer of the ovary have increased from 10,002 in 1973 to 10,800 in 1975. It is estimated that in 1977 there will be 11,000 deaths (Figure 1). The mean age was 63.3 years and the median age was 63.7. The observed median survival time by age from 1955 to 1964 was 1.4 years for all ages, 5.4 years under age 45, 1.8 years from 45 to 54, 1.3 years from 55 to 64, 0.9 years from 65 to 74, and 0.8 years over age 74. Common epithelial ovarian cancers are more frequent in older women. Consequently, the relatively favorable median survival at diagnosis for women under 45 reflects the sur-

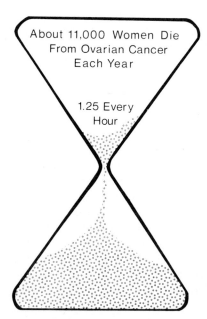

Figure 1.   Ovarian cancer is the leading cause of death from gynecologic cancer.

vival experience of only 17% of all patients. For older women it is important to compare the observed and relative survival rates. The poor results are not nearly as dreary when the observed survival rate is compared to the relative survival rate. For women diagnosed with localized disease, the age gradient is relatively weak.

Cancer of the ovary is the fifth leading cause of *cancer* death in women and is *the leading cause of death from gynecologic cancer.* In the age groups from 30–34 to 65–69 years, cancer of the ovary is the third or the fourth leading cause of death. Among women who are 75 and older, cancer of the ovary is at least the ninth leading cause of cancer death.

The death rates by age for cancer of the ovary increase steadily as the population at risk gets older, until age 70–74, after which there is a slight decline. The nonwhite rates are lower than the white rates in each age group over 20 years. The rates for all ages in white females went slowly and steadily up through the years. The rates for ages over 55 have generally shown an increasing trend. The trends in age-standardized death rates for major sites show that the rate for the ovary is increasing.

STAGE AT DIAGNOSIS

In most reported series, ovarian cancer when first diagnosed is in stages III and IV in about 60 to 80% of the cases. The End Results Section of the National Cancer Institute has reported that the proportion of cases diagnosed with distant metastases has continued to increase since the early 1950s, after a decrease from the 1940s cases to the 1950s cases. After increasing from the 1940s cases to the 1950s cases, the proportion of cases with regional involvement has continued to decrease since the 1950s. The number of cases diagnosed as localized remained approximately the same until recently, when there was a slight decrease. The distribution by stage is now almost the same for blacks and whites.

TREATMENT

The extent of disease or stage for each ovarian cancer patient seems to be the main determinant in choice of therapy. A surgical attack is considered the backbone of therapy, either to completely eradicate the disease or to debulk the cancer. The End Results in Cancer report number 4 reveals that surgery alone was the most frequently used treatment for patients with localized disease diagnosed during 1955 to 1964, but the favorable survival rates for such patients given chemotherapy in addition to surgery seem to have guided clinicians in choosing this combination therapy almost as often as surgery alone in 1965–1969. For patients with regional disease, surgery plus radiation was used most often in the earlier period, but in 1965–1969 the addition of chemotherapy to surgery plus radiation was used as frequently as the earlier treatment. Although survival rates are extremely poor for patients with distant metastases, the use of chemotherapy in combination with surgery seems to yield more favorable results. Currently, radiation is being chosen for a highly selected indication which will be discussed later.

SURVIVAL

The survival rate in 1976 was only slightly better than it was in the previous two decades. This may reflect better management of the complications, earlier cases, and the judicious use of chemotherapy. The overall 5-year survival rate in most series of patients with invasive common epithelial ovarian cancer runs between 15 and 35%.

PERTINENT CONSIDERATIONS

Embryology

Ovarian cancer has been considered as a family of malignancies within the ovary rather than as a single entity. The ovary is complex in its embryology, histology, steroidogenesis, and potential for malignancy. It is made up of germ cells, gonadal stromal cells, and cells of the mesenchymal tissue, each with its own potential to form a tumor. Although sex is determined genetically at fertilization, the ovary passes through its early phases as an indifferent organ with parallel development that could allow it to become an ovary or a testis. Alternations or imbalances during these steps of development may provide the setting for later cellular malfunctioning that produces endocrine imbalances as well as malignancy. The ovary is unique in that it not only gives rise to a great variety of malignancies, but is itself a favorite site for metastases from many other organs.

Phylogenic Development

A review of the phylogenic development as well as the comparative anatomy of the ovary seems indicated in a study devoted to ovarian cancer. It is hoped that a clue might be found that could serve as the Rosetta stone for unravelling the mystery of new growths in the ovary. There are many interesting reports of work that has been done in this field. A brief summary of these condensed reports is incorporated in this discussion.

The protozoan genera plasmodium reproduces, but it is not until the metazoan genera is reached that an identifiable ovary makes its appearance. The female vertebrate species have ovaries, and the process of fertilization becomes more complex.

The ovaries in the bird are interesting in that the left develops into an adult form while the right atrophies (Figure 2). Among fowl the most common spontaneous tumors are lymphosarcoma, leukemia, carcinoma of the ovary, and adenocarcinoma of the intestine. Generally, ovarian tumors affect most species of mammals and birds. Ovarian tumors that develop spontaneously in these animals are epithelial tumors and resemble those found in

COMPARATIVE ANATOMY: CHICKEN

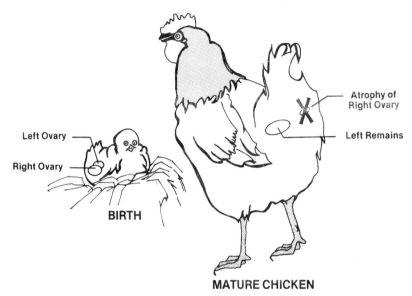

Atrophy of
Right Ovary

Left Remains

Left Ovary

Right Ovary

BIRTH

MATURE CHICKEN

Figure 2.   In birds and chickens the left ovary and oviduct develop to maturity, and the organs on the right side atrophy. Adenocarcinomas and cystadenocarcinomas reported in birds are histologically similar to those found in humans.

the human. However, artificially produced ovarian cancers are always of the granulosa cell tumor type.

It is interesting that one of the most common solid tumors in the bird is carcinoma of the ovary. The peculiar postnatal course of the ovary in the bird makes the problem doubly interesting. Whether there is an abnormal steroidogenesis or a faulty feedback mechanism is difficult to ascertain from the literature. Transferring animal data to interpret a process in the human is fraught with danger, but still there are areas that supply a common ground for consideration. Because ovarian cancer is difficult to diagnose and so deadly in its prognosis, every avenue of approach must be thoroughly investigated.

Conservation or Prophylaxis

Although cancer of the cervix is the most common malignancy in the female pelvis, ovarian cancer is now the leading cause of death from gynecologic malignancy. Six or 7 women in each 100 will require surgery for an ovarian cyst or tumor during their lifetime. One woman in 100 over age 40 will develop a malignancy of the ovary, or to put it another way, 9 or 10 women in each 1,000 will develop a malignancy and only 1 or 2 will be cured. Randall and Hall have reported that about 30 women in 100,000 will develop ovarian cancer before age 45, and that the rate increases to 281 per 100,000 between ages 45 and 60 years. Eight of each 9 malignancies of the ovary develop after the patient's 50th birthday. The ovary may be too old to function, but it is never too old to form a cancer. The reports by Randall cover a period when ovarian cancer was not the serious problem it is today.

A report by Gibbs is more current and documents the problem in a very precise manner. From 1949 to 1969, 236 cases of ovarian cancer were seen at the Butterworth Hospital in Grand Rapids, Michigan. Of these cases, 85.6% had their onset in women over 41. Sixty-nine percent of the ovarian cancers were in stages III and IV. The overall 5-year survival for all stages was 15.7%. Previous operations had been performed in 126 patients. Twenty-eight patients had prior hysterectomies. The expected incidence of ovarian carcinoma following hysterectomy was observed. Ovarian cancer may develop in patients having prior irradiation to the ovaries and breast or gastrointestinal malignancy. Gibbs suggested that a radical approach to pelvic operation (hysterectomy and bilateral salpingo-oophorectomy) beyond age 35 could prevent 20% of all ovarian carcinoma seen.

Barber and Graber have reported an early sign of ovarian cancer that has been most valuable in diagnosis, the postmenopausal palpable ovary (PMPO) syndrome. Simply stated, the palpation of *what is interpreted as a normal sized ovary in the premenopausal woman, represents an ovarian tumor in the postmenopausal woman.* This does not imply that anything palpated in the adnexal area is abnormal, because in certain very thin and relaxed women small atrophic ovaries may be felt. However patients with the PMPO syndrome should not be followed and reevaluated; the presence or absence of an ovarian tumor must be determined promptly. To save more women and diminish the mortality from ovarian cancer, more liberal indications for operation must be accepted. Waiting until one feels a solid tumor mass of up to 5 cm in size and then expecting a cure is an exercise in fancy and futility. As in other cancers, early diagnosis is the most effective way to increase survival rates among women with ovarian cancer. These figures have a sobering effect and emphasize the responsibility shouldered by physicians who are charged with the care of women. Constant vigilance and reevaluation must be pursued.

Early Diagnosis, Treatment, and Terminal Care

The problem of ovarian cancer is best divided into three primary categories—early diagnosis, treatment, and terminal care of patients with advanced or recurrent cancer.

Since it is almost impossible to diagnose ovarian cancer in its early stages, it is impossible to treat it with any predictable degree of certainty for cure. With the present state of knowledge, early diagnosis is the key to successful treatment. The logical question, then, is how can we insure early diagnosis? A high degree of suspicion reinforced by knowledge of the natural history of ovarian cancer is important. Early ovarian cancer is a disease found more often in the community hospitals than in the large medical centers. In cases in which cancer is diagnosed in its early stage, it is considered a surgical disease. The standard treatment is total hysterectomy, bilateral salpingo-oophorectomy, and in some instances omentectomy. There has not been any significant study which clearly demonstrates that removal of the omentum is desirable or necessary. The arguments advanced for its removal are that it may contain microscopic cancer and that the cancer is then in a more advanced stage. In addition, after removal any instilled radioactive substance is better able to come in contact with the peritoneum and therefore to provide better control of ascites. Treatment is covered in detail in other chapters of this book.

OVARIAN TUMORS IN CHILDREN

Ovarian tumors comprise about 1% of all new growths in the field of pediatric gynecology. The problem of diagnosis is surpassed only by the problem and confusion about treatment. In this age group it is difficult to accept the diagnosis of ovarian cancer, and even more difficult for the physician to carry out surgery that will deprive a child of her reproductive potential. Fortunately, more than one-third of ovarian tumors in children are benign cystic teratomas. At Lenox Hill Hospital from 1961 through 1967 there were 12 children with an ovarian cyst and all proved to be benign. This problem can be handled by simple excision of the cyst with preservation of that ovary in most instances. Dysgerminomas and solid teratomas have been found in children more frequently than in later life.

In general, the types of ovarian tumors seen in children are not too dissimilar from those in adults. Therapy must be tailored to the patient and the extent of disease. A malignancy that has spread beyond the ovary should receive radical extirpative therapy. If there is any doubt about the type of tumor or whether it is malignant it is better to do a salpingo-oophorectomy on the side of the tumor if the tumor has an intact capsule and is freely movable. If the tumor proves to be highly malignant, the abdomen may be opened and the remaining reproductive organs excised if this appears to be the best course. In certain low-grade malignancies the previously performed treatment may be considered sufficient to insure a cure.

EFFECT OF SPILL

Often the question is raised of how the prognosis is affected by a rupture of the cyst or tumor which results in spill. The smooth, freely movable cyst which is ruptured accidentally as a result of poor technique or a thin wall will probably have little unfavorable effect on prognosis. The exception may be the mucinous cyst. The nature of the fluid content varies from a stringy, sticky, mucoid secretion to one with the consistency of wet glue. The gelatinous material is tenacious and sticks to everything it touches. It is this adhesive property that creates the pseudomyxoma peritonei sometimes described after rupture or spillage from the cyst. However a poor prognosis can be anticipated with rupture in the presence of a soft vascular ovarian tumor which is densely adherent and directly infiltrating. It is obvious that this poor prognosis is not due solely to the rupture of the cyst, but rather to advanced stage of the disease.

ROLE OF NODE DISSECTION

Should a node dissection be part of planned definitive therapy? The consensus of opinion is that it should not. A survey of its usual spread when the nodes are involved indicates why there has been little enthusiasm for a node dissection in ovarian cancer. The iliac nodes are involved about one-quarter as often as in cancer of the cervix or about 7%. The usual nodal spread is to the upper abdomen. Because the ovary embryologically arises at about T10, it is not surprising that the retroperitoneal nodes in the upper abdomen located around the duodenum, kidney, and celiac axis are involved. From here, the spread advances to the mediastinal and then the supraclavicular areas. Retrograde extension to the inguinal nodes is very infrequent. The natural history of the disease contraindicates a node dissection in most instances.

RADIOACTIVE SUBSTANCES

After all gross disease tissue is removed, a decision must be made about the instillation of radioactive phosphorus (P^{32}). Impressive as the results have been at the Memorial Hospital in the early stages of cancer, most series have not been able to confirm their results. In the presence of positive cells in the pelvis, however, or perhaps after the rupture of a cyst, it may have therapeutic value. Since P^{32} emits only beta rays, it causes very little bowel reaction, whereas the gamma rays of radioactive gold have been associated with late bowel necrosis. The greatest benefit of radioactive substances is in controlling ascites. Their main contribution is their use as palliatives. When nodules are 2 cm or larger, palliation can not be anticipated.

PROPHYLACTIC THERAPY

Guidelines for the use of prophylactic radiation when all gross tumor has been removed are sought constantly. The value of prophylactic radiation cannot be established from a survey of the literature. It has been recommended, however, that radiation therapy be given in highly anaplastic cancers or if there is ascites with positive cells, rupture of a cyst, any question about the complete removal of the tumor, excrescence on the surface of the ovary, or difficulty in establishing planes of dissection. It is reported that a recurrence is biologically more potent, and maximum therapy should be attempted to prevent one. With dysgerminoma that is histologically and serologically proved by a negative pregnancy test, local paraaortic radiation is advisable. Increasing knowledge of the natural history of common epithelial ovarian cancer and the limitation of radiation therapy in controlling ovarian cancer have stimulated an interest in chemotherapy. The plan is to use prophylactic chemotherapy in stages I and II when the disease has been removed, and therapeutically in stages III and IV when the disease persists.

WIDESPREAD DISEASE

When the abdomen is opened and widespread disease has been found, should as much cancer as possible be removed? Graham feels that the tumor mass should be recorded as a percentage and that unless 90% can be removed, the surgical attack should be abandoned and some other therapeutic modality chosen. The consensus of opinion, however, is that as much cancer as possible should be removed without violating good surgical and clinical judgment. Since ovarian cancer is known to spread to the upper abdomen and rarely remains confined to the pelvis, it only lends itself to pelvic exenteration if it violates its natural history.

TERMINAL OVARIAN CANCER

The patient with recurrent and far-advanced cancer presents a real challenge. A balance must be struck between doing too much and doing too little. Therapy should be aimed at relieving symptoms. Since the patient undoubtedly has had several modalities of therapy, including surgery, additional surgery should be reserved for the relief of an intestinal obstruction, drainage of an abscess, or relief from a fistula. Indeed, most of the symptoms arise from the intestine and the problem is best managed by a physician trained in gastrointestinal surgery.

The patient with advanced or recurrent ovarian cancer presents a characteristic clinical picture of inanition and malnutrition. The abdomen is greatly distended while the extremities are thin, giving the impression that the bones are covered with skin without any intervening muscle tissue. The muscle and fat are missing from the hands, resulting in a skeleton-like appearance. The fat has been lost from around the face and the patient seems to have a sardonic smile. The tissue around the eyes has atrophied and the eyeballs appear sunken. The clinical picture is not unlike that associated with the advanced starvation of Nazi concentration camp victims made famous by stories and in pictures (Figure 3). Often spot radiation therapy can be given to the terminal patient to relieve pain. In addition, wisely administered chemotherapy may also achieve palliation. Because the goal is palliative, toxicity must be avoided.

STEROIDOGENESIS IN OVARIAN TUMORS

There has long been a feeling that the finding of abnormal steroidogenesis might supply a key to early diagnosis and management of ovarian cancer, but to date there has been no concrete evidence to support this concept.

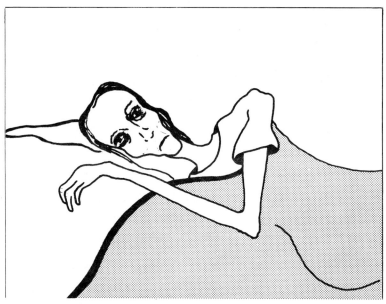

Figure 3. The patient with advanced or recurrent ovarian cancer often has a distended abdomen, atrophic extremities, and loss of facial fat. They are often ravenously hungry, but one bite of food induces marked vomiting.

Cholesterol is considered the keystone upon which steroids are built up from acetate, and for steroid synthesis, endogenous cholesterol is considered the important factor. Preformed cholesterol is reported to play a minor role, but this contention has been challenged. Short has suggested that a higher nutritional plane increases multiple ovulation, which in turn enhances the production of estrogen and progesterone, an effect mediated through the pituitary. The process of steroidogenesis in the adrenal, testis, and ovary is the same up to the point of progesterone formation. At this point the three glands complete the synthesis of their steroids along individual patterns. Androstenedione and testosterone are synthesized as final steps before estrone and estradiol are produced as the main steroids of the ovary. Anything that disturbs the delicate balance of the pituitary-ovarian axis could alter the final step in the formation of estrogens and thus cause an accumulation of intermediate products in the ovary. The Japanese have a low rate of ovarian cancer, while in Denmark the rate is high. The increase of ovarian cancer among Japanese immigrants to the United States may provide a lead to unravel the complex interplay that occurs in steroidogenesis.

Clinical leads often come from animal laboratory experimentation. The Biskinds working with rats and Furth and Sobel with mice, transplanted the gonads into the spleen and produced granulosa cell tumors. Although the menopausal human female has a similar pattern of increased excretion of pituitary gonadotropins, the malignancies formed in the human ovary are not usually the granulosa cell type. The results from animal experimentation are difficult to correlate with clinical findings in the human. When ovarian cancer is produced in animals, the result is usually a functioning tumor, most commonly a granulosa cell tumor, and is associated with continuous unopposed stimulation of the pituitary. In the human, granulosa cell tumor occurs in the young age group and is accompanied by a high estrogen titer with a feedback to control the pituitary. Most ovarian cancers in the human are epithelial tumors and are different from those artificially produced in animals.

SURVIVAL FACTORS

Further evaluation of factors affecting the survival of patients with ovarian cancer may help in the search for earlier diagnosis. Often retrospective studies indicate a point in time when the ovary started its malfunction, much like a cam running off center. A study reported by Wynder et al. included data that seemed to bear out this statement. The incidence of spontaneous abortion, dysmenorrhea, heavy flow, postmenopausal bleeding, and swelling of the breasts was higher than in control series. Sometimes benign cysts may show progressive changes toward precancer and finally cancer. There are reports in the literature of small areas of localized malignancy in benign multilocular cysts. One theory of cystoma etiology reports that there is an invagination of small fragments of the surface germinal epithelium much as in the formation of inclusion cysts. This results in a cyst lined with low cuboidal epithelium as seen in serous cysts, or with a tall columnar epithelium of the mucinous type. These develop pseudostratification with papillary processes, and finally a complex cystadenoma.

STAGING

Staging and detailed histology studies serve as a guide in understanding the natural history of disease. The heterogenous nature of the cancer makes it difficult to establish criteria for histologic staging. The differences in reported 5-year survival rates usually reflect the different criteria used in reporting the material. More attention has recently been directed to establishing rigid histologic and clinical staging for ovarian cancer. Progress will be slow until we establish more accurate histologic criteria that not only help to identify the different cancers, but make it possible for different institutions to compare their material meaningfully.

ROLE OF IMMUNOLOGY

Although immunology has grown to maturity in the field of bacteriology, it is in its embryonic phase in the field of tissue transplant and oncology. Of any of the avenues now being pursued, this approach, though exotic, has the greatest potential for effecting a cure or prophylaxis against the development of a malignancy. Cancer immunology may now be at the threshold of an era in the prevention and treatment of cancer, not unlike that in which the conquest of some major infectious disease was achieved. Studies in the immunology of cancer have the following objectives:

- To determine the antigenic properties of cancer cells
- To understand the details of the mechanisms of immune reactions, particularly those evoked by cancer cells
- To contribute to the knowledge of the etiology of cancer
- To create new and better diagnostic methods to increase the effectiveness of all forms of therapy
- To develop new therapeutic methods based on an immunologic approach
- To establish guidelines to select patients for immunoprophylaxis as opposed to immunotherapy
- To develop new methods to monitor the volume of disease in a patient while under treatment

BIBLIOGRAPHY

Axtell, L.M., Cutler, S.J., Myers, M.H. (eds.): End Results in Cancer, report no. 4. 1972.

Barber, H.R.K.: Foreword—Ovarian Tumors. Clin. Obstet. Gynecol. 12:929, 1969.

Barber, H.R.K., Graber, E.A.: The PMPO syndrome (postmenopausal palpable ovary syndrome). Obstet. Gynecol. 38:921, 1971.

Gibbs, E.K.: Suggested prophylaxis for ovarian cancer. A 20-year report from cases at Butterworth hospital. Am. J. Obstet. Gynecol. 111:756, 1971.

James, P.D.: Epidemiology of ovarian cancer. Lancet 1:412, 1974.

Jones, T.C., Gilmore, C.E.: The ovaries in animals. International Academy of Pathology/Monograph. Grady, H.G. Smith, D.E. (eds.). Williams & Wilkins, Baltimore, 1963, p. 255.

Lingeman, C.H.: Etiology of cancer of the human ovary. J. Natl. Cancer Inst. 53:1603–1618, 1974.

Randall, C.L., Hall, D.W., Armenia, C.S.: Pathology in the preserved ovary after unilateral oophorectomy. Am. J. Obstet. Gynecol. 84:1233, 1962.

Silverberg, E.: Gynecologic Cancer: Statistical and Epidemiological Information. American Cancer Society, Professional Education Publication, 1975.

Stone, M.L., Weingold, A., Sanford, S., Sonnenblick, B.: Factors affecting patients with ovarian carcinoma. Surg. Gynecol. Obstet. 116:351, 1963.

Terz, J.J., Barber, H.R.K., Brunschwig, A.: Incidence of carcinoma in the retained ovary. Am. J. Surg. 113:511, 1967.

West, R.O.: Epidemiologic studies of malignancies of the ovaries. Cancer 19:1001–1007, 1966.

Wynder, E.L., Dodo, H., Barber, H.R.K.: Epidemiology of cancer of the ovary. Cancer 23:352–370, 1969.

2

Anatomy, Embryology, and Comparative Anatomy

The ovaries are solid, slightly nodular, pink-gray bodies, with the approximate proportions of unshelled almonds. They are situated on either side of the uterus, behind and below the uterine tubes. The human ovary undergoes marked changes in size, shape, and position during its lifetime in addition to the histologic changes brought about by various endocrine stimuli. It is important to appreciate the change in size, shape, and consistency that occurs in the ovary in different age groups as well as within any given menstrual cycle. The ovaries are usually not symmetric and the right ovary is often larger than the left.

The size of the ovaries increases slowly but progressively between birth and the seventh or eighth year of life. During this period they lie with their superior poles at the brim of the pelvis and their inferior poles near the uterus. They descend to their final position, which is considerably lower, near the time of menarche. In general they do not show any remarkable change in their gross appearance until 3 or 4 years before the menache, when the pituitary gonadotropins induce increased ovarian function.

The ovary of the newborn is an elongated structure approximately 1.5 cm long and 0.5 cm wide and varies from 1.5 to 3.5 mm in thickness. The ovarian surface is pinkish-white, smooth and glistening. It weighs about 0.3–0.4 g. The ovary gradually grows larger and changes shape and position between birth and puberty. It is developed between the tenth and twelfth segments on the posterior wall near the kidney, then slowly moves into the true pelvis and enlarges to about 3 × 1.8 × 1.2 cm. The weight of both ovaries at puberty is between 4 and 7 g.

The premenopausal ovary measures 3.5 × 2 × 1.5 cm. The menopausal ovary tends to atrophy and shrink when the Graafian follicles and ova disappear. The ovary eventually becomes an inert residue that consists of connective tissue, and it clings to the posterior leaf of the broad ligament. Its pink color becomes pure white. It shrinks to 2 × 1.5 ×0.5 cm, and in some it may be as small as 1.5 × 0.75 × 0.5 cm. Its wrinkled surface resembles the gyri and sulci of the cerebrum. At this point it is almost impossible to palpate it on examination.

In the nullipara the ovary lies in a shallow peritoneal fossa on the lateral pelvic wall known as the fossa ovarica of Waldeyer. Its long axis lies in the vertical plane, so that it has an upper and a lower pole, an anterior and a posterior border, and a medial and lateral surface. The fossa of the ovary lies immediately below the bifurcation of the common iliac artery, and one of the most important relations of the ovary is the ureter, which lies immediately behind it.

During pregnancy the ovaries are lifted out of the true pelvis as the uterus enlarges. In the early part of the first trimester, the corpus luteum may be large and protrude above the ovarian surface. At the time of cesarean section the ovaries are in a resting state and are covered with a shaggy pink material which is a decidual reaction.

Each ovary has two extremities, two surfaces, and two borders. The ovary is attached to the posterior layer of the broad ligament by the mesovarium, to the lateral pelvic wall by the infundibulopelvic fold, and to the uterus by the ovarian ligament. The posterior border is free. The uterine extremity or lower pole is directed inferiorly and is connected through the ovarian ligament to the lateral margin of the uterus. The tubal extremity or upper pole is attached to the peritoneum of the lateral pelvic wall by the infundibulopelvic ligament. The medial surface faces inward and to a great extent is covered by the fimbriated extremity of the Fallopian tube. Usually the lateral surface is in direct contact with the parietal peritoneum overlying the shallow ovarian fossa in the angle between the diverging external iliac and hypogastric vessels. The position of the ovary is therefore likely to be influenced by the movements of the broad ligament and the uterus under normal circumstances (Figure 4).

The relations of the ovary are described in the following paragraphs.

The anterior border is attached to the posterior layer of the broad ligament by a double layer of peritoneum, which forms a mesentery for the ovary. It is known as the mesovarium, and between its two layers the ovarian vessels and nerves enter the hilum of the gland (Figure 5).

The posterior border is directed backward and is free. The ovary is separated by peritoneum from the ureter and the hypogastric artery.

The superior border or tubal pole is in direct contact with the ampulla of the uterine tube, and the infundibulopelvic fold is attached to it.

The inferior border or uterine pole is directed toward the uterus and is attached to it by the uteroovarian ligament.

The medial surface is in contact with the abdominal ostium and fimbriae of the tube.

The lateral surface is in contact with the abdominal ostium and fimbriae of the tube.

The blood supply of the ovary is from the ovarian artery, a branch of the abdominal aorta, which arises immediately below the renal artery. From here it crosses the inferior vena cava and ureter on the right, and on the left it

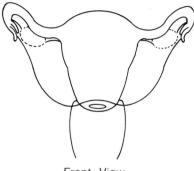

Front View

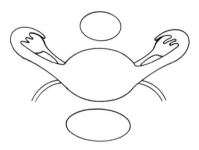

Front View — from the top

Figure 4.   Relationship of the ovaries to the tube and uterus.

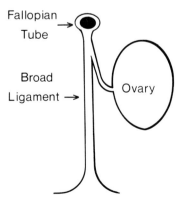

Fallopian
Tube →

Broad
Ligament →

Ovary

Figure 5.   Attachment of the ovary to the broad ligament.

crosses the ureter and the left psoas muscle. Having reached the pelvic brim it crosses the common or external iliac artery and runs between the two layers of the infundibulopelvic fold and enters the broad ligament. It reaches the hilum of the ovary by passing between two layers of mesovarium.

The venous drainage is into a pampiniform venous plexus from which the ovarian vein emerges. On the right side the ovarian vein enters the inferior vena cava at an oblique angle below the renal vein, and on the left side it enters the left renal vein at a right angle (Figure 6).

The nerve supply comes from the level of the tenth thoracic segment. It is derived from the lateral column of gray matter in the spinal cord at this level.

The ovarian artery and vein, nerves, and lymphatic vessels enter the infundibulopelvic fold (ligament), broad ligament, and mesovarium to reach the hilum of the ovary.

Vestigeal remnants of the mesonephric duct and tubules persist within the peritoneal layers of the broad ligament as the epoophoron, the paroophoron, and the duct of Gartner. The epoophoron consists of a longitudinal duct and 8 to 20 small tubes at right angles to it, situated in the lateral aspect of the mesosalpinx. The paroophoron refers to a few scattered tubules medial to the epoophoron and nearer to the uterus. The lower end of the mesonephric duct may persist along the lateral margin of the uterus or vagina as Gartner's duct.

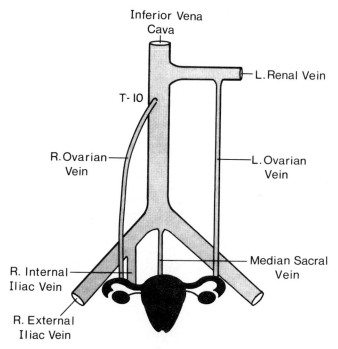

Figure 6. The inferior vena cava and its tributaries constitute the ovary's venous drainage system.

The lymphatic drainage is into the lateral aortic lymph nodes near the kidney, which represents the level of the embryologic origin of the ovary. On the left side, primary nodes may be situated between the left ovarian and left renal veins. On the right side, they may be found between the right renal vein and the inferior vena cava. Shorter lymphatic pathways may also lead to the hypogastric nodes (Figure 7).

Eichner has made a significant contribution to an understanding of the lymphatic system by injecting direct sky blue dye into the ovary and then studying its flow. He also ligated channels at different levels and studied the drainage into anastomotic lymphatic channels.

On injecting the ovary with dye, Eichner observed that normal unobstructive ovarian lymphatics drain through the mesovarian and infundibulopelvic ligaments, then follow the ovarian vessels cephalad.

The various primary pathways were serially ligated to show how lymph might drain if these routes were obstructed by disease. When the infundibulopelvic ligament was ligated, a new pattern of flow developed. The forward progress stopped at the ligature and spread mesially to the Fallopian tube, then by way of the utero-ovarian ligament. It then descended the posterolateral subserosal aspect of the uterosacral ligaments, where it crossed the midline, involved the rectosigmoid at its peritoneal reflection, and encircled the bowel. Although Eichner reported some spread toward the midline on the uterine corpus, none of the dye crossed the midline.

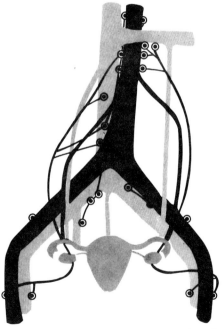

Figure 7. Lymphatic drainage of the ovaries. The dark vessels indicate the arterial system, and the light vessels the venous sytem.

After both the infundibulopelvic and utero-ovarian ligaments were obstructed surgically, the dye spread through the broad ligament to the round ligament, or into the depths of the vessels. The ureteral adventitia was occasionally stained by the latter route. This is an interesting observation. In a study of palliative therapy of advanced ovarian cancer in 67 women at the Memorial Hospital, Lewis found that the clinical problem requiring admission for therapy among 5 patients was related to the genitourinary tract. Three of the patients were admitted for symptomatic obstruction of one ureter, and in 2 others the indication for admission was hemorrhagic cystitis with urinary retention due to clots.

Among patients in whom both the utero-ovarian and infundibulopelvic ligaments were ligated, the obturator and hypogastric nodes as well as the peritoneal reflection of the rectosigmoid and the roots of the uterosacral ligaments were always stained.

Plentl and Friedman summarized the accumulated data on the intrinsic as well as the extrinsic lymphatic supply of the ovary. They reported that the parenchymal lymphatics of the ovary comprise a rich network and that their origin is irregular and mutable, paralleling the cyclic histologic changes of this organ. The tunica albuginea is essentially devoid of lymphatics. The cortex, particularly in the vicinity of the developing follicle, demonstrates a lymphatic network and appears to be dependent upon theca externa cellular activity. The lymphatic network in the vascularis and the medulla formed small collecting tubes which converge upon the hilus without apparent relationship to the blood vessels.

Plentl and Friedman also reported that the lymph from the ovary is drained peripherally by six to eight large collecting chains which leave the ovary by way of the hilus to form the subovarian plexus. Efferent vessels from this plexus drain in a cephalad direction, passing through the infundibulopelvic fold along with the ovarian vessels to the lateral periaortic lymph nodes. On the left side, primary nodes may be situated between the left ovarian and left renal veins. On the right side, they may be found between the right renal vein and the inferior vena cava. Shorter lymphatics may also lead to the hypogastric nodes.

Eichner stated that he was not able to force dye from an ovarian injection into the endometrium. Serosal and superficial myometrial stain could be made at will by forcing the dye, but he failed to produce deeper penetration. He also stated that similar attempts to force extension of endocervical injection into the endometrium, or of endometrial injections to the cervix were unsuccessful.

EMBRYOLOGY

Functionally, the urogenital system can be divided into two entirely different components: the urinary system, which excretes waste products and excess water by means of an intricate tubular system in the kidneys; and the genital system, which assures continuation of the human race by producing germ cells.

Embryologically and anatomically, however, both systems are interwoven. Both develop from a common ridge formed by proliferation of mesoderm along the posterior wall of the abdominal cavity, and the excretory ducts of both systems initially enter a common cavity, the cloaca. Because the urinary and genital systems are so closely related anatomically, and more particularly embryologically, it is almost impossible to study one and ignore the other. However, to keep to the subject of the book, only the embryology of the ovary will be considered.

In the development of both excretory and reproductive organs, mesoderm plays the major part, but entoderm and ectoderm also make important contributions (Figure 8).

Although the sex of the embryo is determined at the time of fertilization, the gonads do not acquire their male or female morphologic characteristics until the seventh week of development.

Almost the entire reproductive and urinary systems of both sexes are formed from the Wolffian body, a large and important structure occupying the posterior or dorsal portion of the primitive peritoneal cavity. The first indication of the gonads appears in a 4-week embryo as a pair of longitudinal ridges, the gonadal or genital ridges, located on each side of the midline between the mesonephros and the dorsal mesentery. They are formed by proliferation of the celomic epithelium or primitive peritoneal epithelium and by condensation of the underlying mesenchyme. There are no germ cells in the gonadal ridge until the sixth week of development. In its early stage it is impossible to determine from histologic examination whether this epithelial mass will be testis or ovary (Figure 9). The impulse that determines male or female development in the sex glands is unknown. Some believe it to be the penetration of the gonadal area by the germ cells migrating along a Keimbahn from a much earlier situs, possibly initially located in the wall of the

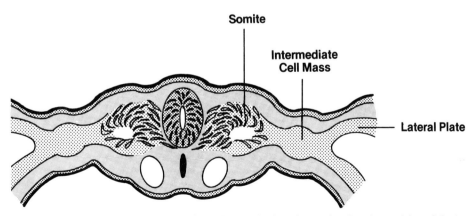

Figure 8.   Cross section of embryo (adapted from chick embryo) showing the position of the intermediate cell mass (nephrotome) between somite and lateral plate.

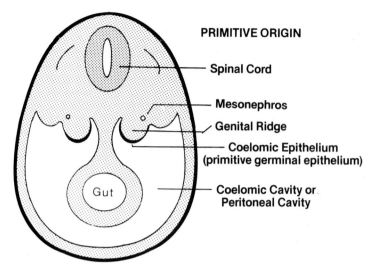

PRIMITIVE ORIGIN

— Spinal Cord

— Mesonephros

— Genital Ridge

— Coelomic Epithelium
(primitive germinal epithelium)

— Coelomic Cavity or
Peritoneal Cavity

Gut

Figure 9. Transverse section through the lower thoracic region showing the early stage in the formation of the gonadal ridge. The coelomic epithelium covering the gonad is thickened to form the germinal epithelium. From this epithelium, sex cords grow into the mesenchyme.

yolk sac close to the allantois (Figure 10). From here they migrate actively along the dorsal mesentery of the hindgut toward the region of the gonadal ridges. In the sixth week of human development, the primordial germ cells enter the ridges and are located partly in the proliferating surface epithelium and partly in the underlying mesenchyme. Germ cells apparently never persist outside the genital ridge.

The genetic sex of the individual is determined at the time of fertilization, but it is not until the embryo has reached the 17 mm stage that it is possible to identify the gonad as either a testis or an ovary.

The ovary is developed from the genital ridge which lies between the root of the mesentery and the Wolffian ridge on the posterior wall of the celomic cavity.

The genital ridge lies on the cranial aspect of the developing suprarenal cortex, and this fact provides an anatomic basis for the hormonal interrelation between the suprarenal cortex and the gonads. The main feature of ovarian development is the progressive importance and increase in size of the cortex at the expense of the medulla. This ridge bulges into the celomic cavity and is formed by a proliferation of the celomic epithelium. The surface epithelium, which is a modified form of peritoneum is called the germinal epithelium. The germinal epithelium (mesothelium) becomes thicker and more prominent. In places, massive clumps of sex cells are visible and cortical sex cords push into the gonad. The cortical cords seem to contain or produce certain somatic cells, which later become the granulosa cells. The first follicles, constituted of ovocytes surrounded by recognizable layers of granulosa cells, appear initially in the central part of the ovary when crown

GERM CELL MIGRATION

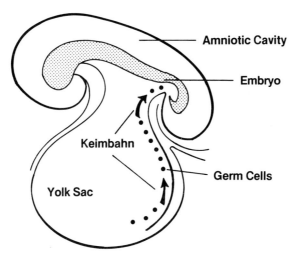

Figure 10. Large round primordial cells appear in the germinal epithelium and sex cords. These cells are believed to come from the endoderm of the yolk sac and to have migrated to the gonad by way of the mesentery (along the keimbahn).

rump length of the fetus measures about 150 mm (slightly younger than 5 lunar months). They are not isolated from the germinal epithelium by the tunica albuginea during fetal life as are the sex glands in the male; indeed this is the earliest distinguishing feature between the ovary and a testis. During cortical differentiation the development of the medullary cords gradually diminishes and the cords are crowded to a central position (Figure 11).

In the male the primitive sex cords are well defined, whereas in the female they are broken up by invading mesenchyme into irregular cell clusters. These clusters, which contain groups of primitive germ cells, are located in the medullary part of the ovary and are later replaced by vascular stroma which forms the ovarian medulla.

The surface epithelium of the female gonad, unlike that of the male, remains thick and continues to proliferate. It gives rise to a second generation of cords, the cortical cords, which penetrate the underlying mesenchyme but remain close to the surface of the gland. These cords are also split into isolated cell clusters, each containing one or more primitive germ cells which have an extragonadal origin and migrate to the indifferent gonad. After arrival in the gonad of the female, the germ cells may be called oogonia. The surrounding epithelial cells, descendants of the surface epithelium, form the follicullar cells. It is generally accepted that the primary medullary cords are a distinctly male feature, whenever the secondary cortical cords are characteristic of the femal gonad (Figure 12).

The oogonia are noted as early as the fifth week, although the gonad cannot be identified as an ovary at that time and may be found through the seventh month of fetal life. They undergo mitotic division with great fre-

DEVELOPMENT OF OVARIES

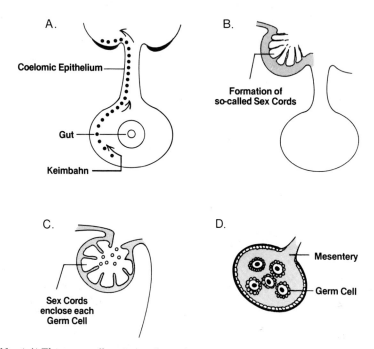

Figure 11. (*A*) The germ cells migrate from the root of the mesentery to the genital ridge. (*B*) The coelomic epithelium growing into the genital ridge forms so-called sex cords. (*C*) The sex cords enclose each germ cell. The germ cells and most of the sex cord cells remain in the superficial part, the future cortex of the ovary. The cords lose contact with the surface epithelium and form small groups of cells with its germ cell, a primitive follicle. Some of the sex cord cells grow into the medulla. These tend to regress and form rudimentary tubules, the rete. (*D*) As the ovary grows it projects increasingly into the peritoneal (coelomic) cavity, thus forming a mesentery.

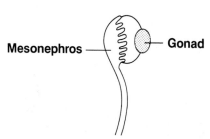

Figure 12.   The relationship of the mesonephros to the developing gonad.

quency, and they are most numerous at the fifth month when their estimated number is about 8 million plus.

The oogonium becomes an oocyte when it enters the first of its two meiotic divisions. The first oocytes can be recognized at about 8 weeks and are most numerous at about 5 months when they number about 4 million. At the time of birth no oogonia remain and the oocytes have been reduced to 2 million. By the seventh postnatal year, only about 300,000 oocytes remain.

The fetal ovary is suspended to the posterior abdominal wall by a mesentery, a double layer of peritoneum containing vessels and nerves. This mesentery is attached to the upper pole of the gland and later becomes the infundibulopelvic fold and the mesovarium. Attached to the lower pole of the kidney is a fibromuscular cord called the gubernaculum, which is also attached to that part of the ventral body wall which will eventually become the large labia. In the female, after the gubernaculum forms, the ovary descends, but not as far as does the testis in the male. The gubernaculum is caught up in the condensed mesenchyme that forms the wall of the uterus, so as to become divided into two parts: the ligament of the ovary passes from the ovary to the uterus (utero-ovarian ligament), and the round ligament of the uterus ends in the outer genital swelling or labium majus. The ligament of the ovary shortens as the ovary assumes its adult position in the pelvis (Figure 13).

The ovary is developed between the tenth and twelfth thoracic segments, on the posterior abdominal wall near the kidney. This accounts for its long attenuated blood supply, its venous drainage, its nerve supply from a plexus adjacent to its origin, and also its lymphatic drainage into nodes lying adjacent to the renal veins.

A supernumerary ovary is one that is independent of and the same size as the normal ovary. It is an extremely rare condition.

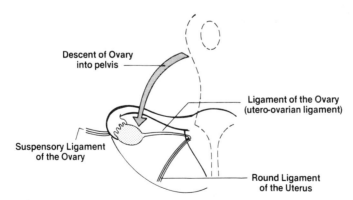

Figure 13. In the female the gubernaculum forms and the gonad descends, but not so far as does the testis in the male. The gubernaculum is caught up in the condensed mesenchyme that forms the wall of the uterus, and thus it becomes divided into two parts: the ligament of the ovary passing from the ovary to the uterus, and the round ligament of the uterus which ends in the outer genital swelling or labium majus. The ligament of the ovary shortens as the ovary takes up its adult position in the pelvis.

An accessory ovary is usually attached to the normal gland by peritoneal bands in the mesovarium or adjacent part of the broad ligament, near the hilum of the ovary. They have clinical significance if they undergo pathologic changes or when bilateral oophorectomy is carried out; their presence may result in continued ovarian activity. Accessory ovaries occur in about 3% of women.

Ectopic ovaries may be congenital or acquired, but the acquired type is much more common. Congenital displacement may be caused by nondescent of the ovary which remains above the pelvic brim. It may also result when the ovary is pulled into the inguinal canal or labium majus by the gubernaculum. The acquired type of displacement is quite common and is very liable to occur after pregnancy, when the ovary may prolapse into the cul-de-sac.

COMPARATIVE ANATOMY

Jones and Gilmore have presented a brief review of the comparative anatomy of the ovary. They report that the amphioxus has gonadal tissue distributed in various tissues of its body, and that the lowest form in which the ovary is concentrated in one organ is the lamprey. In higher vertebrates the gonads are not segmented and are intraabdominal. It is interesting that in the bird the left ovary and oviduct develop to maturity and the organs on the right side atrophy, whereas in some bats the reverse is true. Among birds that live long enough, adenocarcinoma of the ovary similar to that found in man is not uncommon. Lower vertebrates generally produce many ova surrounded by an abundant yolk sac; thus their ovaries are large and nodular in appearance. The ovaries of most mammals have ova with little or no yolk. Reptiles have ovaries with a large central cavity surrounded by germinal epithelium, while birds have an intricate network of spaces rather than a central cavity.

There is a great variation in size among the ovaries of different animals. The ovary of a whale may reach 40 cm in length and weigh more than 1500 g, whereas a shrew may have an ovary that is less than a millimeter in maximum dimension. Despite this great difference, the ovary in each has similar histologic features and essentially the same physiology.

Jones and Gilmore reported that tumors occur in the ovaries of many different animals. Granulosa tumors have been noted with some frequency in the ovaries of cows and dogs. Adenocarcinomas and cystadenocarcinoma have been found in birds, and not infrequently if they live a long life. Dysgerminoma and Sertoli cell tumors have been reported in the dog, and dermoid cysts have been reported in the ovary of the dog. Arrhenoblastomas have also been reported, but the documentation is not adequate for unqualified acceptance.

Aside from the ova and their attending follicular apparatus, the tissues found in the ovary are the corpus luteum, a mesothelium covering the external surface of the ovary, and a stroma comprised of connective tissue, blood vessels, and nerves. In the human ovary the stromal matrix consists of whorls of spindle-shaped cells enmeshed in reticular fibers. The presence of a cortex and a medulla has been established in the ovaries of man and other mammals. In the cortex a tunica albuginea is represented by a condensation of the stroma just beneath the germinal epithelium. In the medulla only loose connective tissue, elastic fibers, and smooth muscle are found.

HISTOLOGY

The histology of the ovary is described in detail in standard textbooks on gynecology. However a resume of significant points is appropriate here for background purposes. The histology of the ovary must be described with reference to its hormonal function. The ovary produces ova as well as important hormones, i.e., estrogen and progesterone. Since the histologic patterns of the ovary vary with sexual activity, and the time of the menstrual cycle, it is not possible to give a simple description of the ovary in all its phases.

The ovary is generally divided into a cortical zone and a medulla. The cortical zone contains stroma, ova, and (depending on age) those bodies (corpora lutea, corpora albicantia, etc.) that form after the discharge or degeneration of the ovum. During reproductive life the cortex is broad and makes up one-half to two-thirds of the depth of the ovary. The stroma is made up of spindle-celled connective tissue, placed very compactly. Beneath the germinal epithelium there develops with advancing age a connective tissue layer of increasing density called the tunica albuginea, containing collagenous (van Gieson-red) fibers. These fibers are almost absent from the rest of the cortical stroma, which is peculiar in that, besides blood vessels, lymphatics, and nerves, it shows an abundance of short and long spindle-shaped nuclei. The cell bodies to which these nuclei belong are difficult to discern in ordinary sections, and silver methods reveal reticular fibers between them. This richly nucleated stroma is very characteristic of the human ovary, is established long before puberty, and remains fairly constant in its nuclear density up to old age.

The ovarian medulla contains many blood vessels, in particular spirally running arteries, lymphatics, and nerves embedded in fibrous tissue, and all of these structures are continuous at the hilum with those present in the mesovarium. Because the medulla may contain such structures as the rete ovarii and hilus cells, many look on it as primarily potentially androgenic instead of estrogenic like the cortex. In the hilus there are often remnants of certain embryonic structures, especially the rete ovarii and the parovarian tubules. The latter are of Wolffian origin and appear as clusters of small lumina lined by cuboidal epithelium and surrounded by a thick muscular zone. The rete tubules are zigzagged in arrangement, lined by flat epithelium, and have no surrounding muscle tissue.

The ovary is covered by a low cuboidal epithelium called the germinal epithelium, which is modified peritoneum. It is derived from the celomic epithelium and joins the flat serosal cells of the peritoneum at the mesovarium. The epithelium is easily detached on handling the organ and may be found in the postmenopausal ovary, although only in patches. It may be invaginated and occasionally it penetrates the underlying stroma by tubular formations. Sometimes its cells are cubical or even flat, especially when overlying large growing structures such as a maturing follicle or a corpus luteum.

The sympathicotrophic or hilus cells are often seen in the hilus of the ovary. They are usually polyhedral or ovoid and arranged in a type of mosaic pattern. Since Reinke crystals have been found in these cells and are identical to those found in Leydig cells, a relationship between these two cells has been proposed. Tumors arising from these cells have produced a virilizing effect similar to that found with the Sertoli-Leydig (arrhenoblastoma) cell tumors.

The development of the follicles, the formation of a corpus luteum, the atretic follicles, and ovarian changes of pregnancy are discussed in detail in standard textbooks of gynecology.

SUMMARY

A knowledge of the embryology and anatomy is important in understanding the clinical findings and the pathologic picture accompanying an ovarian malignancy. The ovary originates at the level of the 10th to the 12th thoracic segments (T-10 to T-12) and migrates to the pelvis. In prepubertal girls, the ovary is an abdominal structure; it only becomes a pelvic structure at puberty. The origin of the ovary may offer an explanation for the gastrointestinal symptoms of ovarian cancer and may also explain its propensity to spread to the upper abdomen.

It is interesting that in the bird the left ovary and oviduct develop to maturity, and the right ovary and tube atrophy. In birds that live long enough, an adenocarcinoma similar to that seen in man is not an uncommon finding.

BIBLIOGRAPHY

Dodds, G.S.: The Essentials of Human Embryology. Third edition. Wiley, New York, 1947.

Eichner, E.: In vivo studies on the pelvic lymphatics in women, *in* Progress in Gynecology. Vol. III. Edited by Meigs and Sturgis. Grune & Stratton, New York, 1957.

Griffith, C.T.: The Ovary in Gynecology. Principles and Practice. Second edition. Edited by R.W. Kistner. Year Book Medical Publishers, Chicago, 1975, p. 323.

Haines, R.W., Mohinddin, A.: Handbook of Human Embryology. Third edition. Williams & Wilkins, Baltimore, 1965.

Jacoby, F.: Gynecological and Obstetrical Anatomy. Edward Arnold, 1948.

Jones, T.C., Gilmore, C.E.: The ovaries in animals, *in* The Ovary. Edited by H.G. Grady and D.E. Smith. International Academy of Pathology Monograph. Williams & Wilkins, Baltimore, 1963.

Langman, J.: Medical Embryology. Williams & Wilkins, Baltimore, 1963.

Lewis, J.L., Jr.: Palliative therapy of advanced ovarian cancer. Clin. Obstet. Gynecol. 12:1038, 1969.

Netter, F.H.: The Ciba Collection of Medical Illustrations. Vol. 2. Ciba Pharmaceutical Products, Summit, New Jersey, 1954.

Novak, E., Jones, G.S., Jones, H.W., Jr.: Gynecology. Condensed from Novak's Textbook of Gynecology. Ninth edition. Williams & Wilkins, Baltimore, 1975.

Novak, E., Woodruff, J.D.: Novak's Gynecologic and Obstetric Pathology. Fifth edition. Philadelphia and London, 1962.

Plentl, A., Friedman, E.: Lymphatic System of the Female Genitalia: The Morphologic Basis of Oncologic Diagnosis and Therapy. Saunders, Philadelphia, London, Toronto, 1971.

Reiffenstuhl, G.: The Lymphatics of the Female Genitalia. Lippincott, Philadelphia, 1964.

3

Epidemiology of Cancer of the Ovary

E tiology and epidemiology are often intertwined and therefore an introductory discussion is devoted to these subjects.

CANCER ETIOLOGY

The goal of cancer etiology is cancer prevention. Three types of agents have now been shown to cause cancers: chemicals, radiation, and viruses. Of these, two—chemicals and radiation—clearly cause cancer in man. The third, viruses, are highly suspect on the basis of present knowledge.

CANCER EPIDEMIOLOGY

Cancer epidemiology seeks to correlate differences in the incidence of different types of cancer with differences in the external or internal environments of persons developing these cancers. The correlation between cigarette smoking and lung cancer is an established example.

Recent investigations have raised some intriguing questions that call for further study. These include the sevenfold higher incidence of breast cancer and ovarian cancer among Americans compared to Japanese women; the much greater incidence of colon cancer in the United States than in certain areas of Africa; and the spotty geographic distribution of esophageal cancer throughout Africa.

So far the results of epidemiologic research strongly suggest that variations in social practices and in exposure to environmental agents are largely responsible for variations in the incidence of cancers among different groups of people. Therefore, if such environmental exposures and social practices could be identified and eliminated, most cancers in man might be prevented. Because of the complexity of the relationship between man and his environment and the long latent period of cancer development, the identification of particular cancer-inducing factors is extremely difficult. But there is no other area of cancer research that holds more promise for cancer prevention.

The ovary is the sixth leading site for cancer in females in the United

States. It accounts for about 5% of all female cancer deaths. Age-adjusted death rates for malignant neoplasms of the ovary show that the Danes have the highest rate and the Japanese the lowest. The white American female is about in the middle of the group. The urban incidence is slightly higher than the rural. Studies among American Indians show that their rates are lower than those of whites and other non-Indians, but this result may be related to the lack of longevity in this group.

A number of epidemiologic factors are suspected of being linked with ovarian cancer. Among these are nulliparity, infertility, marked premenstrual tension, abnormal breast swelling, marked dysmenorrhea, increased abortion rate, early menopause, group A blood, irradiation of pelvic organs, environmental factors, industrial products such as asbestos and talc, higher socioeconomic status, celibacy, breast cancer, and resistance to mumps parotitis.

There are seven major demographic leads:

1.   Ovarian cancer, particularly in postmenopausal women, is less common in Japan than in the Western world. Compared with Caucasian women, Oriental women, who have a low incidence of breast and ovarian cancer, have a high estriol titer between ages 15 and 19. It has been accepted that estriol acts as an antagonist of carcinogenic activity of estradiol-estrone. As each group moves toward age 40, the difference decreases until it is negligible. Because there is little difference at the time that cancer in these organs begins to develop, it must be concluded that estriol was protecting the immature cell.

2.   Among first-generation Japanese women in the United States, ovarian cancer occurs more commonly than in Japan.

3.   Not only has there been an increase in the incidence of ovarian cancer in the Western world, there has also been some increase in Japan.

4.   Cancer of the ovary tends to be somewhat more common in upper than in lower income groups in the West.

5.   Ovarian cancer in New York City is more common among Jews than other religious groups, particularly in postmenopausal women.

6.   There is a positive correlation between the incidence pattern of ovarian, mammary, and endometrial cancers.

7.   In several studies ovarian cancer is more commonly reported among single and nulliparous women.

EVIDENCE OF INCIDENCE

Estimates of the incidence of cancer show that cancer of the ovary is the sixth leading cancer in women. About 1.4% or 1 of every 70 newborn girls will develop cancer of the ovary during their lives. The incidence rates have been reported in greater detail in chapter 1 (Figure 14).

It is still questionable whether the observations on the incidence pattern of various cancers are valid. Cancer of the ovary is one of the inaccessible cancers that are difficult to diagnose. Confirmation of the presence of the

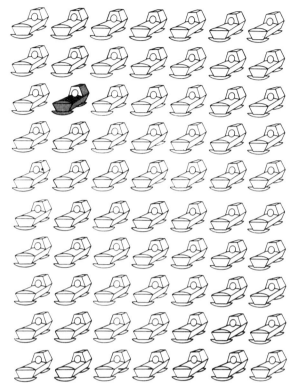

1.4 %– 1 of every 70 Newborn Girls will develop
Ovarian Cancer

Figure 14.   The Third National Cancer Survey found that 1 of every 70 newborn girls (1.4%)
will develop ovarian cancer.

disease almost always requires surgery and expert pathologic interpretation.
Part of the increase of ovarian cancer in the United States may be attributable to improved diagnostic facilities and increased awareness of the
disease. However, when the increase in population and the increase in the age
of the population are taken into account, there is still an increase in incidence
that has not been explained.

Ovarian cancer appears to be more often diagnosed in individuals to
whom better medical care is available, and data on this factor from specific
hospitals must therefore be cautiously evaluated in respect to socioeconomic
status as well as educational level. For socioeconomic and educational
distributions, the vital statistics of a city or a national population are more
meaningful than those of any individual hospital.

The incidence among single women is difficult to evaluate, but the effects
of other demographic factors have been ascertained. Studies of the death rate
in New York City suggest that ovarian cancer is somewhat more common
among Jewish women. The data suggest that the disproportionate number of

Jewish women with cancer of the ovary may be the result of increased susceptibility in postmenopausal women of that group.

The low rate of ovarian cancer in Japan is real, because diagnostic
facilities and vital statistics are equal to those of the Western world. It is also
noteworthy that the incidence of ovarian cancer increases among Japanese
women when they migrate to the United States, a finding which suggests
that environmental rather than genetic factors are partially responsible for
the low rates of this cancer among the Japanese.

RADIATION

Studies by Speert and West showed no relationship between irradiation
and ovarian cancer. Speert followed 958 patients who had received
radiotherapeutic menopause: only one developed cancer of the ovary. He also
followed 343 consecutive patients with ovarian cancer and 247 consecutive
patients with cystadenomas of the ovary. Of these 590 women, 17 had a
record of previous pelvic radiation for benign conditions. One of the variables
examined by West was the milliroentgens delivered to ovaries by diagnostic
and therapeutic x-irradiation. The results of his study did not warrant the
conclusion that exposure to x-ray, particulary diagnostic x-rays, influences
the production of ovarian malignancies. West noted that calculations were
based only on whether or not the patient and the control had received x-irradiation over the abdomen; the question of who may have had more was not
considered. On this scale there was no significant difference between the patients and the group with benign ovarian tumors.

Endocrinologic considerations: The apparently normal endocrinologic
status of the ovarian cancer patient stands out more than any marked variation from the general female population. Wynder and associates have
challenged this observation. However the few marked differences that have
been shown by their study, particularly in menstrual history, even if real,
provide less of a lead than the different rates among ethnic groups and
especially the changing rates among non-Americans who immigrate to the
United States.

The ovary is complex in its embryology, histology, steroidogenesis, and
potential for malignancy. It is made up of germ cells, cells of sex cord, and
cells of the mesenchymal tissue. Although sex is genetically determined at
fertilization, the ovary passes through its early phases as an indifferent
organ with parallel development that could allow it to become a testis or an
ovary. Alterations or imbalances during these steps of development may provide the setting for later mesenchymal functioning, and cell nests may give
rise to a clinically dramatic picture.

Clinical leads often come from animal experimentation. The Biskinds
working with rats, and Furth and Sobel with mice, transplanted the gonads
into the spleen and produced granulosa cell tumors. Although menopausal
women have a similar pattern of increased excretion of pituitary
gonadotrophins, the malignancies formed in the human ovary are not usually
the granulosa cell type.

In addition to our findings on the rarity of ovarian cancer among women in Japan and its increase among Japanese immigrants to the United States, another important epidemiologic clue comes from the facts that prostatic cancer is also increasing among Japanese immigrants and that mammary cancer appears to be increasing much more slowly. Japanese immigrants provide much data to suggest that environmental factors may affect the development of the steroid-related cancers.

Cholesterol is considered the keystone upon which steroids are built. It is apparently built up from acetate, and endogenous cholesterol is the important factor for steroid synthesis. Prefabricated cholesterol is reported to play a minor role, although Frosham believes that exogenous cholesterol may affect steroid production.

Bulbrook's findings in this area merit attention. Among female Japanese immigrants living in Vancouver, the more Canadian food they eat, the more similar become their 5a/5b ratios to those of Canadian women. (The 5b derivatives are not androgenic; however the 5a derivative is extremely potent. Indeed, dihydrotestosterone (DHT), the 5a derivative, is probably the principal androgenic hormone formed in target tissue from testosterone. Thus, testosterone has been reduced to a prehormone, the circulating precursor for DHT.) Short has suggested that a higher nutritional plane increases multiple ovulation, which in turn enhances the amount of estrogen and progesterone produced, an effect mediated through the pituitary. Lutwak-Mann has recently reviewed some aspects of the influence of diet on ovarian function. This important area certainly needs further exploration.

The process of steroidogenesis in the adrenal, testis, and ovary is the same up to the point of formation of progesterone. At this point the three glands complete the synthesis of their steroids along individual patterns. Androstenedione and testosterone are synthesized as final steps before estrone and estradiol are produced as the main steroids of the ovary. Anything that disturbs the delicate balance of the pituitary-ovarian axis could alter the final step in the formation of estrogens and thus cause an accumulation of intermediate products in the ovary. A number of publications document that these intermediate products are not innocuous, but their exact role in the problem under discussion remains to be seen.

Dysmenorrhea, heavy menstrual flow, and relatively early onset of menopause were the only gynecologic findings in which there were any differences between the study and control patients. Dysmenorrhea is a complex disorder which can be divided into two classifications. Primary dysmenorrhea is characterized by an absence of recognizable pathology and characteristically is rarely seen in the absence of ovulation. It may disappear spontaneously or persist without change. Secondary dysmenorrhea is related to discernible pathology and frequently gets progressively worse, as in endometriosis.

The many theories advanced to explain the mechanism of dysmenorrhea substantiate the subtle nature of this problem. All investigators agree that a strong psychogenic factor makes it difficult to compare the severity of dysmenorrhea.

This study suggests some relation of dysmenorrhea to ovarian cancer, although the findings may be related to an artifact. Ovarian cancer patients tended to experience dysmenorrhea both before and during menstrual flow, whereas the controls were affected more often during the flow. However a considerable number of women with ovarian cancer did not give any history of dysmenorrhea. We must also consider whether our findings may have been influenced by a greater awareness of gynecologic complaints among women with ovarian cancer than among those without gynecologic disease.

Certain observations by Bell and Loraine are relevant to a discussion of dysmenorrhea. Among patients with intractable dysmenorrhea, these investigators found excretion levels of estrogen that were lower than in women without intractable dysmenorrhea. The total gonadotrophin levels, however, were within the normal range for women during reproductive life. It is interesting to speculate on the significance of low estrogen excretion in the presence of dysmenorrhea.

Although there was a higher incidence of heavy vaginal bleeding among the ovarian cancer patients, the subjective interpretation associated with this finding makes it difficult to evaluate. The bleeding was of average duration.

The age of spontaneous menopause among the ovarian cancer patients is slightly earlier than in the controls and in other controls reported in the literature. Could this finding reflect an earlier reduction of estrogen production? It is important to establish the age of menopause so that there is a point of reference. Barnes reported that the average age of the last menstrual period is 50 years. Data published by the National Center for Health Statistics confirm this observation. A further breakdown of data from the Center indicates that natural menopause occurred in 25% of women by age 47, in 50% by age 50, in 75% by age 52, and in 95% by age 55. The exact 50% point for age at natural menopause is 49.7 years. This study also revealed that between 25 and 30% of women in the United States experience surgical menopause.

A major point of interest is the relative incidence of ovarian cancer in Japanese and American women. Among postmenopausal Japanese women in particular, there is very little ovarian cancer. Further study of this finding should include a review of the known endocrinology in the postmenopausal period. The observation in postmenopausal women, for whom there is more repeatedly confirmed evidence, is that there is estrogen hypoexcretion and excess gonadotrophin excretion. Although estrogen excretion may persist in reduced amounts for a considerable time after menopause, daily vaginal smears indicate that the cyclic patterns disappear within 6 months after the last menstrual period.

Randall and coworkers have found that women experiencing normal menopause appear to have a better estrogenic status than those who have undergone oophorectomy. Oophorectomy in postmenopausal women did not alter estrogen levels, but adrenalectomy in previously oophorectomized women resulted in a rather prompt and pronounced decrease in estrogen. The reduction in urinary estrogen excretion following oophorectomy in the premenopausal woman and the further decrease after adrenalectomy establish the ovary and adrenal as the main sources of estrogen secretion.

Rosenberg and Engel found that gonadotrophin secretion tended to be stimulated by low doses of estrogenic substances and to be suppressed by larger doses. Between ages 60 and 70 (in the late menopause) there is a marked reduction in gonadotrophic excretion, related to the length of time after menopause, and this reduction is undoubtedly a pituitary reflection of progressive generalized tissue senility. Gonadotrophins in the menopausal patient are quantitatively more potent with regard to FSH than LH activity. There is also a diminished output of 17-ketosteroids and 17-hydroxycorticosteroids in this age group. Thyroid function decreases a little but is not reflected in the PBI or BMR values. However, the I^{131} uptake decreases after menopause.

Plotz and Friedlander have shown that the postmenopausal ovary appears to secrete predominantly androgens rather than estrogens. The postmenopausal ovary does not always produce estrogen per se, but it is more frequently indirectly involved in estrogen production in the adrenals by adding significant amounts of estrogen precursors, androgens, to the plasma pool.

Since ovarian cancer is bilateral in at least 50% of the cases and appears to be more in the nature of simultaneous primaries than metastases, a common endocrine denominator influencing the etiology must be sought.

West reported that the second variable in his study was the unusual interest in the therapeutic rise of hormones. Particular interest was directed during the interview toward eliciting any history of natural or synthetic hormones including estrogen, progesterone, testosterone, thyroid, ACTH, and cortisone or its derivatives. He concluded that there is no significant difference in the use of cortisone or thyroid and, when all endocrines are considered together, significant differences are not apparent.

MUMPS

West suggested that mumps might offer some protection against ovarian cancer. He interpreted his data in two ways: (1) Having mumps in childhood may help to protect against getting an ovarian cancer in later years. (2) Some unknown factor that gives a patient resistance against a clinically recognizable case of mumps at the same time decreases one's resistance to ovarian malignancy. In a study by Wynder, Dodo, and Barber, no meaningful difference was noted. However it was concluded that because of the relationship of the mumps virus to the gonad, this disease deserves further exploration.

ROLE OF STRESS

A considerable amount of literature has linked stress to hormonal secretion as mediated via the hypothalamus in man and experimental animals. No precise evidence of increased stress could be deduced from marital status and occupation background in a study group by Wynder and coworkers, although these factors were not investigated in detail. The role of stress deserves further controlled study.

DOUBLE PRIMARIES

Observations of women with multiple primary neoplasms contribute to the evidence that cancers of the ovary and breast share common etiologic determinants. Women with breast cancer have twice the risk of subsequently developing a separate primary cancer of the ovary. Death rates among patients with cancer of the ovary and breast have a positive correlation. The greater tendency for mammary cancer to be antecedent probably reflects the better chance of survival with this disease than with ovarian cancer. Clark, Moertel, and associates reported that most double primary ovarian cancers involved antecedent mammary cancer. Although this cannot be evaluated in terms of relative risks for the general population, the breast-ovary cases appear more numerous when compared with the frequency of double lesions involving ovarian and other types of cancer. In analysis, it is important to consider the age distribution and the relatively poor survival of ovarian cancer patients, as well as the admission practices of a hospital.

CAUSATIVE CARCINOGENS

The search for causative carcinogens should logically be focused on the immediate environment, such as food, personal customs, or other influences that have been introduced to an affluent, pleasure-oriented American society.

Several chemical carcinogens have been shown to induce ovarian cancer in rodents, but there is no firm evidence that these substances cause cancer in women. Cancer of the ovary is not among those neoplasms reported in the few women exposed industrially to dyes, tars, soots, and other products containing anthracenes and related compounds that have resulted in cancer. Of the main industrial products known or suspected to have human carcinogenic activity, only asbestos and talc have been seriously considered as possible causes of ovarian cancer. Could these substances be introduced by means of contraceptive diaphragms that have been dusted with talc that may contain asbestos? The millions of women who have been exposed in this manner would logically produce more cancers if this were a cause-and-effect relationship. Studies of women with occupational exposure indicate that the observed rate is slightly higher than the expected rate of cancer of the ovary as well as of the lung and mesotheliomas of pleura and peritoneum. Evidence linking ovarian cancer to asbestos exposure is disputed because of the few women studied and because of difficulty in distinguishing primary carcinoma of the ovary and peritoneal implants from mesotheliomas originating in the peritoneum.

FAMILY HISTORY

A review of family histories indicated no positive association with ovarian or any other cancer, including cancer of the breast. Nevertheless, it is possible that there might be unusual instances of a familial trend to ovarian cancer. There are several reported cases of women with ovarian cancer whose mothers or sisters had also developed this cancer.

BLOOD GROUP

Osborne and DiGeorge have reported on the ABO blood groups and neoplastic disease of the ovary. They selected diseases of the ovary for their study of the ABO blood group because (1) the ovaries are subject to a great variety of both benign and malignant neoplasms; (2) mucinous cysts of the ovary contain the ABO (H) group-specific substances in women who also secrete these substances in their saliva; and (3) carcinoma of the ovary has been reported to associate with the ABO blood group system.

In a volunteer donor control they found that the frequency of blood group O is 42.82% and that that of blood group A is 38.58%. In patients with ovarian disease the percentage of group O is 39.97 and that of group A is 44.04. The 1.22% frequency of ovarian disease in group A relative to the 1% frequency in group O is statistically significant ($P = 0.025$). In analyzing the 19 different classifications of ovarian disease, they observed that only six classifications (four benign and two malignant) contribute to the increased frequency of ovarian disease in women of blood group A. These are mucinous cysts, endometriosis cysts, dermoids, simple cysts, papillary adenocarcinoma, and secondary carcinoma.

The conclusions drawn from this study are that ovarian neoplasms which associate with blood group A have a glandular type of epithelium, have either a cystic or papillary structure, and include development of some atypical or extraovarian type of epithelium. In contrast, the ovarian diseases which do not appear to associate with blood group A are solid rather than cystic and, if of an epithelial origin, they are entirely of an ovarian type. There is one finding which, if verified, is significant, and that is that there is a four- to sixfold excess of secondary carcinomas of the ovary in women of blood group A compared to women of blood group O.

It is interesting to review the correlation between CEA and blood group A. Scientists have been taking apart bits of the CEA molecule to find out why its activity appears to be similar to that of blood group A substance. When the CEA molecule is split enzymatically, the fractions with high CEA activity seem also to have a high level of group A activity. And by breaking down the molecule chemically, the Montreal group under the direction of Gold has found a repeating unit of n-acetyl glucosamine—a substance familiar to blood group chemists—which seems to be partly responsible for the antigenicity of CEA.

NUTRITION AND CANCER

It is becoming apparent that there are dietary associations with particular cancers. Logically, much of a country's cancer risk must be attributable to diet. It is accepted that no major cancer is common everywhere in the world. More importantly, we know that high rates are rarely genetic, because migrants from one culture to another characteristically evidence a shift in cancer patterns once they have settled in the new country. An increased incidence of skin cancer has been reported among Europeans migrating to Australia, to new working habits and new sexual mores. It has been reported that migrants to the United States develop more bowel cancer, and eventually more breast, endometrial, ovarian, and prostate cancer when they come from less affluent regions where these cancers are uncommon. These cancers alone comprise over 40% of all nonskin cancers in this country, so priority is being given to the investigation into what environmental factors produce this high level of risk.

Ovarian cancer, breast cancer, and endometrial cancer follow bowel cancer as the most common problems in the affluent westernized populations. Environmental factors are involved because migrants from low-risk countries eventually acquire high risks in highly industrialized countries. Naturally there is a correlation between risk for these cancers and the average consumption of dietary protein and fat.

Because cancers in each of these target organs can be produced in animals by specific carcinogens, the possibility of a dietary carcinogen or precursor certainly must be considered. On the other hand, no chemical produces ovarian, endometrial, and breast cancers in animals. An alternative possibility, for which there is no direct animal parallel, is that the same factors that produce growth and early menarche in Americans also overstimulate the endocrine target epithelium to make the ovary particularly vulnerable to cancerous change. Much work remains to be done on the correlation between nutrition and ovarian cancer.

EPIDEMIOLOGIC LIMITATIONS

The major epidemiologic difficulties of an ovarian cancer study relate to certain subjective questions, mostly in the gynecologic area, as well as to the appropriate choice of controls.

Questions relating to menstruation, for example, history of dysmenorrhea and amount of menstrual bleeding, are subjective. Though this applies to both study and controls, it could be that the patient with an ovarian cancer may have a bias different from that of other comparison groups. Reliability of recall must also be considered. Where the comparison groups are concerned, benign ovarian diseases might have been chosen. However some factors may apply to all ovarian diseases, so these may not be appropriate controls. Other hormone-related and gynecologic cancers obviously do not make adequate control groups. These restrictions reduce the number of available controls in a cancer hospital. In choosing controls from other hospitals, certain diseases, like rheumatoid arthritis, particularly in the young, have an unusual epidemiologic background and therefore cannot be included. Also, when subjects are drawn from a cancer detection center they may represent a biased population because of their socioeconomic and religious background, and because of medical and surgical histories, particularly of gynecologic disorders. To reduce bias, data from one control group were compared with those from another before they were combined. Ideally, women from the general population should be interviewed, but it is difficult to find an appropriate group willing to answer the questions required in this study.

As Lingeman points out, epidemiologic evidence strongly suggests that environmental variables are major etiologic factors in ovarian cancer. The finding that the highest rates for ovarian cancer are recorded in highly industrialized countries suggests that physical or chemical products of industry are major causes of these neoplasms. A major exception is highly industrialized Japan, which has one of the lowest rates in the world. Thus the causative factors must be postulated to be more highly concentrated in the United States environment than in Japan. This higher concentration is evident from the increased rates of cancer of the ovary in Japanese migrants in the United States and in their offspring.

A problem in most epidemiologic studies is the number of cases available for analysis. Although most studies are large enough to permit analysis of single variables, the modules in a study of a relatively uncommon disease are usually too small to permit an adequate crossing of variables. A large-scale relationship may appear, but it is less likely that a small association can be statistically verified.

FUTURE STUDIES

Future investigations into the epidemiology of ovarian cancer should interrelate the epidemiologic findings with chemical data on steroid excretion. Because the progress of the disease may alter the steroid pattern, it is worthwhile to obtain more steroid data prospectively, as Bulbrook and Hayward are now trying to do. Pathologists might also more carefully examine the adrenal and pituitary glands of patients who have died from ovarian malignancies.

Additional laboratory investigations should include routine blood cholesterol levels and glucose tolerance tests. It would be particularly interesting to conduct prospective studies to follow the incidence of ovarian cancer among women on long-term oral contraception.

Steroid excretion patterns should be explored in greater detail in women of different weights. The relation of diet to steroid formation based on the major leads provided by studies on Japanese immigrants to the United States should be studied also, because an increase in the overall fat consumption in this group is paralleled by increased blood cholesterol levels, an increase of hormone-related cancers, and an increase of other diseases suspected to be related to dietary fats.

Another area that merits more detailed exploration is that of target-organ response. Certain women have a different response in each breast after the administration of either endogenous or exogenous hormones. Should no major hormone differences be determined for ethnic groups who have different rates of hormone-related cancers, the target organ response to a given hormone or its intermediary products might be explored with success. Target organ responses may be influenced by a change in diet, especially in lipid components.

SUMMARY

Epidemiology of ovarian cancer depends primarily on accurate diagnosis. For example, a specific tumor, a specific histologic type within a single organ may point to a particular causal factor. When accurate diagnosis is not possible, epidemiologic work is handicapped, and Berg and Baylor have disclosed just such a situation in ovarian cancer. Nowhere is accurate diagnosis more important than with ovarian tumors. These tumors are difficult to manage and have a high mortality rate. Moreover, ovarian cancers differ from country to country, and it is from these differences that important etiologic factors may emerge. The Danes have a high incidence of ovarian cancer, whereas Japanese women in their homeland have relatively low rates. The Danes eat a high dairy product diet and therefore a high cholesterol diet, while the Japanese diet is low in cholesterol. Studies in nutrition and hormones among these two groups have contributed little toward finding a possible etiologic factor. The descendants of the Japanese who have moved to the United States have an increased rate of ovarian cancer, and in some reports it is higher in their offspring than in American women.

An acceptable classification is needed for correlation of all parameters associated with ovarian cancer. Despite the lack of agreement in classification, remarkable differences between populations are evident. In a collected series the overall incidence varies from 14.4 to 3.3 per 100,000 per annum, as well as in tumor types. Reports suggest that Africans are affected much more commonly than others by Burkitt's lymphoma involving the ovary. They have more dysgerminomas, granulosa-cell tumors, and Brenner tumors as well as embryonal rhabdomyosarcoma type. The biggest obstacle in studying ovarian cancer is the lack of uniform classification and nomenclature for tumors, and a comprehensive, precise definition of terms.

Wynder, Dodo, and Barber reported that ovarian cancer patients often have a long history of heavy periods, more premenstrual tension, more breast swelling, more miscarriages, and an early menopause. It would seem that the ovary is like a cam running off center—never completely normal.

BIBLIOGRAPHY

Bell, E.T., Loraine, J.A.: Hormone excretion patterns in patients with dysmenorrhea. Lancet 2:519–521, 1966.
Berg, J.W.: Nutrition and cancer. Semin. Oncol. 3:17, 1976.

Berg, J.W., Baylor, S.M.: The epidemiologic pathology of ovarian cancer. Hum. Pathol. 4:537, 1973.

Biskind, M.S., Biskind, G.R.: Development of tumor in rat ovary after transplantation into the spleen. Proc. Soc. Exp. Biol. Med. 55:176–179, 1944.

Buell, P.: Changing incidence of breast cancer in Japanese-American women. J. Natl. Cancer Inst. 51:1479–1483, 1973.

Bulbrook, R.D., Hayward, J.L.: Abnormal urinary steroid excretion and subsequent breast cancer. A prospective study in the island of Guernsey. Lancet 1:519, 1967.

Cook, P.J., Burkitt, D.P.: Cancer in Africa. Br. Med. Bull. 27:14–20, 1971.

Doll, R., Muir, C., Waterhouse, J. (eds.): Cancer Incidence in 5 Continents. Vol. 2. International Union Against Cancer. Springer Verlag, Berlin, 1972.

Graham, J., Graham, R.: Ovarian cancer and asbestos. Environ. Res. 1:115–128, 1967.

Haenszel, W.: The United States Network of Cancer Registries. Recent Results Cancer Res. 50:52–58, 1975.

Higginson, J., Muir, C.S.: Epidemiology, in Cancer Medicine. Edited by J.F. Holland and E. Frei. Lea & Febiger, Philadelphia, 1973, pp. 241–306.

Hinderson, W.J.: Talc and carcinoma of the ovary and cervix. J. Obstet. Gynecol. Br. Commun. 78:266–272, 1971.

Jackson, S.M.: Ovarian dysgerminoma in three generations. J. Med. Genet. 4:112–113, 1967.

James, P.D.: Epidemiology of ovarian cancer. Lancet 1:412, 1974.

Keal, E.E.: Asbestosis and abdominal neoplasms. Lancet 2:1211–1216, 1960.

Kolstad, P., Beecham, J.C.: Epidemiology of ovarian neoplasia. Proceedings of the American-European Conference on the Ovary, Montreux, Switzerland. Excerpta Medica, International Congress Series No. 364, 1974, p. 56.

Lewis, A.C., Davison, B.C.: Familial ovarian cancer. Lancet 2:235–237, 1969.

Li, F.P.: Familial ovarian carcinoma. J.A.M.A. 214:1559–1561, 1970.

Liber, A.F.: Ovarian cancer in mother and five daughters. Arch. Pathol. 49:280–290, 1950.

Lingeman, C.H.: Etiology of cancer of the human ovary. J. Natl. Cancer Inst. 53:1603–1618, 1974.

Lynch, H.T., Krush, A.T.: Carcinoma of the breast and ovary in three families. Surg. Gynecol. Obstet. 133:644–648, 1971.

MacMahon, B., Pugh, T.F.: Epidemiology: Principles and Methods. Little Brown, Boston, 1970, p. 1.

McCrann, D.J., Marchant, D.J., Bardawil, W.A.: Ovarian carcinoma in three teen-age siblings. Obstet. Gynecol. 43:132–137, 1974.

Molloy, W.B.: Identical ovarian malignant disease in two sisters. Aust. N.Z. J. Obstet. Gynecol. 10:265–268, 1970.

Newhouse, M.L.: A study of the mortality of female asbestos workers. Br. J. Ind. Med. 29:134–141, 1972.

Osborne, R.H., DiGeorge, F.V.: The ABO blood groups in neoplastic disease of the ovary. Am. J. Hum. Genet. 15:380–388, 1963.

Staszewski, J.: Cancer registry data versus mortality data. Recent Results Cancer Res. 50:103–110, 1975.

West, R.O.: Epidemiologic study of malignancies of the ovaries. Cancer 19:1001–1007, 1966.

Wynder, E.L., Dodo, H., Barber, H.R.K.: Epidemiology of cancer of the ovary. Cancer 23:352–370, 1969.

4

Histologic Classification of Ovarian Tumors

O ne of the prerequisites for comparative studies is agreement on histologic criteria for the classification of cancer types and a standardized nomenclature. All too often, different terms are used for the same pathologic entity, and indeed the same term is sometimes applied to lesions of different types. It is most important to have an internationally accepted classification of tumor. A committee of the International Federation of Gynecology and Obstetrics (FIGO) formulated a classification of the common epithelial tumors of the ovary, and more recently a group of pathologists appointed by the World Health Organization suggested a WHO classification. The World Health Organization currently lists 19 different cell types and 27 subtypes for benign and malignant primary ovarian tumors based on histogenesis. The histogenetic classification has provided a parameter to judge prognosis. Unfortunately, it has not been applicable to all ovarian tumors. Approximately 90% of ovarian carcinomas originate from the epithelial (mesothelial cells) surface of the ovary. These classifications are presented in this chapter.

Most histologic classifications are based primarily on morphology and histogenesis. Although it is admittedly imperfect because of the imprecision of current embryologic knowledge and the difficulties in identifying specific cell types, it has the advantages of grouping together closely related ovarian tumors, which may be mixed or difficult to distinguish from one another, and of separating neoplastic types that have a dissimilar prognosis and require different therapy.

Ovarian tumors are often composed of a combination of several types that may vary in their biologic behavior, and it is important that the diagnostic terms chosen include all the varieties encountered and indicate as accurately as possible the proportion and distribution of each.

Grading of malignant tumors (a neoplasm is named from its most differentiated portion and graded from its least differentiated part) has been widely recommended. In general it has proved to be of prognostic value in evaluating some but not all ovarian tumors.

The ovarian stroma is specialized and may be stimulated by the growth of

43

a variety of tumors, either benign or malignant, primary or secondary. It can assume the morphologic appearance of steroid-hormone-secreting tissue and may produce androgens, estrogens, and rarely progestogens. Therefore it is important to describe the stroma. When the stroma is endocrinologically active, it has been occasionally designated as "tumors with functioning stroma." This term is not included in the present classification.

In 1961 a committee of the International Federation of Gynecology and Obstetrics (FIGO) formulated a classification of common epithelial tumors of the ovary which was adopted in 1971. The World Health Organization (WHO) has also prepared an International Histologic Classification of Ovarian Tumors. WHO made an effort to conform to the classification of common epithelial tumors proposed by FIGO and subsequently used in publications from several large centers. Broad categories of tumors have been divided into numerous subtypes throughout the classification. This subtyping was done to stimulate the investigation of smaller and possibly distinctive groups as well as general classes. In addition to the epithelial ovarian tumors, WHO includes germ cell tumors, hormone-producing tumors (gonadal stromal), and metastatic carcinoma.

A brief outline is presented for purposes of orientation:

I.   Tumors of surface epithelium and ovarian stromal origin
    A.   Serous
    B.   Mucinous
    C.   Endometrioid
    D.   Clear cell
II.   Germ cell tumors
    A.   Dysgerminoma
    B.   Tumors in the teratoma group
        1)   Extraembryonal group
        2)   Embryonal teratomas, solid and cystic
        3)   Adult teratomas, solid and cystic
        4)   Struma ovarii
        5)   Carcinoid
III.   Gonadoblastoma
IV.   Gonadal stromal tumors (sex cord—mesenchymal)
    A.   Granulosa
    B.   Sertoli-Leydig
V.   Tumors not specific for the ovary
    A.   Burkitt's
    B.   Lymphoma
VI   Metastatic tumors
VII.   Sarcomas

The Cancer Committe of FIGO reported that although ovarian carcinoma is a common malignant tumor, it cannot be regarded as an entity. Therapeutic statistics on ovarian cancer have limited value if attention is not paid to the histologic type of growth. Experience has shown that there is no clear correlation between clinical and histologic malignancy in ovarian tumors. This tenet holds valid for various types of neoplasms, but especially for epithelial tumors, granulosa cell tumors, and virilizing tumors.

According to the FIGO recommendations on the histologic classification of ovarian tumors, cases of germ cell tumors, hormone-producing neoplasms, and metastatic carcinomas should be excluded from therapeutic statistics on ovarian epithelial tumors. The FIGO classification is presented below.

Histologic Classification of the Common
Primary Epithelial Tumors of the Ovary
(To Be Used from January 1, 1971)

I.   Serous cystomas
    A.   Serous benign cystadenomas
    B.   Serous cystadenomas with proliferating activity of the epithelial cells and nuclear abnormalities but with no infiltrative destructive growth (low potential malignancy)
    C.   Serous cystadenocarcinomas
II.   Mucinous cystomas
    A.   Mucinous benign cystadenomas
    B.   Mucinous cystadenomas with proliferating activity of the epithelial cells and nuclear abnormalities but with no infiltrative destructive growth (low potential malignancy)
    C.   Mucinous cystadenocarcinomas
III.   Endometrioid tumors (similar to adenocarcinomas in the endometrium)
    A.   Endometrioid benign cysts
    B.   Endometrioid tumors with proliferating activity of the epithelial cells and nuclear abnormalities, but with no infiltrative destructive growth (low potential malignancy)
    C.   Endometrioid adenocarcinomas
IV.   Mesonephric tumors
    A.   Benign mesonephric tumors
    B.   Mesonephric tumors with proliferating activity of the epithelial cells and nuclear abnormalities, but with no infiltrative destructive growth (low potential malignancy)
    C.   Mesonephric cystadenocarcinomas
V.   Concomitant carcinoma, unclassified carcinoma (tumors that cannot be allotted to groups I–IV)

It has been proposed that cases which according to the above classification are tumors of low potential malignancy, i.e., IB, IIB, IIIB, and IVB, should be called borderline cases. The Cancer Committee of the Federation cannot accept this term, especially because histologically unquestionably benign tumors of papillary nature may give rise to implantation of metastases which spontaneously disappear after removal of the primary growth. Such tumors should not be included among cases of IB, IIB, IIIB, or IVB. The Cancer Committee is aware of the fact that ovarian neoplasms allotted to the group "low potential malignancy" may be of different biologic behavior. However there is presently no method to subdivide these cases.

The World Health Organization includes not only the common epithelial tumors, but also the germ cell tumors, hormone-producing tumors (gonadal stromal), and metastatic carcinomas. The Histologic Classification of Ovarian Tumors proposed by the WHO follows.

Histologic Classification of Ovarian Tumors

I.   Common "epithelial" tumors
    A.   Serous tumors
       1) Benign
          a) Cystadenoma and papillary cystadenoma
          b) Surface papilloma
          c) Adenofibroma and cystadenofibroma
       2) Of borderline malignancy (carcinomas of low malignant potential)
          a) Cystadenoma and papillary cystadenoma
          b) Surface papilloma
          c) Adenofibroma and cystadenofibroma
       3) Malignant
          a) Adenocarcinoma, papillary adenocarcinoma, and papillary cystadenocarcinoma
          b) Surface papillary carcinoma
          c) Malignant adenofibroma and cystadenofibroma
    B.   Mucinous tumors
       1) Benign
          a) Cystadenoma
          b) Adenofibroma and cystadenofibroma
       2) Of borderline malignancy (carcinomas of low malignant potential)
          a) Cystadenoma
          b) Adenofibroma and cystadenofibroma
       3) Malignant
          a) Adenocarcinoma and cystadenocarcinoma
          b) Malignant adenofibroma and cystadenofibroma
    C.   Endometrioid tumors
       1) Benign
          a) Adenoma and cystadenoma
          b) Adenofibroma and cystadenofibroma
       2) Of borderline malignancy (carcinomas of low malignant potential)
          a) Adenoma and cystadenoma
          b) Adenofibroma and cystadenofibroma

        3) Malignant
           a) Carcinoma
              (i) Adenocarcinoma
              (ii) Adenoacanthoma
              (iii) Malignant adenofibroma and cystadenofibroma
           b) Endometrioid stromal sarcomas
           c) Mesodermal (Müllerian) mixed tumors, homologous and heterologous

  D. Clear cell (mesonephroid) tumors
        1) Benign: adenofibroma
        2) Of borderline malignancy (carcinomas of low malignant potential)
        3) Malignant: carcinoma and adenocarcinoma

  E. Brenner tumors
        1) Benign
        2) Of borderline malignancy (proliferating)
        3) Malignant

  F. Mixed epithelial tumors
        1) Benign
        2) Of borderline malignancy
        3) Malignant

  G. Undifferentiated carcinoma
  H. Unclassified epithelial tumors

II. Sex cord stromal tumors
  A. Granulosa-stromal cell tumors
        1) Granulosa cell tumor
        2) Tumors in the thecoma-fibroma group
           a) Thecoma
           b) Fibroma
           c) Unclassified

  B. Androblastomas; Sertoli-Leydig cell tumors
        1) Well differentiated
           a) Tubular androblastoma; Sertoli cell tumors (tubular adenoma of Pick)
           b) Tubular androblastoma with lipid storage; Sertoli cell tumor with lipid storage (folliculome lipidique of Lecène)
           c) Sertoli-Leydig cell tumor (tubular adenoma with Leydig cells)
           d) Leydig cell tumor; hilus cell tumor
        2) Of intermediate differentiation
        3) Poorly differentiated (sarcomatoid)
        4) With heterologous elements

  C. Gynandroblastoma
  D. Unclassified

III. Lipid (lipoid) cell tumors

IV. Germ cell tumors
    A. Dysgerminoma
    B. Endodermal sinus tumor
    C. Embryonal carcinoma
    D. Polyembryoma
    E. Choriocarcinoma
    F. Teratomas
       1) Immature
       2) Mature
          a) Solid
          b) Cystic
             (i)   Dermoid cyst (mature cystic teratoma)
             (ii) Dermoid cyst with malignant transformation
       3) Monodermal and highly specialized
          a) Struma ovarii
          b) Carcinoid
          c) Stuma ovarii and carcinoid
          d) Others
    G. Mixed forms

V. Gonadoblastoma
    A. Pure
    B. Mixed with dysgerminoma or other forms of germ cell tumor

VI. Soft tissue tumors not specific to ovary

VII. Unclassified tumors

VIII. Secondary (metastatic) tumors

IX. Tumor-like conditions
    A. Pregnancy luteoma
    B. Hyperplasia of ovarian stroma and hyperthecosis
    C. Massive edema
    D. Solitary follicle cyst and corpus luteum cyst
    E. Multiple follicle cysts (polycystic ovaries)
    F. Multiple luteinized follicle cysts and/or corpora lutea
    G. Endometriosis
    H. Surface-epithelial inclusion cysts (germinal inclusion cysts)
    I. Simple cysts
    J. Inflammatory lesions
    K. Parovarian cysts

Norris and Chorlton have divided the functioning ovarian tumors into five basic categories. The largest group is derived from the specialized gonadal stroma—granulosa cell tumors, thecomas, Sertoli-Leydig tumors, and Sertoli tumors. Most lipid cell tumors, regardless of the cytologic features, arise from stromal cells. Some germ cell tumors qualify as functioning ovarian tumors inasmuch as certain ones give rise to gonadotrophin production and some teratomas form tissues that have an associated endocrine effect. Rare primary epithelial tumors of the ovary have an associated endocrine effect caused by steroid production from adjacent supporting stroma. Some metastatic carcinomas do the same thing. The gonadoblastoma contains elements of both the germ cell and the gonadal stromal tumors in almost equal proportions. Included in this classification is a group of neoplasms which are not derived from germ cells or gonadal stromal, and which are associated with a wide variety of paraendocrine syndromes. The classification of functioning ovarian tumors by Norris and Chorlton follows.

Classification of Functioning Ovarian Tumors

1.   Tumors of gonadal stroma
     A.   Granulosa-theca tumor
     B.   Sertoli-Leydig tumor (arrhenoblastoma)
     C.   Sertoli tumor (folliculoma lipidique)
     D.   Lipid cell tumors
     E.   Unclassified gonadal stromal tumors
2.   Tumors with functioning stroma
     A.   Brenner tumor
     B.   Adenofibroma
     C.   Cystadenoma
     D.   Cystadenocarcinoma
     E.   Metastatic carcinoma
3.   Functioning germ cell tumors
     A.   Choriocarcinoma
     B.   Teratomas with endocrine components
4.   Mixed germ cell and stromal tumors
     A.   Gonadoblastoma
5.   Nonendocrine tumors with endocrine effect
6.   Tumorous hyperplasias simulating neoplasms
     A.   Nodular theca-lutein hyperplasia of pregnancy
     B.   Hilus cell hyperplasia

SUMMARY

These classifications are based primarily on the microscopic characteristics of the tumors and thus reflect the nature of morphologically identifiable cell types and patterns. The definitions and discussions of the different categories of tumors are reviewed in chapter 5.

The main problem in ovarian cancer is that of early diagnosis. At present, early diagnosis is a matter of chance rather than a scientific method. However, until such methods are available it is important to study the natural history of disease by all means available. By accumulating material from many investigators treated by a variety of methods, some progress may be achieved in salvaging additional patients.

It is obvious that the interpretation of data concerning ovarian tumors is difficult and limited by the small numbers from any one series. However, as the material accumulates and is reported according to stage, grade, and histologic criteria that are universally acceptable, a meaningful and profitable study will result. The acceptance and use of the clinical staging and histologic classification established by the World Health Organization and the International Federation of Gynecology and Obstetrics has helped compare therapeutic results among institutions around the world. It has led to a greater insight into the natural history of ovarian cancer and has resulted in a more rational approach to therapy with anticipated improved results.

BIBLIOGRAPHY

Barber, H.R.K., Sommers, S.C., Snyder, R., Kwon, T.: Histologic and nuclear grading and stromal reactions as indices for prognosis in ovarian cancer. Am. J. Obstet. Gynecol. 121:795, 1975.

Cancer Committee of the General Assembly of International Federation of Obstetrics and Gynecology. Int. J. Gynecol. Obstet. 9:172, 1971.

Jimerson, G.K.: Germ cell tumors of the ovary: The role of pathology in diagnosis and management. Clin. Obstet. Gynec. 17:229, 1974.

Norris, H.J., Chorlton, J.: Functioning tumors of the ovary. Clin. Obstet. Gynecol. 17:189, 1974.

Santesson, L., Kottmeier, H.L.: General classification of ovarian tumors, in Ovarian Cancer. U.I.C.C. Monograph Series. Vol. II. Edited by F. Gentil, A. C. Junqueira. Springer-Verlag, Berlin, 1968.

Santesson, L: Cited by Kraus, F.T.: Gynecologic Pathology. Mosby, St. Louis, 1967.

Scully, R.E.: Recent progress in ovarian cancer. Cancer 1:73, 1970.

Serov, S.F., Scully, R.E., Sobin, L.H.: Histologic typing of ovarian tumors. International Histological Classification of Tumors, No. 9. World Health Organization, Geneva, 1974.

Teilum, G.: Classification of endodermal sinus tumor (mesoblastoma vitellinum) and so-called "embryonal carcinoma" of the ovary. Acta Pathol. Microbiol. Scand. 64:407, 1965.

Woodruff, J.D.: Pathophysiology of the ovary. Clin. Obstet. Gynecol. 17:169, 1974.

5

Definitions and Discussions of the Histologic Typing of Ovarian Tumors

COMMON EPITHELIAL OVARIAN TUMORS

The word *common* has been used because approximately 75 to 80% of ovarian tumors belong in this general category. They arise from the basic germinal epithelium or mesothelium and can be designated as mesotheliomas with varying amounts and activities of the gonadal mesenchyme. The latter is known as the ovarian stroma and contains two elements—the potentially functioning element or theca, and the supporting connective tissue: thus all ovarian tumors are potentially hormone producing.

Between the obviously benign and the obviously malignant there is a common epithelial tumor that is termed a tumor of borderline malignancy or a carcinoma of low malignant potential. No matter how abnormal the epithelium appears, unless it invades the stroma, the tumor must be placed in this category. The assessment of stromal invasion in the serous tumors is usually easy, but the diagnosis in the mucinous tumors may present some difficulty. The mucinous tumors are multilocular and parvilocular, and it is difficult to determine whether these outpouchings represent invasion or not. These outpouchings may get pinched off and appear to be islands of tumor in the stroma, and as such they compound the difficulty of making an accurate diagnosis. A set of differential-diagnostic criteria has been proposed that appear to be more reliable than the determination of the presence or absence of invasion alone: (1) if there is unquestionable invasion, the tumor is classified as carcinoma: and (2) if invasion is uncertain, the diagnosis depends on the height of the atypical proliferating epithelium—if the epithelium is less than four cells in thickness, the tumor is borderline; if it is four cells or greater, a diagnosis of invasive carcinoma is made. Benign, borderline, and malignant forms of any of the neoplastic types listed below may coexist in any one tumor.

51

Tumors of borderline malignancy occasionally implant on the peritoneum and, although such implants may be invasive, distant metastases are rare. The diagnosis must be morphologically objective and, to have prognostic significance, it must be based exclusively on an examination of the ovarian tumor without consideration of whether spread beyond the ovary has taken place.

The descriptive prefixes *adeno-* and *cystadeno-* and the adjective *papillary* should be added to the more specific designation of a tumor whenever appropriate. The suffix *-fibroma* should be used when a tumor, with the exception of the Brenner tumor, is composed predominantly of stroma derived from the ovarian stroma. If the neoplastic epithelium is growing primarily on the peritoneal surface of the ovary, the word *surface* is an appropriate addition to the diagnostic term. The adjective indicating the epithelial cell type should generally be placed first among the descriptive words.

SEROUS TUMORS

The epithelial cells of the serous tumors resemble to varying degrees those of the Fallopian tube. Papillae, ciliated cells, and psammoma bodies are commonly encountered. Ciliated cells are rarely found in the invasive serous carcinomas. The tumors may form mucin which is extracellular.

Julian and Woodruff have indicated there is a borderline low-grade type of papillary malignancy characterized by excessive papillary growth and a tendency to implant on the peritoneal surfaces with the production of ascites, although the lesion would still have to be called histologically benign. They speak of this as grade 0 papillary serous cystadenocarcinoma, which is characterized by very infrequent mitoses and a remarkably high salvage. The salvage decreases as the mitosis count increases (Figure 15).

MUCINOUS TUMORS

The epithelium may resemble endocervical or enteric epithelium and occasionally contains argentaffin cells and Paneth cells. This raises the question of whether these tumors should be classified with the teratomas. The epithelial elements include prominent components of mucin-filled cells (Figure 16).

An unusual variant of the mucinous cystadenoma is pseudomyxoma ovarii. In this type there are extremely thin connective tissue septa between the cystic spaces. There is often disruption of these thin septa with fusion of the cysts filled with mucinous material.

Mucinous tumors may be associated with pseudomyxoma peritonei, which may be associated with a malignancy of the ovary or a mucocele of the appendix. When both are present the ovarian mass is recorded as the primary tumor.

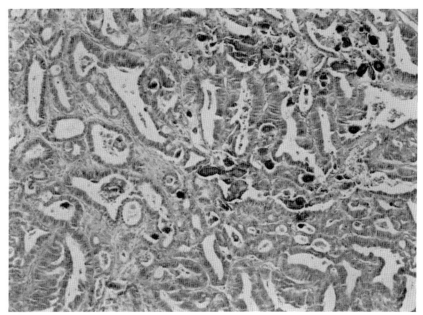

Figure 15. Serous tumors are composed of epithelium resembling that of the Fallopian tube or the surface epithelium of the ovary. Psammoma bodies may be present but do not in themselves indicate malignancy. The tumor cells may produce considerable mucin, which is almost entirely extracellular. They may be unilocular or multilocular.

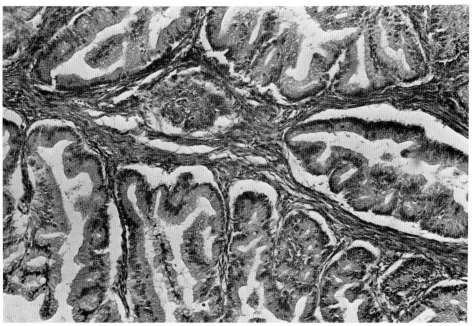

Figure 16. Mucinous tumors may be unilocular of multilocular. They are lined by tall columnar epithelium resembling that of the cervix or large intestine. Microscopically, the tumor has an outer fibrous capsule from which extend septa supporting the walls of the cyst. The walls are lined by tall columnar epithelium with basal nuclei and contain a gelatinous glycoprotein or mucin. Malignancy in a mucinous cyst is characterized by the formation of areas of solid carcinoma in the wall. The cells are columnar, show mitoses, and tend to form glandular structures.

ENDOMETRIOID TUMORS

The endometrioid tumor was first described by Sampson. Santesson, Long, and Taylor have studied this tumor and reported on it in detail.

Tumors of the endometrioid group have the microscopic features of one or more of the typical forms of endometrial neoplasm. Some of the endometrioid tumors have been shown to have arisen in endometriosis, but the demonstration of such an origin is not required for the diagnosis.

The histologic criteria used by Long and Taylor to differentiate endometrioid tumors from serous cystadenocarcinomas are as follows: (1) The cellular arrangement is glandular or acinar with varying resemblance to primary endometrial carcinoma, depending upon the differentiation of the tumor. (2) Papillae, when present, should be blunt in contrast to the finer branching papillae of serous tumors. (3) The growing border of the tumor should be even, without the papillary projections of serous tumors. (4) Squamous metaplasia may be present. (5) With differential staining techniques, glycoprotein and nonspecific mucin can be distinguished in the apical regions of the epithelial cell and abundant extracellular mucin can be seen (Figure 17).

One-third of these tumors are accompanied by a carcinoma of the endometrium which is similar in microscopic appearance. Many of the

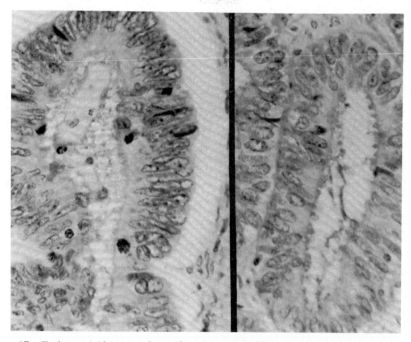

Figure 17.   Endometrioid tumors have the microscopic features of one or more of the typical forms of endometrial neoplasia. They may be adenoacanthomas. These tumors arise in endometriosis, but the demonstration is not required for the diagnosis. Endometrioid carcinomas may have a marked papillary pattern, which is unusual in carcinomas of the endometrium.

associated uterine tumors are very small. When both organs are involved, the evidence suggests separate primaries under the following conditions: (1) When dysplastic lesions are found in the endometrium containing a small carcinoma, the implication is that the latter arose in situ and was not a metastasis from an accompanying ovarian cancer. (2) The patient is classified as ovarian if she presented with clinical manifestation of ovarian cancer, and she is classified as endometrial if the symptoms first related to the uterus. (3) When the endometrial cancer is less than 2 cm in diameter, well differentiated, and no more than minimally invades the myometrium, it is practically certain that the accompanying ovarian tumor is primary. (4) When the uterine cancer is larger than 2 cm, poorly differentiated, grade III, and more invasive into the myometrium, there is a strong possibility that the ovarian cancer represents a metastases. (5) Endometrioid cancers of the ovary may have a markedly papillary pattern, which is unusual in carcinomas of the endometrium (Figure 18).

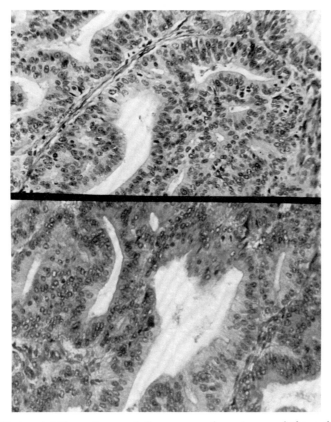

Figure 18. Endometrioid carcinoma of the ovary and carcinoma of the endometrium are associated in about one-third of the cases. In general, they have a similar microscopic appearance. It is difficult to make a judgment about whether a double primary is present or whether one is primary and the other is metastatic.

CLEAR CELL TUMORS (MESONEPHROID)

These tumors are composed of clear cells containing glycogen and resembling those of the renal cell carcinoma (Figure 19). They are large epithelial cells with abundant clear cytoplasm. The cells may be arranged in sheets or cords. The hobnail or peg-shaped cell is considered characteristic of the tumor. The cell is characterized by scant cytoplasm and large nuclei that project into the lumen. The hobnail cell is a clear cell that may have discharged its contents into a lumen. Mucus may be secreted by neoplastic cells but does not accumulate in their cytoplasm.

Occasionally, a renal cell carcinoma metastasizes to the ovary and may be confused with a primary clear cell carcinoma. The tumor must be distinguished from endodermal sinus tumor, the dysgerminoma, and the lipid cell tumor.

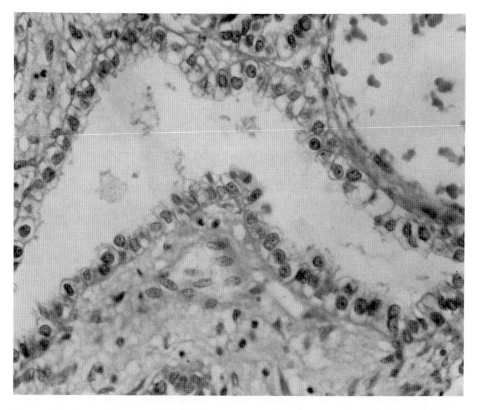

Figure 19. Clear-cell (mesonephroid) tumors are composed of clear cells containing glycogen and resembling those of renal cell carcinoma. They may have hobnail or peg-shaped cells lining small cysts and tubules. Hobnail cells have scant cytoplasm and large nuclei which project into the lumen.

BRENNER TUMORS

The Brenner tumor is composed mainly of fibrous tissue with small islands of clear epithelial cells of squamous appearance (Figure 20). Sometimes the islands become cystic and the epithelial cells become mucinous. The designation *malignant Brenner tumor* is used when carcinomatous change has taken place in the predominant cell type, with the development of either transitional cell or squamous cell carcinoma.

MIXED COMMON EPITHELIAL TUMORS

The tumor should be classified according to the predominant element. In general, the ultrastructural study of various types of ovarian carcinoma has shown heterogeneity within the same tumor with coexistence of more than one cell type and with variations from differentiation to anaplasia. The coexistence of serous and mucinous cells in ovarian carcinoma, also noted by Gondos, can be satisfactorily explained by the histogenetic theory to the multipotential ovarian surface germinal epithelium.

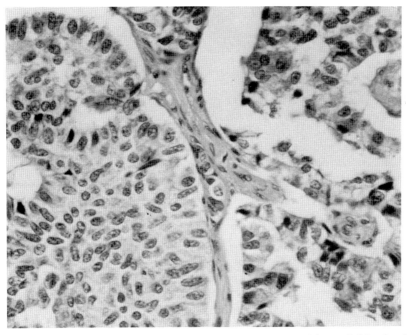

Figure 20. The Brenner tumor is composed of fibrous tissue with small islands of clear epithelial cells of transitional or urethelial type cells. The cells often contain grooved, "coffee bean" nuclei. The term *malignant Brenner tumor* is used when carcinomatous change has taken place in the predominant cell type with the development of either a transitional cell or squamous cell carcinoma.

GERM CELL TUMORS

Structures may be derived from any or all of the three embryonic layers—ectoderm, mesoderm, and endoderm. In some tumors extraembryonic structures predominate; in others, immature and/or mature structures may be derived from any or all embryonic layers. There are four main types of germ cell tumor: (1) dysgerminoma, (2) tumors of tissues found in the embryo or adult—the teratoma, (3) tumors of dysgenetic gonads—commonly a gonadoblastoma, and (4) tumors of extraembryonic tissues such as choriocarcinoma.

Dysgerminoma

The ovarian homologue of seminoma testis is a pure monocellular entity composed of uniform vesicular cells arranged in the form of strands or nests and separated by a variable amount of connective tissue stroma. Stroma and parenchyma commonly show lymphocyte infiltration, one of the most striking histologic characteristics of the tumor. In summary, microscopically it consists of masses of large clear epithelial cells with large nuclei, resembling primitive germ cells, in the cords or alveoli. Fine connective tissue infiltrated by lymphocytes separates the bundles of epithelial cells. The malignancy varies, but many appear to be relatively benign and do not recur. Those in childhood appear to be more malignant (Figure 21).

The dysgerminoma is considered to arise from the germ cells of the sexually indifferent stage in gonadogenesis. Morphologically and histologically, the dysgerminoma cells are identical with primordial germ cells.

Embryonal Carcinoma

Embryonal carcinoma is generally predominantly solid but may contain many small cysts or may be primarily cystic with solid areas in its wall. Microscopically, it is characterized by the presence of embryonal and adult tissues derived from all three germ layers. The polyembryoma is a form of embryonal carcinoma (polyembryonic embryoma). It is a teratomatous tumor of the gonads containing myriads of embryonal bodies comparable to normal presomite embryos (Figure 22).

Endodermal Sinus Tumor

The endodermal sinus tumor (Teilum) is a highly malignant germ cell tumor showing a selective overgrowth of yolk sac endoderm intimately associated with the extraembryonic mesoblast. There are distinctive perivascular structures resembling the endodermal sinuses of the rat placenta, and both intracellular and extracellular hyaline globules, giving a periodic acid Schiff reaction. The hyaline bodies resemble Russell bodies. These tumors are thus extraembryonic derivatives of yolk sac endoderm from embryonal carcinoma (Figure 23).

The yolk sac tumor (endodermal sinus tumor) may contain cysts resembling yolk sac vesicles (polyvesicular vitelline pattern). The polyvesicular

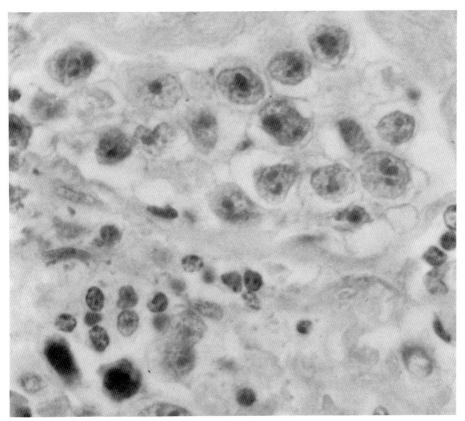

Figure 21. Dysgerminoma is a tumor of uniform appearance. Microscopically, it consists of masses of large clear epithelial cells with large nuclei, resembling primitive germ cells, in cords or alveoli. Fine connective tissue infiltrated by lymphocytes separates the bundles of epithelial cells; granulomas, which may contain Langhans' giant cells, are often present. The cytoplasm of the tumor cells contains glycogen, the presence of which may be an aid in diagnosis.

vitelline tumor (Teilum) is a distinctive type of highly malignant yolk sac tumor, but histologically it is characterized by a myriad of blastocyst-like yolk sac (endoblast) vesicles. It is important to distinguish the endodermal sinus tumor from the clear cell (mesonephroid) carcinoma. The clear cell carcinoma has a different pattern, lacks endodermal sinuses and hyaline bodies, typically occurs in older women, and has a much better prognosis.

Choriocarcinoma

This very rare, highly malignant tumor is composed of both cytotrophoblast and syncytiotrophoblast. It may be associated with sexual precocity. The primary ovarian choriocarcinoma is a derivative of embryonal carcinoma and, in contrast to the tumor originating in a pregnancy in the uterus, it does not respond to chemotherapeutic agents as well (Figure 24).

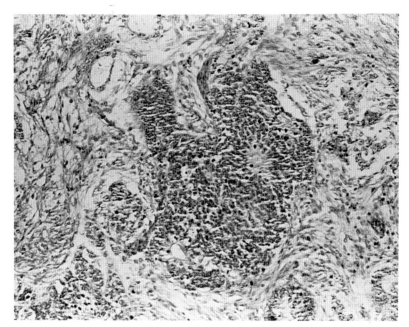

Figure 22. Embryonal carcinoma is a tumor composed of anaplastic embryonal cells of epithelial appearance growing in a variety of patterns, i.e., acinar, tubular, papillary, and solid. Teilum reports that the term *embryonal carcinoma* is restricted to tumors composed of undifferentiated neoplastic embryonal cells representing the undifferentiated forms of extraembryonic as well as embryonic types.

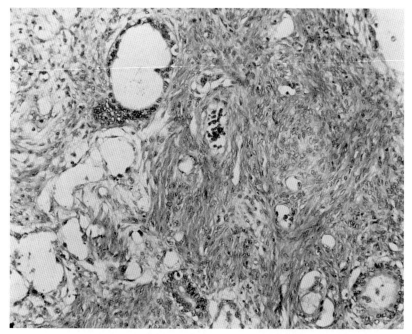

Figure 23. The endodermal sinus tumor is characterized by the presence of a loose vacuolated network of embryonal cells and distinctive perivascular structures resembling the endodermal sinuses of the rat placenta. They contain both intracellular and extracelluar hyaline globules giving a positive periodic acid Schiff reaction. When it contains cysts resembling yolk sac vesicles, it has a polyvesicular vitelline pattern.

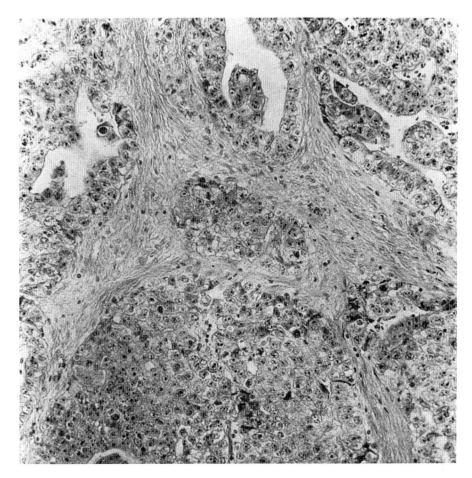

Figure 24. Choriocarcinoma is an extremely rare tumor of the ovary. Syncytiotrophoblast is always present, but sometimes cytotrophoblast is also formed. The hormones produced are those normally associated with chorionic tissue—chorionic gonadotropin, estrogens, etc.

Solid Adult Teratoma

The solid adult teratoma is a rare tumor composed entirely of adult tissues derived from all three germ layers. When it is diagnosed according to strict criteria, the results from appropriate therapy are excellent.

Cystic Adult Teratoma

These cysts are composed of all three germinal layers, although epithelial structures predominate (Figure 25). Studies of nuclear sex chromatin in ovarian teratomas have uniformly shown a female pattern. They are positive for sex chromatin and therefore indicate the presence of XX sex chromosomes; this has been confirmed by chromosomal studies. The presence of nuclear sex chromatin also suggests that these cells are haploid. However a significant portion of teratomas in the male have shown the sex chromatin pattern of females. This discrepancy can be explained if we accept

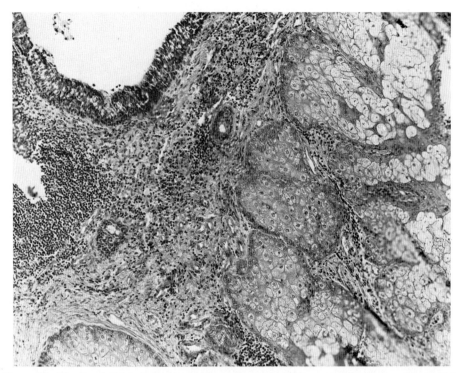

Figure 25.   Cystic adult teratoma (dermoid cyst) is a cyst with a rounded eminence from which hairs grow and on or in which teeth may be found. The eminence may contain sweat glands, teeth, hair, nervous tissues, cartilage, bone, respiratory and intestinal epithelium, and thyroid gland tissue. Thick yellow sebaceous material fills the cyst. The tumor often contains other ectodermal, especially neuroectodermal, derivatives; elements of endodermal and mesodermal origin are also found with great frequency. Occasionally, respiratory epithelium or glia forms a portion of the cyst lining. Squamous cell carcinoma is the usual form of malignant change; adenocarcinoma and sarcoma are much less common, and melanoma is very rare.

the explanation that teratomas in males are derived from haploid germ cells by a process of autofertilization or fusion of adjacent haploid cells. The result would be a diploid chromosome number with either XX or XY chromosomes. The same process in the female could result only in XX diploid cells. Some teratomas in the male have shown a mosaic pattern with sex chromatin-positive and sex chromatin-negative cells, suggesting that their origin may be multicentric rather than from a single germ cell. The microscopic examination may reveal all types of mature ectoderm, mesoderm and entodermal elements. It is not uncommon to find gastrointestinal mucosa, stratified squamous epithelium, hair follicles, sebaceous glands, cartilage, and nervous and respiratory elements. Giant cells and pseudoxanthoma cells are often seen. Occasionally, an overgrowth of thyroid tissue results in a struma ovarii which may function.

Although 2% of cystic tumors are complicated by malignancy, the malignant change is confined usually to one ovary, and patients with squamous carcinoma within the cyst have a much better survival rate than do the patients with the other forms of malignancy, i.e., sarcoma, carcinoids, and adenocarcinoma.

Struma ovarii may complicate a dermoid but is not so designated unless thyroid tissue is the main or sole teratoid component. About 10% of patients with these tumors show evidence of thyrotoxicosis, and only a few prove to be malignant.

Carcinoid tumors (argentaffinomas) of the ovary may arise in the wall of a dermoid cyst either from intestinal or bronchial epithelium. The characteristics of the syndrome resulting from this tumor include intermittent flushing, cyanosis, diarrhea, and asthmatic attacks. The clinical manifestations are attributed to the production of excessive quantities of 5-hydroxytrypamine (serotonin) by the argentaffin cells of the tumor. The argentaffin granules may be identified with appropriate silver stains even in neoplasms of apparent bronchial origin. These tumors occasionally metastasize.

GONADOBLASTOMA

Gonadoblastoma is composed of a mixture of germ cells (dysgerminoma) and gonadal stromal cells (granulosa-Sertoli). Since the tumor had previously been reported only in intersexual individuals, it was called dysgenetic gonadoma. In most cases in which sex chromatin studies have been done, the nuclear pattern has been negative in the patient (46 XY) or may have a sex chromosome mosaicism (XO/XY). Most patients with a gonadoblastoma are intersexual with a phenotype female habitus, are amenorrheic, and may be virilized. Grossly, the tumor ranges from a solid mass of gray to cream-colored, fleshy tissue resembling a dysgerminoma to a firm, fibrous mass. A characteristic feature is calcification, which may be evident on x-ray examination of the pelvis. Microscopically, there are masses of large germ cells which wrap themselves around granulosa-like cells. Between the nests of cells, there are a large number of cells suggestive of Leydig cells. Calcification is often encountered. Bilateral involvement occurs in approximately one-third of the cases. The malignant potential of pure gonadoblastoma has not been established, and it may well depend on the mixture of gonadoblastoma with other germ cell tumors present, such as dysgerminoma or endodermal sinus tumor. These patients often reveal eunuchoidal features or signs of Turner's syndrome and sterility, and the tumor has the potential of developing a malignancy (Figure 26).

GONADAL STROMAL TUMORS
(SEX CORD-MESENCHYME TUMORS)

Female Cell Type

Gonadal stromal (sex cord-mesenchyme) tumors make up the category of tumors which includes gonadal stromal tumors of the female cell type, such as the granulosa or granulosa-thecoma type, or of the male cell type, such as

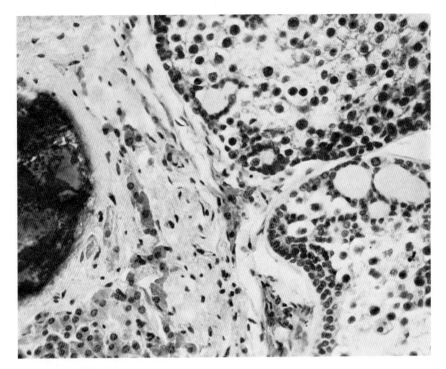

Figure 26. Gonadoblastoma is a tumor associated with dysgenetic gonads, usually streak gonads. Commonly there is a sex chromosome anomaly such as XO/XY. The patient is a phenotypic female. The tumor is composed of two types of cell: (A) a large primitive germ cell, and (B) small cells of the granulosa cell type. Call-Exner bodies (small rosettes) may be seen in the latter. These two types of cell form epithelial islands in a stroma which may contain Leydig-like cells. Sometimes the germ cells may undergo rapid proliferation and give rise to a dysgerminoma. Some of the dysgerminata in children may arise in this way. [Courtesy of Dr. R. E. Scully. Reprinted from *Progress in Gynecology, Vol. 5.* Grune & Stratton, New York, 1970, chap. 3.]

Sertoli-Leydig cell (arrhenoblastoma) and Sertoli and hilus (Leydig) cell tumors. These are not as common as the germ cell tumors, nor are they as malignant.

1. Granulosa Cell Tumors—Although there are approximately 100 granulosa tumors among children reported in the literature, only three have proved to be malignant. Hertig has called them the most glamorous of all neoplasms. Granulosa cell tumors in childhood are infrequent and account for few cases of precocious puberty. The startling secondary sexual changes that they produce in children are dramatic. From 5 to 10% of the tumors occur before the patient reaches the age of puberty. However they may function and produce a feminine habitus, maturation of the genitalia, and enlargement of the breasts. Pubic hair is scant and vaginal bleeding may occur. However precocious puberty is usually constitutional, and only about 2% result from an ovarian tumor. More often the diagnosis is made after an abdominal or pelvic mass is discovered. The tumors are bilateral in about 5% of the cases.

The tumor has a good prognosis. The malignancy rate in adults is about 25%, but only about 3 to 6% in children. The recurrences are usually local, and distant metastases are rare. Recurrences may occur at any time, but the rate of recurrence is very slow and it often takes many years to develop. The histologic appearance of a tumor of this group is no index of its final behavior (Figure 27).

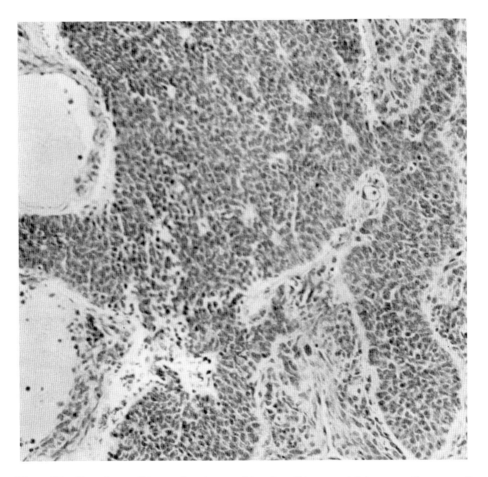

Figure 27. Granulosa cell tumor is a tumor of female cell type containing more than a small component of granulosa cells. The cells may be arranged in a variety of patterns, including follicular (microfollicular and macrofollicular), trabecular, insular, and diffuse (sarcomatoid). The microfollicular pattern is characterized by the presence of distinctive Call-Exner bodies. The most specific diagnostic feature of the granulosa cell tumor, in addition to its characteristic patterns, is the appearance of its nuclei, which may be either irregular in shape, with their long axes directed haphazardly, or round and uniform. Although mitoses may be numerous, the nuclei typically lack the pleomorphism and hyperchromatism of the nuclei of adenocarcinoma and undifferentiated carcinomas. The presence of nuclear grooving in granulosa cells is often helpful in the differential diagnosis.

Sertoli-Leydig Cell Tumor—This term has been selected instead of the more familiar term, *arrhenoblastoma*, because many of these tumors are nonfunctioning or have estrogenic effects rather than masculinizing tendencies. In those tumors with a predominance of functioning Sertoli cells, the effect may be that of a feminizing tumor. However, if the Leydig cells are predominant and function, the patient first is defeminized (atrophy of breasts, loss of female contour, amenorrhea) then masculinized (hirsutism, hypertrophy of clitoris, and voice changes). The tumor usually affects women of the childbearing age and is very rare in childhood. The tumor is bilateral in only 5% of the cases. From 3 to 20% of these tumors demonstrate malignant behavior, which is usually manifested by intraabdominal spread rather than by distal metastasis (Figure 28).

Mixed Type (Gynandroblastoma)—Gynandroblastoma should contain typical aggregates of granulosa cell with Call-Exner bodies and either hollow tubules or Leydig cells containing crystalloids of Reinke. There are no reports of this tumor in childhood, but there is no reason to believe that it will differ in its behavior from granulosa cell or Sertoli-Leydig cell tumors (Figure 29).

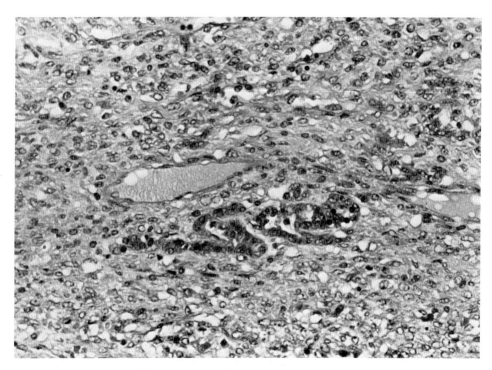

Figure 28.   Sertoli-Leydig cell tumors (arrhenoblastomas) contain Sertoli and Leydig cells of varying degress of maturity. Histologically they consist of primitive tubules surrounded by Leydig cells which may be crystalloids of Renke. These are rod-shaped structures in the cytoplasm of Leydig cells and are said to be diagnostic of these cells.

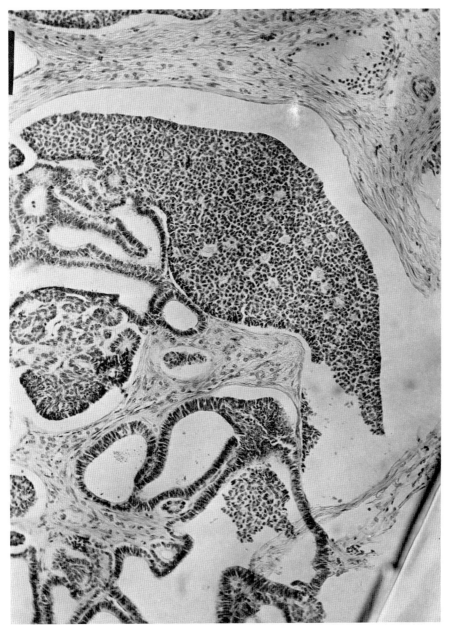

Figure 29. Gynandroblastoma is a very rare tumor in which collections of granulosa cells with typical Call-Exner bodies coexist with hollow tubules lined by Sertoli cells. Although the two cell types need not be present in equal amounts in order to bear the name *gynandroblastoma*, they should be present in at least a 70/30 ratio. This tumor is also known as a sex cord stromal tumor of mixed cell types. [Courtesy of Dr. R. E. Scully. Reprinted with permission from *The Ovary*, Int. Acad. Path. Monograph No. 3. Williams & Wilkins Co., Baltimore, 1962, chap. 9.]

Tumors Not Specific For the Ovary

The ovary may be involved as part of disseminated Hodgkin's disease. These tumors are usually found in adults, but ovarian involvement has been reported among children suffering from Burkitt's tumor. It is interesting that the first virus to be suspected of causing a human cancer was isolated as a result of epidemiologic observations made in populations of tropical Africa, particularly in those with Burkitt's tumor. The particular distribution of the tumor from the geographic and ecologic standpoint as well as its age distribution were typical of an infectious disease, and thus they led to the suspicion that Burkitt's tumor may be caused by an infectious agent. A concerted effort resulted in the isolation of a virus (EB virus) from Burkitt's tumor cells (Figure 30). Lymphoma of the ovary is rare (Figure 31).

Miscellaneous

Fibroma and sarcomas fall into this category. Ovarian sarcomas occur more frequently in children than in adults. Grossly these tumors are solid, lobulated, or soft growths. They grow rapidly and fill the abdomen. The cut surface of the cellular sarcomas are soft and fleshy, whereas the more fibrous ones are firm and somewhat granular when sectioned. Azoury and Woodruff reported on 47 primary sarcomas of the ovary. The most common symptoms

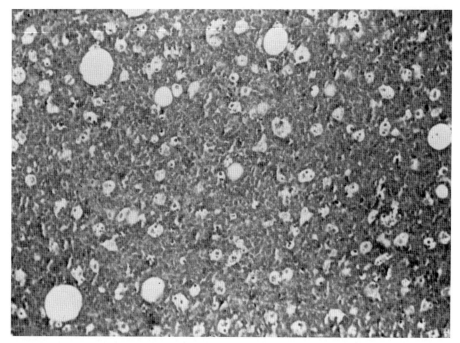

Figure 30. Burkitt's lymphoma is characterized by proliferation of a primitive lymphoreticular system. It presents a histologic picture of stars in the heavens.

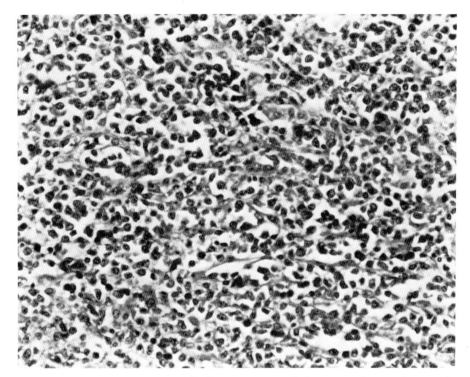

Figure 31. Lymphoma is an exceedingly rare tumor of the ovary. It may be mistaken microscopically for a granulosa cell tumor or a dysgerminoma, because growth in the dense ovarian stroma may result in a pseudocarcinomatous pattern. It may grow diffusely or in the form of well-defined nests and cords of cells, simulating the pattern of a carcinoma.

were abdominal pain and swelling. Regardless of therapy, survival is poor (Figure 32).

METASTATIC CANCER

Approximately 10% of ovarian cancers are metastatic and the survival rate is very low. Most arise from the bowel, breast, or thyroid. Since cancer of the colon is on the increase among women and is the second most common cancer, the incidence of metastasis to the ovary from the colon is also increasing. Careful sectioning of the ovaries has revealed that approximately 25% of patients with colon cancer have metastases to the ovary. Metastatic breast cancer is rarely detected clinically because the patient usually dies from widespread disease before the ovaries have become large enough to produce symptoms. However the results of prophylactic oophorectomies have disclosed that over 40% of patients will have metastases to the ovary if multiple sections are taken.

Krükenberg tumor is an unusual type of malignancy which usually arises in the gastrointestinal tract and metastasizes to the ovary. It is often bilateral, is typically solid, and retains its shape. There a few cases reported

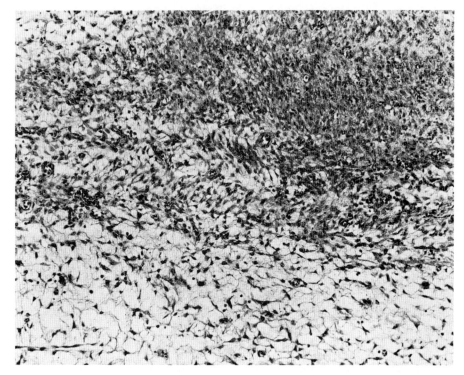

Figure 32. Sarcoma of the ovary is a very rare tumor. Grossly the tumors are solid, lobulated, or soft growths. The cut surface of the cellular sarcomas are soft and fleshy, whereas the more firm ones are firm and somewhat granular when sectioned. The ovarian sarcomas are divided into three groups: teratoid, mesenchymal, and mixed tumors. The sarcomas have bizarre nuclei; some are larger and more irregular than those seen in normal tissue. The number of mitoses is increased. The old entity known as *stromatous endometriosis*, characterized by ectopic endometrial stroma without endometrial glands, is today considered the etiologic factor in ovarian sarcoma, carcinosarcoma, and mixed mesodermal tumors whether homologous or heterologous.

among children. Krükenberg tumors are characterized histologically by large, swollen, signet-ring-like cells which lie in clumps within areas of mucoid degeneration, and these are scattered through an edematous stroma-like matrix. Only tumors meeting these criteria should be so designated (Figure 33).

SUMMARY

Many classifications for ovarian tumors have been proposed over the years. None have been completely satisfactory, and it has been difficult to get the medical profession to adopt a common classification for reporting results. In 1961 a committee of the International Federation of Gynecology and Obstetrics proposed a classification for ovarian tumors, and more recently a committee of the World Health Organization has formulated a more detailed classification. The new classifications have grouped closely related

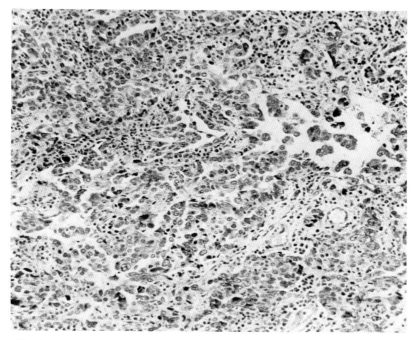

Figure 33. Krükenberg is a rare secondary carcinoma of the ovary. Histologically, it has a characteristic appearance. There is a very cellular stroma, resembling a sarcoma, in which large epithelial cells lie singly or in alveoli. These epithelial cells have a clear cytoplasm with a crescentric nucleus pushed to one side, resulting in a typical signet ring appearance. The cytoplasm is full of mucin.

ovarian tumors. Because current embryologic knowledge is imprecise and because it is difficult to identify specific cell types, the present classifications have inherent weaknesses. In spite of these shortcomings the new classifications have been accepted and material is being reported according to them.

It is important to standardize the parameters used in studying ovarian cancer. The editors of the journals should insist upon a common method of presenting data. By accumulating material from many investigators using the same parameters for their studies, it would be possible to identify the best form of treatment. Progress may then be achieved in salvaging additional patients.

BIBLIOGRAPHY

Barber, H.R.K., Graber, E.A.: Gynecological tumors in childhood and adolescence. Obstet. Gynecol. Surv. 28:357, 1973.

Barber, H.R.K., Graber, E.A., Kwon, T.: Ovarian cancer (monograph). Ca-A Cancer Journal for Clinicians. American Cancer Society, Professional Education Publication, 1975.

Janovski, N.A., Paramanandhan, T.L.: Ovarian Tumors: Tumors and Tumor-Like Conditions of the Fallopian Tubes and Ligaments of the Uterus. Saunders, Philadelphia, 1973.

Julian, C.G., Woodruff, J.D.: Low-grade papillary cystadenocarcinoma of the ovary. Obstet. Gynecol. 40:860, 1972.

Morris, J.M., Scully, R.E.: Endocrine Pathology of the Ovary. Mosby, St. Louis, 1958.

Scully, R.E.: Recent progress in ovarian cancer. Hum. Pathol. 1:73, 1970.

Serov, S.F., Scully, R.E., Sobin, L.H.: Histological typing of ovarian tumors. International Histological Classification of Tumors, No. 9. World Health Organization, Geneva, 1973.

Teilum, G.: Special Tumors of Ovary and Testis and Related Extragonadal Lesions. Munksgaard, Copenhagen, 1971.

6

Histologic, Nuclear, and Stromal Grading

According to Decker and coworkers, within a given stage of ovarian epithelial carcinoma, regardless of the histologic cell type, the increasingly higher grades have an increasingly poor prognosis. This finding suggests that more intensive therapy be considered for all patients with ovarian epithelial carcinomas than is currently undertaken. Decker also restated that epithelial ovarian cancer has always been difficult to treat successfully. The concept of a "scale of malignancy" was suggested by Virchow as long ago as 1858, but its application to ovarian carcinoma classification systems has not been implemented. Reports by Decker have demonstrated the value of grading tumors for prognostic significance, and the International Federation of Gynecology and Obstetrics (FIGO) has now recognized that grading has value in the classification of carcinoma of the endometrium. It is anticipated that increased attention will be directed to the grading of ovarian cancers. Barber and associates reported on histologic and nuclear grading and stromal reactions as indices for prognosis in ovarian cancer. This report provides the basis for this chapter.

Ovarian cancer is one of the most frustrating problems in gynecology. Each year about 17,000 new cases are diagnosed in the United States, and almost 11,000 patients die from ovarian cancer. The incidence comprises 24% of all gynecologic cancers, but the dramatic figure is that it causes more than 47% of gynecologic cancer deaths. The challenge presented is that the results in 1976 were no better than they were in the previous two decades. Early diagnosis, of which there is none, and prophylaxis, to which there is resistance, offer the only hope of improving the lot of these unfortunate patients. Until major advances are made in the areas of early diagnosis and treatment with predictable promise for cure, attention must be directed to study of the natural history of the disease and its histologic patterns, cell type, and stromal reactions. This approach should further validate end results and in the future help improve the survival rate in ovarian carcinoma. This chapter explores the relationships among the staging, grading, and stromal reactions of the tumors as they relate to survival.

In 1961 a committee of FIGO formulated a classification of common epithelial tumors of the ovary which was adopted in 1971. The World Health Organization (WHO) has also prepared an International Histologic Classification of Ovarian Tumors. WHO tried to conform to the classification of common epithelial tumors proposed by the FIGO and subsequently used in publications from several large centers. Broad categories of tumors have been divided into numerous subtypes throughout the classification in order to stimulate the investigation of smaller and possibly distinctive groups as well as general classes. In addition to the epithelial ovarian tumors the WHO classification includes germ cell tumors, hormone-producing tumors (gonadal stromal), and metastatic carcinomas. This classification is discussed in chapter 4.

The patients treated in the early part of the study were staged in a retrospective manner based on physical examination, on laboratory and pathologic reports, as well as on operative records. Although it provides an outline for comparison of material between different centers, it has inherent weaknesses. Cases are included in the invasive group only if there is in-filtrative destructive growth into the stroma, regardless of the extent of the proliferative activity of the epithelial cells and nuclear abnormalities. Because mucinous tumors are commonly both multilocular and parvilocular, it is often impossible to determine accurately whether glandular structures lying within the stroma are the result of budding from a larger gland or cyst, or whether they indicate invasion of the stroma. In this study an attempt was made to determine whether documentation of histologic and nuclear grading as well as of stromal response would help establish whether these tumors are low-grade malignant or not.

MATERIALS AND METHODS

The patients reported were those with epithelial ovarian cancers who were treated at Lenox Hill Hospital in New York from 1963 to 1973. During the early part of the study the treatment employed was to remove the cancer or as much as possible, if this could be done, without an inordinate amount of morbidity and death. During those years, postoperative pelvic and ab-dominal radiation was added in those patients whose disease was not com-pletely removed or in those patients considered to be at risk for recurrence due to the size of the tumor. In the last part of the study a protocol had evolved that served as the basis for treatment. Most of the patients were treated by a small group of gynecologists and by only two radiation therapists.

Histologic Grading

The Broders classification, devised by A.C. Broders of the Mayo Clinic, consists of four numerical grades (I, II, III, and IV) for both epidermoid car-cinoma and adenocarcinoma of the cervix. It is the most commonly used classification in the United States. The basis for this classification is the well-known observation that the degree of malignancy keeps pace with the degree of cell differentiation; thus grade I is the most highly differentiated and grade IV the most immature.

The original Broders grading method was cumbersome, because as many as 13 different cytologic characteristics had to be observed and evaluated. In estimating the grade of an epidermoid carcinoma, the following factors are recorded for each grade: epithelial pearls, individual keratinized cells, intercellular bridges, tumor giant cells, and mitosis per high-power field. It is obvious that pathologists differ in the weight they assign to each of these factors. One axiom in use is that a neoplasm is named from its most differentiated portion and graded from its least differentiated parts. Most pathologists now use a simplified version.

Ewing influenced many pathologists when he presented his material using only three grades. In Ewing's scheme, Broders' grades III and IV are combined and called grade III. This is the histologic classification followed in this report. It is based on the uniformity or lack of uniformity of the cells, on whether the nucleus is regular or not, and on the ratio between the nucleus and cytoplasm, the number and size of the nucleoli, and the number of mitoses per high-power field (Figures 34–36).

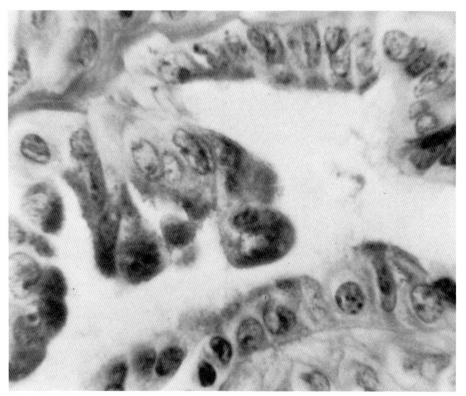

Figure 34.   Grade I is the most highly differentiated cell type. The cells are fairly uniform, the nucleus is quite regular, and there is little increase in the number of nucleoli.

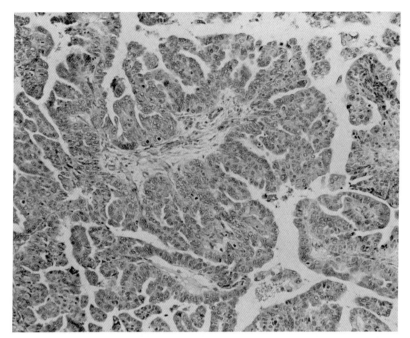

Figure 35. Grade II is intermediate between grade I, which is near normal, and grade III, in which the cells are very immature.

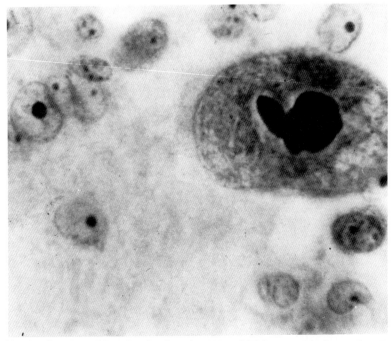

Figure 36. Grade III combines Broders' grades III and IV into one grade, grade III. In this grade the cells are immature and lack uniformity, the nucleus is irregular and enlarged, and the nuclear/cytoplasm ratio is altered so that the nucleus makes up a large part of the cell. The number and size of the nucleoli are increased, as is the number of mitoses per high-power field.

Nuclear Grade

The nuclei of the tumor cells were graded from 1 to 3 according to the classification of Black and Speer: grade 1—markedly enlarged, irregular in outline with chromatin clumping and prominent nucleoli; grade 2—intermediate degree of differentiation; grade 3—similar in size and appearance to each other and to normal ovarian tissue when present. It should be noted that in the histologic grading the better differentiated tumors are grade I and that grade III is the least differentiated, whereas in grading the nuclei grade 1 is the most anaplastic and grade 3 the least anaplastic (Figures 37–39).

Stromal Reactions

Chabon, Takeuchi, and Sommers employed a stromal evaluation in a breast study and have adapted this method of grading for the ovarian cancers in this study. The stroma of each epithelial ovarian cancer was graded according to the number of lymphocytes, plasma cells, and polymorphonuclear leukocytes present. Lymphocytes, plasma cells, and polymorphonuclear infiltration in the stroma and around small veins were graded 0 to 3: 0—none; 1—minimal; 2—moderate; and 3—marked (Figures 40–42).

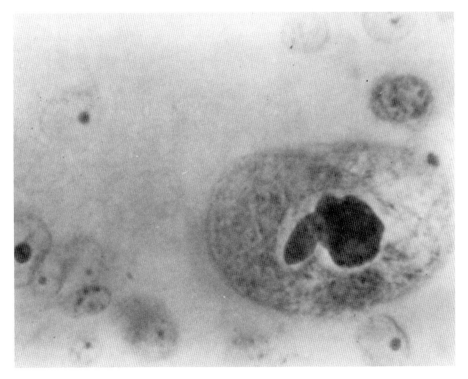

Figure 37.   Nuclear grade 1 is characterized by nuclei that are markedly enlarged and irregular in outline, with chromatin clumping and prominent nucleoli. It is the most anaplastic grade.

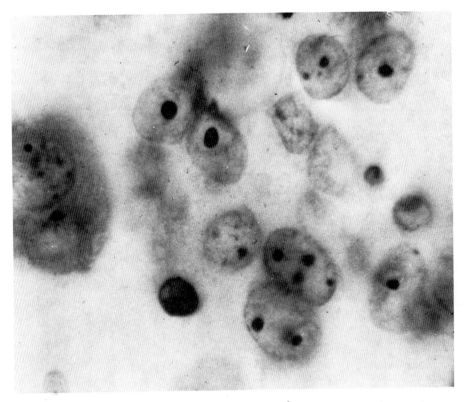

Figure 38. Nuclear grade 2 is intermediate in differentiation between grades 1 and 3.

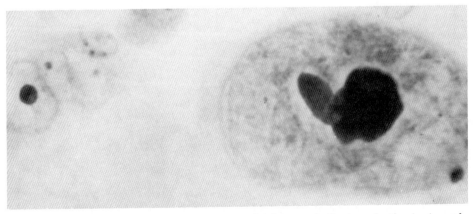

Figure 39. Nuclear grade 3 is characterized by nuclei that are similar to each other in size and appearance, and similar to normal ovarian tissue when present.

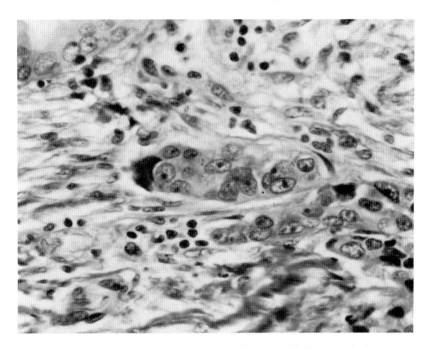

Figure 40. Lymphocytes, plasma cells, and polymorphonuclear infiltration in the stroma and around small veins were graded 0 to 3.0 = none; 1= minimal (Figure 40); 2 = moderate (Figure 41); and 3 = marked (Figure 42).

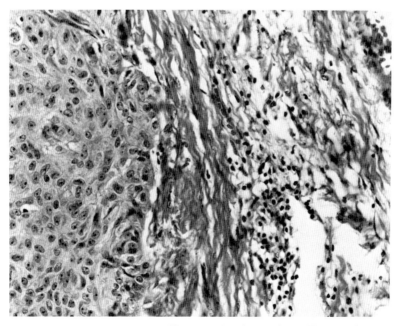

Figure 41. Moderate infiltration. (See the caption to Figure 40.)

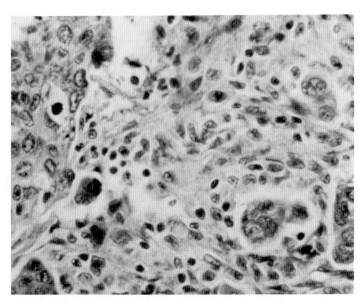

Figure 42.   Marked infiltration. (See the caption to Figure 40.)

RESULTS

The cancers of the ovary studied include those of 182 patients seen from 1963 to 1973. Eight were lost to follow-up, so only 174 could be followed for the entire study. However 5 of the 8 were available for 2 years of the study. Since therapy and prognosis in ovarian cancer depend largely on the extent of disease and of the penetration of the capsule, all patients have been staged according to the stage-grouping for primary epithelial cancer of the ovary as established by FIGO. The staging is discussed in chapter 11. Although the major part of the paper is related to prognosis relative to the findings of staging and grading, a discussion of the over-all material is indicated. The type and number of epithelial cancers were as follows: serous 88, mucinous 26, endometrioid 38, clear cell 10, undifferentiated 20. The age distribution of the 182 patients is listed in Table 1.

Each slide was reviewed by a panel of pathologists consisting of not less than two or more than four members. If there was any disagreement on whether a tumor was invasive, or if discussion indicated that clear-cut criteria for cancer were not evident, the case was not included in the study. Many slides contained more than one cell type and were included in the group having the predominant histologic type.

The study included only patients with epithelial ovarian tumors who received their primary treatment at Lenox Hill Hospital. A few who had exploratory laparotomies and biopsies elsewhere and were then referred on for definitive therapy are included as fresh cases. The patients with recurrent epithelial tumors that were referred for additional treatment as well as those with nonepithelial ovarian cancers are not included in this study.

Table 1. Age Distribution of Ovarian Cancer

	Papillary Serous Cystadeno Cancer	Mucinous Cystadeno Cancer	Endometrioid Cancer	Clear Cell Cancer	Undifferentiated Cancer
Mean age alive	54.6	51.9	50.5	58.3	64.0
Mean age dead	58.6	61.0	65.0	60.6	62.9
Total	57.4	56.9	59.5	59.9	63.1
Range	20–81	23–78	32–86	35–87	46–82

Survival Related to Histologic and Nuclear Grading and Stromal Reaction

The histologic grades range from I to III, with III being the least differentiated, and the nuclear grades from 3 to 1, with 1 being the most anaplastic. The histologic and nuclear grades for serous cystadenocarcinoma are outlined in Table 2. Among those patients in histologic grades I and II, 29 were living at 2 or more years and 23 died during this interval. In the group of patients in the less favorable histologic grade III, 5 of 30 were living at 2 or more years and 25 were dead. There were 52 patients in the more favorable histologic grades I and II, and among those in nuclear grades 3 and 2, 24 were living at 2 or more years and 16 were dead. In nuclear grade 1, five were living and 7 were dead. There were no cases with favorable nuclear grade 3 in the unfavorable histologic grade III group. One of 10 and 4 of 15 with nuclear grades 2 and 1, respectively, were living at 2 or more years.

The endometrioid cancers listed in Table 3 show that in the more favorable histologic grades I and II, 14 of 26 were living at 2 or more years and 12 were dead, whereas in the less favorable histologic grade III, 2 of 12

Table 2. Serous Cystadenocarcinomas—All Patients

Histologic Grade	Nuclear Grade	Stage I IA	IB	IC	Stage II IIA	IIB	Stage III	Stage IV	Total
I	3	2	2	1				(1)	5 (1)
	2	2 (1)					1		3 (1)
	1								
II	3						1		1
	2	3	1	(1)	3 (1)	1	6 (9)	1 (3)	15 (14)
	1	3 (1)			(1)		2 (2)	(3)	5 (7)
III	3								
	2				1 (1)		(6)	(3)	1 (10)
	1		2		1 (1)		1 (8)	(6)	4 (15)
Total		16 (3)			6	6 (4)	11(25)	1 (16)	34 (48)

Cases in parenthesis were dead at 2 years. Six were lost to follow-up and not included.

Table 3. Endometrioid Cancers—All Cases

Histologic Grade	Nuclear Grade	Stage I IA	IB	IC	Stage II IIA	IIB	Stage III	Stage IV	Total
I	3	1					(1)	(1)	1 (2)
	2	1							1
	1								
II	3								
	2	4	1 (1)				4 (4)	(3)	9 (8)
	1	1					1 (1)	1 (1)	3 (2)
III	3								
	2						(4)	(1)	(5)
	1	2					(3)	(2)	2 (5)
Total		10 (1)			0 (0)		5 (13)	1 (8)	16 (22)

Cases in parenthesis were dead at 2 years.

were living at 2 or more years and 10 were dead. In histologic grades I and II, 20 of 26 patients were in nuclear grades 2 and 3; 11 were living at 2 or more years, and 10 were dead; in nuclear grade 1, 3 of 5 patients were living and 2 were dead. In the less favorable histologic grade III there were no cases with the favorable nuclear grade 3. Of 12 patients with nuclear grades 2 and 1, 2 were living at 2 or more years and 10 were dead.

The results in mucinous cystadenocarcinoma, undifferentiated carcinoma, and clear cell carcinoma are listed in Tables 4, 5, and 6 respectively. As anticipated among the undifferentiated, there were no cases in the favorable histologic grade I and none in the favorable nuclear grade 3 among the 20 patients. This study did not determine whether documentation of histologic and nuclear grading as well as stromal response might help establish whether a given mucinous carcinoma was of low-grade malignancy or not. However among the 24 cases only 1 was in the less favorable histologic grade III and only 2 were in the unfavorable nuclear grade 1, results suggesting that these are less aggressive tumors than the other epithelial ovarian cancers.

Table 4. Mucinous Cystadenocarcinoma

Histologic Grade	Nuclear Grade	Stage I			Stage II		Stage III	Stage IV	Totals
		IA	IB	IC	IIA	IIB			
I	3	2			1			1	4
	2	3					1		3 (1)
	1	1							1
II	3						1 (1)		1 (1)
	2	3				(1)	2 (3)	(2)	5 (6)
	1	1							1
III	3								
	2							(1)	(1)
	1								
Total		9			1 (1)		4 (5)	1 (3)	15 (9)

Cases in parenthesis were dead at 2 years. Two were lost to follow-up and not included.

Table 5. Undifferentiated Carcinoma—All Cases

Histologic Grade	Nuclear Grade	Stage I			Stage II		Stage III	Stage IV	Total
		IA	IB	IC	IIA	IIB			
I	3								
	2								
	1								
II	3								
	2								
	1				(1)				(1)
III	3								
	2	(1)					(2)		(3)
	1				(1)	(1)	2 (4)	(8)	2 (14)
Total		(1)			(2)	(1)	2 (6)	0 (8)	2 (18)

Cases in parenthesis were dead at 2 years.

Table 6. Clear Cell Carcinoma

Histologic Grade	Nuclear Grade	Stage I		IC	Stage II		Stage III	Stage IV	Total
		IA	IB		IIA	IIB			
I	3	(1)							(1)
	2	1							1
	1								
II	3								
	2				(1)	1			1 (1)
	1			(1)			1 (1)		1 (2)
III	3			(1)					(1)
	2			(1)					(1)
	1						(2)		(2)
Total		1 (1)		(2)	(1)	1	1 (3)	0 (0)	3 (7)

Cases in parenthesis were dead at 2 years.

The stromal reaction is reported in Table 7. Among those dead before 2 years, 23 had no lymphocytes and 61 no plasma cells. It should be noted that there is overlap among these groups because some patients had neither lymphocytes nor plasma cells in their stroma. Of those patients living 2 or more years, 15 had no lymphocytes in their stroma and 45 had no plasma cells. An evaluation of Table 7 shows that in the early stages there was less of a combined lymphocyte and plasma cell reaction than in the more advanced stages. Although stromal reaction with lymphocytes and plasma cells is considered a favorable reaction, the results in this series did not bear out this observation. There may be other factors that are more important, or perhaps the ovary does not attract lymphocytes and plasma cells to the degree that tumors in other organs do, at least in the early stages. The number of cases may not be sufficient to permit study of the stromal reaction, but in a group of this size it is anticipated that the heterogenicity of the immune state should indicate that the body defenses are active. The lack of documentation may be attributable to the failure of the ovary to mobilize its immune defense as rapidly as defenses are mobilized in breast cancer. However the stromal reaction among the ovarian cancers did increase with the stage of disease. Although the stromal reaction was minimal in the early stages when each histologic type was grouped together (stages I through IV), a marked lymphocyte, plasma cell, and stromal reaction was observed.

Certain observations can be made from Tables 4–7. The greatest number of survivals were in the more favorable histologic grades I and II, as well as the more favorable nuclear grades 3 and 2. The least anaplastic histologic and nuclear grades are found in the early stages, and the more anaplastic tumors in the more advanced stages. The correlation is particularly evident among the undifferentiated tumors. In this group the fact that there were no cases in the favorable histologic grade I or favorable nuclear grade 3 confirmed the malignant potential of this histologic type. Although the histologic and nuclear grades and stromal reaction added little in determining the degree of malignancy for a given mucinous cancer, the grading and stromal reaction

Table 7. Stromal Reactions (Overall)

Stages I Through IV

Stromal Reactions	IA	IB	IC	IIA	IIB	III	IV	Total
Lymphocytes								
0	7 (2)	1 (1)	(2)	(2)	1	5 (13)	1 (3)	15 (23)
1+	21 (1)	3	(1)	3 (2)	1	10 (26)	1 (17)	39 (47)
2+	2 (1)	2	1	3 (2)	(2)	7 (13)	1 (15)	16 (33)
3+				(1)				(1)
Plasma cells								
0	22 (4)	4 (1)	(3)	3 (4)	2	12 (32)	2 (17)	45 (61)
1+	6	1		(1)	(1)	3 (8)	(9)	11 (19)
2+	2	1	1	3 (2)	(1)	6 (9)	1 (9)	13 (21)
3+						1 (3)		1 (3)
Polymorphonuclear leukocytes								
0	24 (4)	5 (1)	1 (2)	6 (5)	2 (2)	18 (37)	2 (35)	58 (86)
1+	4	1	(1)	(1)		2 (10)		7 (12)
2+	2			(1)		2 (4)	1	5 (5)
3+						(1)		(1)
Total	90 (12)	18 (3)	3 (9)	18 (21)	6 (6)	66 (156)	9 (105)	210 (312)

Cases in parenthesis were dead at 2 years.

did indicate that as a group the mucinous cancers are a less aggressive tumor than the other epithelial ovarian cancers. For the common epithelial ovarian tumors, grading correlated with prognosis in the early stages but was less reliable in the more advanced cancers. There were differences in the malignant potential among cancers in the same stage of disease.

Our results parallel those reported by Decker. He presented his material by graph for each stage, breaking the tumors down into grades 1, 2, and 3. He commented that the importance of grading tumors to date has been controversial. The analysis of data presented by him supports the following conclusions: (1) All epithelial ovarian carcinomas are equally lethal when compared by stage and grade. (2) The low-grade tumors become increasingly lethal as the stage increases. (3) High-grade, low-stage tumors should be treated differently from low-grade, low-stage tumors. (4) When therapy is uniform within a stage, grading is of prognostic value to both the patient and physician. In general, mucinous cystadenocarcinomas and endometrioid adenocarcinomas tend to be low-grade and low-stage, and serous cystadenocarcinomas and solid adenocarcinomas tend to be high-grade, high-stage. In the past when tumors were evaluated only by histologic features without regard to stage and grade, greater malignant potential was erroneously attributed to a tumor type. Decker's conclusions are summarized in the following paragraphs.

We have included a fourth category—the "solid" tumor—in our evaluation of epithelial ovarian tumors. This tumor probably represents one of the other three that has been prolific enough to have obliterated any cystic component.

These studies from the literature and results of the present analysis indicate that valid and reliable evaluation of ovarian carcinoma cannot be achieved unless both grade and stage are considered. A specific, carefully done staging regimen should be adhered to. The extent of peritoneal involvement, nodal involvement, subdiaphragmatic surface status, and peritoneal cytology also should be noted carefully at the initial surgery. Such detailed analysis probably would (1) lead to the finding of more high-stage lesions, (2) explain some of the poor results with low-stage lesions, and (3) lead to more appropriate treatment than has heretofore been offered to these patients.

Histologic grading of tumors should be routine, and such grading would have significant prognostic value regardless of the stage or histologic cell type, especially when the lesion is a low-stage lesion. If the criteria specified by Malloy and colleagues are applied strictly, the borderline lesion category should be eliminated. A useful addition to the FIGO classification is grading by either the Broders scale or a similar grading system with designations by stage, substage, and grade. Once this type of classification has been adopted, the effectiveness of therapeutic modalities can be compared within an institution and among institutions.

The histologic type of the tumor has been included in the FIGO classification in which the common epithelial tumors of the ovary are concerned. The serous, mucinous, and endometrioid lesions are well defined. The unclassified group—the group we designated as the "solid" lesion—represents one of the other groups of epithelial malignancies that has lost its structural identification. This is consistent with the finding of more higher grade lesions in this category.

The data presented here show that, in general, low grade is associated with low stage and that more mucinous and endometrioid lesions than serous or solid lesions are low-grade and low-stage. Further, if serous and mucinous lesions are compared stage for stage and grade for grade, they are of equal lethal potential. There were insufficient data to develop such comparisons for the endometrioid or solid lesions. The data suggest that more intensive treatment than is currently being given for stage I disease is indicated for all histologic cell types when the lesion is other than FIGO stage IA, Broders' grade 1, intracystic, nonruptured, nonadherent, and without extracystic excrescences.

Our current approach to therapy of all epithelial ovarian carcinomas is dictated by the stage and, in some instances, by the grade of the lesion. For lesions of stage IA, grade 1, that are intracystic, nonadherent, and nonruptured, a unilateral oophorectomy with biopsy of the contralateral ovary may be offered if childbearing is important. Otherwise, total abdominal hysterectomy and bilateral salpingo-oophorectomy with omentectomy, without further therapy, are done. For all other stage I lesions, total abdominal hysterectomy and bilateral salpingo-oophorectomy with omentectomy are performed, followed by intraperitoneal radioisotopes or chemotherapy for 6 months, depending on the specific situation.

For stage II disease, total abdominal hysterectomy and bilateral salpingo-oophorectomy with omentectomy are performed, followed by 12 months of therapy with an alkylating agent. A reexploration is made at 12 months, and if the patient is clinically free of disease and absence of disease is confirmed, chemotherapy is stopped. If disease is demonstrated, chemotherapy is continued.

For stages III and IV disease, treatment involves total abdominal hysterectomy with bilateral salpingo-oophorectomy and omentectomy and removal of as much tumor as possible. These procedures are followed by chemotherapy with an alkylating agent. If the patient is clinically free of disease, and if this is confirmed at reexploration at 2 years, therapy is stopped. Demonstrated disease warrants further chemotherapy. Patients who do not respond to therapy with alkylating agents are considered candidates for second-line or investigational drugs.

This concludes the report by Decker.

Cases Grouped Together—Stages I–IV

An overall view is possible by grouping together the cases from stages I through IV in order to study the percentage of histologic and nuclear grades and stromal reaction within each type of epithelial ovarian cancer (Table 8). Thus there are enough cases for study of serous cystadenocarcinoma and endometrioid carcinoma. The percentage distributions by histologic grade, nuclear grade, and stromal reaction are similar. In each instance, histologic grade II and nuclear grade 2 account for 51 to 61% of the cancers. From the data in Table 8, it is not possible to determine if the nuclear and histologic grades are closely correlated for a given case.

Relatively speaking, mucinous cystadenocarcinoma was characterized by the greatest percentage of highly differentiated tumors (38% histologic grade I and 25% nuclear grade 3).

The relationship of stage, histologic grade, nuclear grade, and stromal reaction in short-term survivors compared with longer-term survivors was reviewed in the two groups with the more adequate sample sizes—serous cystadenocarcinoma (88) and endometrioid carcinoma (38). There were only 3 survivors with endometrioid carcinoma at 5 years, and thus detailed study of multiple prognostic factors was impossible.

When the 88 patients were divided into subgroups by stage of disease, neither histologic grade, nuclear grade, nor stromal reaction, when analyzed independently, is significantly predictive of long-term (5 or more years) survival. When the cases are grouped together, however, grading did correlate with prognosis.

Life-table Method in Analyzing Survival

Table 9 summarizes the material from this study. The direct method for calculating a survival rate does not utilize all information available. The actuarial, or life-table, method utilizes all survival information accumulated up to the closing date of the study and describes the manner in which the patient group was depleted during the total period of observation. This method provides a better insight into the nature of the disease and the effect of therapy than does one specified end point. For example, the overall 5-year survival by the direct method does not tell whether all patients died at 1 year or 4 years or by a fixed percentage rate for each year during the 5-year period. However with the life-table method it is obvious that of the patients who died after treatment, most were dead at 2 years. The number alive between 5 and 10 years is not appreciably different from the percentage surviving 5 years.

Figure 43 shows the survival rates for stages I through IV, including the entire group of 182 patients. The survival rate at 2 years is 43.5% and the standard error is ±3.7%. The survival rate at 5 years is 34.6% and the standard error is ±3.7%. When the standard error is multiplied by 2, and when this number in each instance is added and subtracted from the survival rates at 2 years (±7.3%) and 5 years (±7.2%) respectively, the 95% confidence limit is established. Enough cases were studied at 2 and 5 years to allow us to make a valid statement about the findings. Figure 44 summarizes the survival time for each group of epithelial tumors according to the life table method of analyzing survival rates.

Comment

The main problem in ovarian cancer is early diagnosis. At present, early diagnosis is a matter of chance rather than a scientific method. However,

Table 8. All Stages

| | Histologic Grade | | | | | | Nuclear Grade | | | | | | Stromal Reaction | | | |
| | I | | II | | III | | 1 | | 2 | | 3 | | Lymphocytes + Plasma Cells L+P+ | | Polymorphonuclear Leukocytes P+ | |
	No.	%	No.	%	No.	%	No.	%	No.	%	No.	%	No.	%	No.	%
Clear cell carcinoma	2	(20)	5	(50)	3	(30)	5	(50)	4	(40)	1	(10)	4	(40)	1	(10)
Undifferentiated carcinoma			1	(5)	19	(95)	16	(80)	4	(20)			17	(85)	3	(15)
Serous cystadenocarcinoma	10	(12)	42	(51)	30	(37)	32	(39)	43	(52)	7	(9)	65	(79)	13	(16)
Endometrioid carcinoma	4	(11)	22	(58)	12	(32)	12	(32)	23	(61)	3	(8)	30	(79)	3	(8)
Mucinous cystadenocarcinoma	9	(38)	14	(58)	1	(4)	2	(8)	16	(67)	6	(25)	18	(75)	5	(21)

Table 9.   Computation of the 5-Year Survival Rate and Its Standard Error

Years After Treatment	Alive At Beginning Of Treatment	Died During Interval	Lost To Follow-up	Withdrawn Alive During Interval	Effective No. Exposed to Risk of Dying	Proportion Dying	Proportion Surviving	Cumulative Proportion Surviving*
0–1	182	68	3	2	179.5	0.379	0.621	0.621
1–2	109	32	2	2	107.0	0.2990	0.701	0.435
2–3	73	3	3	10	66.5	0.045	0.955	0.416
3–4	57	6	0	10	52.0	0.115	0.855	0.355
4–5	41	1	0	6	38.0	0.026	0.974	0.346
5–6	34	3	0	6	31.0	0.097	0.903	0.313
6–7	25	2	0	4	23.0	0.087	0.913	0.285
7–8	19	1	0	2	18.0	0.056	0.944	0.269
8–9	16	0	0	9	11.5	0.000	1.00	0.269
9–10	7	0	0	2	6.0	0.000	1.00	0.269

*Cumulative proportion surviving from beginning of treatment through end of interval.

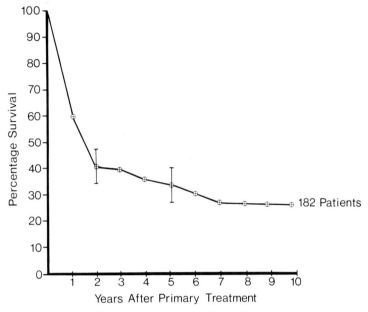

Figure 43. Survival for all stages with 95% confidence limits expressed at 2 and 5 years.

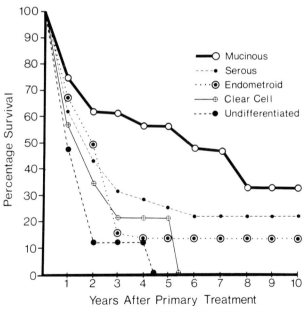

Figure 44. Survival for all stages according to life table analysis of survival.

91

until such methods are available, it is important to study the natural history of the disease by all means available. By accumulating material from many investigators treated by a variety of methods, some progress may be achieved in salvaging additional patients.

It is obvious that the interpretation of data is difficult and limited by the small numbers from any one series. However, as the material accumulates and is reported according to stage, grade, and histologic criteria that are universally acceptable, a meaningful and profitable study will result. The acceptance and use of the clinical staging and histologic classification established by the World Health Organization and the International Federation of Gynecology and Obstetrics have helped compare therapeutic results among institutions around the world. It has led to greater insight into the natural history of ovarian cancer, resulting in a more rational approach to therapy with anticipated improved results. In addition, careful grading of the tumor both for the epithelial elements as well as the stroma should validate end results.

The material reviewed indicates that staging and grading are both important and should be used to establish therapy. It is obvious that they are not competitive but rather complementary. The importance of grading in endometrial and cervical cancer has been established and accepted. But a universal grading system for ovarian cancer has yet to be adopted. This study shows that the grade was important in predicting prognosis in the early stages of ovarian cancer but was a less reliable guide in the more advanced cancers. In general, stage of disease was more important than histologic or nuclear grades.

Within each stage there is a great deal of variation, making it difficult to compare results between institutions. Because there are varying degrees of malignancy in groups of a particular stage, it is important to examine tumor tissues microscopically to determine their grade or degree of malignancy according to the histologic and nuclear grade as well as the stromal reaction. Staging is determined clinically and estimates the extent of the disease and the size of the tumor, whereas histologic type and grading provide its microscopic character. From the present study there are indications that in any stage there is considerable variation, and it is suggested that certain tumors are more potent than others within a given stage. Accepting this, treatment should be tailored to the cancer rather than to the stage of disease.

Host resistance is considered an important factor in cancer control. It can be studied by examining the lymphocytes and plasma cells that infiltrate the area where the tumor is growing. A marked lymphocyte and plasma cell response is interpreted as the body's mounting of a defense against the tumor. In certain tumors, especially in breast cancer, this has been repeatedly confirmed. In the present series the number of lymphocytes and plasma cells were not as great as anticipated in stage I, especially since this stage had the best survival rate. However the number of lymphocytes and plasma cells increased as the disease became more advanced and may indicate that the tumor has to grow to a certain volume or a certain potency before it can stimulate a local immune response. If a correlation is observed between lymphocytic and plasma cell response and long-term survival when large series are accumulated, perhaps immunotherapy can be employed to stimulate an immume response of this type.

The histologic grade remained fairly constant in a given tumor, and cell differentiation suggested the degree of malignancy, especially in the early stages. In the early stages, classification based on tumor grade provided a satisfactory means for the determination of prognosis.

Large numbers of subgroups must be studied for many years before there is enough information to make a statistically valid statement about prognosis. By lumping variables into a small number of arbitrary groups, a statistically significant number of patients can be amassed for study in each group. However the information on a single or individual factor is lost. To study a great number of variables in a small group of patients as presented here would be statistically invalid. It is difficult for any one institution to accumulate a large number of untreated ovarian epithelial cancers. Generally, when cases from different institutions are pooled there are so many variables that findings become useless in adapting therapy for a given stage and grade of ovarian cancer. Not infrequently, within each institution treatment is subject to change within a given 5-year period. However, as the microscopic criteria become more widely accepted and groups of institutions agree to work from a common protocol, some of the confusion will be resolved. In this way meaningful statistics with multiple variables will be available to guide the clinician in his management of ovarian cancer. A documentation of the histologic and nuclear grades as well as the stromal reaction adds another parameter in establishing treatment.

SUMMARY

Among the prerequisites for comparative studies of cancer, and particularly ovarian cancer, are international agreement on histologic criteria for the classification of cancer types and a standardized nomenclature. An internationally agreed upon classification of ovarian tumors, acceptable to gynecologists, pathologists, radiologists, and statisticians would enable workers in ovarian cancer in all parts of the world to compare their finding and to promote collaboration.

It was mutually agreed by a committee appointed by the World Health Organization to have three separate classifications: (1) anatomic site, (2) histologic type, and (3) degree of malignancy. In 1963 the World Health Organization International Reference Center for Histological Classification of Ovarian Tumors was established.

It is obvious that the classification will require study and modification as experience accumulates. Although there is disagreement on certain points, it provides an overall classification and a starting point for an internationally agreed upon classification of tumors. The classification is based primarily on the microscopic characteristics of the tumors and thus reflects the nature of morphologically identifiable cell types and patterns. Previously used and widely accepted terms have usually been retained, unless they were considered to be seriously misleading. Occasionally it was necessary to adopt controversial histogenetic designations, when they were the most convenient terms available. The World Health Organization has made an effort to conform to the classification of common epithelial ovarian tumors proposed by the International Federation of Gynecology and Obstetrics and used by many of the large centers. The classification has subdivisions to include the obviously benign and the obviously malignant tumors, as well as a large group of potentially malignant (borderline) tumors.

The World Health Organization has expanded the classification to include germ cell tumors, gonadal stromal tumors, gonadoblastomas, tumors not specific for the ovary, unclassified tumors, and secondary metastatic tumors.

The material in this chapter directs itself to the histologic and nuclear grading and stromal reactions as indices for prognosis in ovarian cancer. The neoplasm was named from its most differentiated portion and graded from its least differentiated parts.

It was observed that certain tumors are more potent than others within a given stage and that undifferentiated cancers were generally in the unfavorable histologic grades. Studies at Lenox Hill Hospital determined that it was in the best interest of the patient to tailor the treatment to the cancer rather than to have a standard treatment for a given stage of ovarian cancer. Although the histologic grade and nuclear grade are important in determining prognosis, stage of disease was the most important parameter in judging prognosis.

The use of life-table analysis, and particularly the slope of the curve as opposed to the relative 5-year survival result, are very significant. This slope–survival comparison is most important in studying the results of different therapeutic modalities in the management of ovarian cancer.

A plan for standardizing the parameters used in studying ovarian cancer should be proposed and adopted. The editors of the journals could insist upon a common method of presenting data. By accumulating material from many investigators using the same parameters for their studies, some progress may be achieved in salvaging additional patients.

BIBLIOGRAPHY

Barber, H.R.K., Sommers, S.C., Snyder, R., Kwon, T.: Histologic and nuclear grading and stromal reactions as indices for prognosis in ovarian cancer. Am. J. Obstet. Gynecol. 121:795-807, 1975.

Broders, A.C.: Carcinoma: Grading and practical application. Arch. Pathol. 2:376-381, 1926.

Decker, D.G., Malkasian, G.D., Jr., Taylor, W.F.: Prognostic importance of histologic grading in ovarian cancer. Symposium on Ovarian Carcinoma. J. Natl. Cancer Inst. Monograph 42, 1975.

Dyson, J.L., Beilby, J.O., Steele, S.J.: Factors influencing survival in carcinoma of the ovary. Br. J. Cancer 25:237-249, 1971.

Long, M.E., Sommers, S.C.: Staging, grading and histochemistry of ovarian epithelial tumors. Clin. Obstet. Gynecol. 12:937–954, 1969.

Long, M.E., Taylor, H.C., Jr.: Nucleolar variability in human neoplastic cells. Ann. N.Y. Acad. Sci. 63:1095, 1956.

Malkasian, G.D., Jr., Decker, D.G., Webb, M.J.: Histology of epithelial tumors of the ovary: Clinical usefulness and prognostic significance of the histologic classification and grading. Semin. Oncol. 2:191, 1975.

Report presented by the Cancer Committee to the General Assembly of FIGO: New York, April 1970. Int. J. Gynecol. Obstet. 9:172-179, 1971.

Silverberg, E.: Gynecologic Cancer: Statistical and Epidemiological Information. American Cancer Society, Professional Education Publication, 1975.

Sommers, S.C., Long, M.E.: Ovarian carcinoma: Pathology, staging, grading and prognosis. Bull. N.Y. Acad. Med. 49:858, 1973.

7

Symptoms, Signs, and Diagnosis

I t is commonly stated that ovarian malignancies are frequently asymptomatic; subjective complaints occur only after complications arise or, in the case of carcinoma, after dissemination is widespread. Therefore it is accepted that of all aspects of ovarian cancer, the symptomatology is the least satisfactory. If there are no early symptoms of malignant ovarian tumors, then this fact is partly responsible for the very poor results achieved, because one of the important factors in prognosis in ovarian cancer is the extent of disease at the time of treatment. Specific symptoms depend on the size, location, and type of tumor, as well as on complicating factors such as torsion, hemorrhage, infection or rupture. Among the germ cell or gonadal stromal tumors, symptoms may relate to the hormone secreted by the tumor.

The usual presenting symptoms of patients with ovarian cancer are pain or discomfort, abdominal swelling, abnormal uterine bleeding, and gastrointestinal and urinary complaints. Unfortunately, these are late symptoms and signs.

The insidious onset of ovarian cancer needs no elaboration. It is time, however, to change the generally accepted notion that there are no early symptoms of ovarian cancer. Symptomatology includes vague abdominal discomfort, dyspepsia, increasing flatulence, a sense of bloating, particularly after ingesting food, mild digestive disturbances, and pelvic unrest which may be present for several months before diagnosis. Unfortunately, for the patient, a work-up at that time including a gastrointestinal series and/or a barium enema often reveals no definitive information. Continued symptoms without a definite diagnosis frustrates both patient and doctor. All too often the patient is considered a middle-aged crock who goes to too many cocktail parties and eats too many hors d'oeuvres. Thus many ovarian cancers are nurtured in a sea of bicarbonate of soda and antacids. It is imperative, therefore, to rule out ovarian cancer in women between 40 and 60 who present with persistent gastrointestinal symptoms that cannot be definitely diagnosed. In terms of function it must be emphasized that a variety of paraendocrine effects, such as hypercalcemia, hypoglycemia, and Cushing's syndrome as well as disorders such as hemolytic anemia, may rarely be related to the presence of an ovarian tumor.

The peak incidence of the common epithelial ovarian cancer is in women between 40 and 60 plus years of age. The ovary may get too old to function, but it never gets too old to form tumors. Women at high risk usually have a long history of ovarian imbalance or dysfunction, including increased premenstrual tension, heavy menstruation with marked breast tenderness, a tendency for spontaneous abortion, infertility, and nulliparity, as well as an early menopause. The ovary is like a cam running off center.

The author has established a triad that serves as a guide in making an early diagnosis of ovarian cancer:

1. Patients between ages 40 and 60 plus years who are in the high risk groups to develop common epithelial ovarian cancer.
2. A history of ovarian dysfunction characterized by increased premenstrual tension, heavy menstruation with marked breast tenderness, a tendency to spontaneous abortion, infertility, and nulliparity, as well as an early menopause.
3. Vague abdominal discomfort and mild digestive symptoms that persist, including dyspepsia, flatulence, and distension, especially after ingesting food. The symptoms are only helped to a slight degree by antacids and bicarbonate of soda.

When the triad is present it is important to think of the diagnosis of ovarian cancer and systematically to carry out all diagnostic measures that are outlined elsewhere in the book (chapter 8).

There is no definite and specific explanation for the early gastrointestinal symptoms that so often accompany early ovarian cancer. Cancer of the ovary spreads over surfaces, and in the advanced stages it coats the bowel and interferes with peristalsis. However in the early stage this is not present. McGowan has reported that, compared with the peritoneal fluids from women with benign ovarian tumors those from women with ovarian cancer had significantly higher indexes for calcium, inorganic phosphorus, urea nitrogen, uric acid, cholesterol, total protein (not albumin), total bilirubin, lactic dehydrogenase (LDH), and glutamic-oxaloacetic acid transaminase (G-OT), and a pH of 7.43. The altered peritoneal fluids may irritate the bowel. Another point that may be relevant concerns the embryologic origin of the ovary. It arises at about the level of the 10th thoracic vertebra (T-10) and migrates to the pelvis. Pain originating in the ovary may be referred to the abdomen and secondarily give rise to gastrointestinal symptoms. This is a theoretical explanation and lacks documentation at this time. It is interesting to speculate whether the origin of the primitive germ cells in the fetal yolk contributes to the early gastrointestinal symptoms in ovarian cancer. Unless the primitive germ cells are able to migrate to the ovary, there is lack of ovarian development.

DIAGNOSIS

The early diagnosis of ovarian cancer is a matter of chance and not a triumph of the scientific approach. The means of early detection are very limited. In most cases the finding of a pelvic mass is the only available method of diagnosis, with the exception of functional tumors which may manifest endocrine activity even with minimal ovarian enlargement. In some cases the pelvic findings may be uncertain even late in the disease. The tumor may be deep in the pelvis, the patient may be obese, heavily muscled, and uncooperative. The elderly patient may have an inelastic and conical vagina complicated by marked atrophy. Occasionally, there may be widespread metastases in the presence of minimal pelvic findings. The usual signs and symptoms as well as physical findings associated with ovarian cancer all represent an advanced cancer of the ovary. An abdominal mass or distension or both are a prime diagnostic feature. However ovarian cancers seldom give symptoms until they grow to 15 cm, and they cannot be palpated abdominally until they get this large. Pain in the early stage is associated with a complication, such as torsion or rupture. Later, pain occurs when there is infiltration of adjacent organs or nerve sheaths by tumor. Menstrual disorders may be seen with endocrine-producing tumors. In the menopausal patient, vaginal bleeding may occur and has been attributed to the functioning stroma in the tumor. Ascites with positive cells is a sign of advanced disease, and 5-year survival is reported in only about 8% of these patients.

Pelvic Examination

Routine pelvic examination will detect only one cancer in 10,000 examinations of asymptomatic women. Ovarian tumors cannot be palpated abdominally until they reach 15 cm in size. Pelvic findings are often minimal and not helpful in making a diagnosis, even in patients with advanced disease.

The pelvic findings are of limited help in making the diagnosis. However, combined with a high index of suspicion, they may help alert the physician to the diagnosis. There are nine pelvic signs:

1. A mass in the ovarian area
2. Relative immobility due to fixation and adhesions
3. Irregularity of the tumor
4. Shotty consistency with increased firmness
5. Tumors in the cul-de-sac described as a handful of knuckles
6. Relative insensitivity of the mass
7. Increasing size under observation
8. Bilaterality (70% in ovarian carcinoma versus 5% in benign cases)
9. In late disease, common findings of nodular hepatomegaly, ascites, and palpation of the omental cake.

The diagnostic procedures include the Pap smear, which has been reported to be positive in 40% of patients with advanced disease, as well as a 90% incidence of positive cells on cul-de-sac taps. The author's results are very poor when compared to these figures.

The question of the value of laparoscopy remains to be determined. It may be most useful in following the patient during prolonged chemotherapy regimens.

A complete work-up in suspected cases should include:

1. A careful history
2. A complete physical examination, including careful rectal and pelvic examinations
3. Pap smear
4. Proctoscopy as deemed indicated
5. CBC and urinalysis
6. SMA-12
7. Chest x-ray
8. Intravenous pyelogram
9. GI series
10. Barium enema
11. Optional paracentesis, laparoscopy, and lymphangiogram

This work-up will help document the extent of disease, and indeed may determine whether the cancer is primary or metastatic to the ovary. About 5–10% of ovarian cancers are metastatic. A complete diagnostic evaluation is included in chapter 8.

Gusberg and Frick's indications for an exploratory laparotomy are listed below, with a slight modification by the addition of number six:

1. Any pelvic mass that has appeared after the menopause, particularly if it is an adnexal mass
2. An adnexal mass that progressively enlarges beyond 5 cm while under observation in a woman of any age
3. Appearance or persistence of an ovarian mass while the patient is on the combined contraceptive pill.
4. Any adnexal mass 10 cm or larger
5. Inability to determine accurately whether the mass is a fibroid or an ovarian tumor
6. The palpation of what appears to be a normal-sized ovary in a patient 3–5 years postmenopausal, is indicative of an ovarian tumor

SUMMARY

The symptoms, signs, and diagnosis must be based on a knowledge of the natural history of ovarian cancer.

Natural History of Ovarian Cancer

Because our ability to diagnose ovarian cancer early is limited, we must resort to the knowledge of its natural history in trying to identify the patient at high risk. We do know some facts, however, and we should be alert to them: Most ovarian cancers (epithelial) occur after the age of 35, most commonly between the ages of 40 and 60. The diagnosis of ovarian cancer, as with all other malignancies, is most beneficial to the patient when it is made while a tumor is still localized. For ovarian carcinoma, this means identifying it when the only physical finding is an enlarged ovary.

It is also possible that the diagnosis can be based on hormonal activity of the ovarian tumor, but this is much less specific. Unfortunately, most ovarian carcinoma is diagnosed only after the patient develops symptoms due to the spread of tumor. When a woman in the 40 to 60 age group appears with vague gastrointestinal symptoms that are difficult to diagnose, consider that the problem may be ovarian. The English gynecologist Stanley Way says that most ovarian cancers are nurtured in a sea of sodium bicarbonate for months before the diagnosis is established.

Diagnosis

Early diagnosis has been more a matter of chance than a scientific approach, so we must begin to use any clue we have. An enlarged ovary should always be evaluated regardless of the patient's age, because when ovarian cancer is found in this way, cure rates are very high. On the other hand, when disease has already spread throughout the abdomen before the diagnosis—as it does in 70% of ovarian cancer patients—the 5-year survival rate is less than 20%. The chances of improving these dismal figures would be immeasurably better if we could find ways to uncover the borderline or potentially malignant cases.

Cytology

Some investigators claim good results in detecting ovarian cancer by means of vaginal and cervical cytology, but our own experience has not been good. Cytology is also used to diagnose cells taken from the posterior cul-de-sac by way of culdocentesis, but we have not found this to be of much benefit either. Not only do patients find the procedure painful, but in our hands the results have not been very reliable. Besides, by the time an ovarian cancer has spilled malignant cells that can be identified in cytologic smears, it may no longer be in an early stage of growth. Also, if an inflamed mesothelial cell appears in the smear, it looks like a malignant cell, in which case surgery is almost mandatory.

We find cytologic diagnosis to be of value in elderly, poor-risk patients in whom there is every evidence of advanced ovarian cancer, including pelvic and abdominal masses and ascites, and in whom laparotomy would be too dangerous. In these patients a presumptive diagnosis of cancer may be made on the basis of cells obtained by paracentesis. Treatment can then begin.

Clinical Clues

A pattern suggestive of ovarian carcinoma may warn you of difficulty. Although symptoms are certainly not specific, these gastrointestinal complaints are not uncommon:

- Loss of appetite
- Indigestion
- "Gas"—with concomitant distention

And do not neglect any gynecologic or hormonal disorders. Ovarian carcinoma patients often have a long history of heavy periods, more premenstrual tension, more dysmenorrhea, more breast swelling, and more miscarriages. It seems that the ovary is like a cam running off center—never completely normal.

The following triad of findings should arouse the suspicion of ovarian cancer:

1. A woman in the high risk age group between 40 and 60 plus years
2. A history of ovarian dysfunction
3. Vague gastrointestinal symptoms such as dyspepsia, indigestion, gas with concomitant distension.

BIBLIOGRAPHY

Barber, H.R.K., Graber, E.A.: Surgical aspects of ovarian tumors, *in* Selected Topics of Cancer Current Concepts. Symposia Specialists, Miami, 1974, p.163.

Barber, H.R.K., Graber, E.A., Kwon, T.: Ovarian cancer (monograph). American Cancer Society, 1975.

Barber, H.R.K.: Ovarian cancer: Still an enigma. Dr. 1:17, 1975. Medcom, New York.

DiSaia, P.J., Morrow, C.P., Townsend, D.E.: Synopsis of Gynecologic Oncology. Wiley, New York, 1975.

Griffiths, C.T.: The ovary, *in* Gynecology Principles and Practice. Edited by R.W. Kistner. Year Book Medical Publishers, Chicago, 1975, p.335.

Rutledge, F., Boronow, R.C., Wharton, J.T.: Gynecologic Oncology. Wiley, New York, 1976.

Way, S.: Malignant Disease of the Female Genital Tract. Blakiston, Philadelphia, 1951, p.183.

8

Diagnostic Evaluation and Preoperative Work-up

Cancer of the ovary is the leading cause of death from gynecologic cancer. Early diagnosis is a matter of change rather than a scientific approach. The inability to diagnose ovarian cancer is evident from reports showing that 60 to 70% are in stages III and IV at the time of diagnosis. The physician must have a high index of suspicion, use any and all clues, and evaluate an enlarged ovary regardless of the patient's age. Our chances for improving the low 5-year survival would be immeasurably better if we could find ways to uncover the borderline or potentially malignant cases. The means for diagnosis are nonspecific but will be reviewed.

CYTOLOGY

Some investigators claim good results in detecting ovarian cancer detection by means of vaginal and cervical cytology, but my experience with cytology has not been good. The Grahams reported that the Pap smear was positive in 40% of patients *with advanced disease.* Cytology is also used to diagnose cells taken from the posterior cul-de-sac by culdocentesis, but this has not been found to be of much benefit either. Not only do patients find the procedure painful, but in our hands the results have not been very reliable. By the time an ovarian cancer has spilled malignant cells that can be identified in cytologic smears, it may no longer be in an early stage of growth. Also, if an inflamed mesothelial cell appears in the smear, it looks like a malignant cell, in which case surgery is almost mandatory. Positive cells from cul-de-sac taps have been reported in 90% of patients with ovarian cancer. My results are very poor when compared to these figures.

Cytologic diagnosis has limited application. It is valuable in the elderly, poor-risk patient in whom there is every evidence of advanced ovarian cancer, including pelvic and abdominal masses and ascites, and in whom laparotomy would be considered too dangerous. In these patients a presumptive diagnosis of ovarian cancer may be made on the cells collected by paracentesis. Treatment can then begin.

CHEMISTRIES

Although carcinoembryonic antigens (CEA), alpha fetoprotein (AFP), and lactic dehydrogenase (LDH) do not help in making the diagnosis, if elevated, they serve to monitor the patient's response to therapy.

Some investigators have raised the possibility that lactic dehydrogenase elevation may be valuable as a screening test. In a prospective study I did not find it useful as a preoperative screening test. Total serum LDH is moderately elevated in most cancer patients with extensive hepatic metastases. The increase is usually associated with minor changes in the isoenzyme pattern, particularly an increase in LDH 3 and LDH 5 (the faster moving isoenzymes). The LDH titer is higher in pleural and peritoneal effusions with malignant cells than it is in the serum. When the association of LDH and advanced ovarian cancer was raised, a review of our data failed to confirm a correlation of the LDH level with the extent of disease.

Our laboratory has routinely performed CEA tests with ovarian cancer patients, but we have not confirmed the reports that CEA has been identified in the plasma of 35% of these patients. I believe that more cases and more time will be required before a definite statement can be made on the relationship between CEA and ovarian cancer. In a study from our laboratory neither the heterologous nor the homologous antibody against the common epithelial tumors cross-reacted with CEA. In view of our clinical findings and the laboratory data, I doubt that CEA will play a significant role as a prognostic screening test. However in certain patients it may serve to monitor progress during treatment of the cancer.

Serum alpha fetoprotein (AFP) assays have currently gained an important place in the diagnosis of hepatocellular and testicular tumors as well as the endodermal sinus tumors. The observation that AFP may be elevated before tumors are detected by other means has important implications. In addition, successful therapy is associated with a decline in AFP levels to normal, and a subsequent rise when the tumor recurs. AFP is known to be a product of the human fetal liver, gastrointestinal tract, and yolk sac. It has been shown that the endodermal sinus tumor, which is of vitelline origin, invariably gives a positive test for AFP.

Investigators from the National Cancer Institute have shown that malignancies other than trophoblastic disease produce elevated chorionic gonadotropin titers. Significantly, 30% of common epithelial tumors and up to 90% or more of the embryonal ovarian carcinomas are associated with measurable amounts of this hormone, Although the findings of these substances does not identify the kind of malignancy—or in some cases whether the patient has a malignancy at all—it certainly indicates high risk and warrants investigation.

Changes in the levels of humoral immunoglobulins in blood serum of patients with ovarian cancer have been recorded and used to monitor progress with chemotherapy. The level of IgG, IgA, and IgM was regularly examined in 18 patients with ovarian carcinoma during the time of chemotherapy. The IgG level dropped at least 10% in 10 patients, while the IgA and IgM levels dropped in 9 patients. In long-term chemotherapy the level of IgG and IgA was more changed than the level of IgM.

Melnick and Barber studied the cellular immunologic responsiveness to extracts of ovarian epithelial tumors. The leukocyte migration inhibition assay was employed in an attempt to detect cellular immunologic responsiveness to a solubilized extract of pooled, epithelially derived ovarian carcinomas. In 6 of 7 patients with cystadenocarcinomas of the ovary, leukocyte migration inhibition was noted in the presence of the ovarian tumor extract in our tissue culture system when compared to the migration test of leukocytes that were not exposed to the ovarian extract. Compared to control leukocytes, those from patients with nonepithelial ovarian cancers, benign ovarian neoplasms, and other genital tract cancers showed no inhibition of migratory behavior when exposed to the ovarian tumor extract. Cells from normal pregnant and nonpregnant females, as well as male subjects, also showed no inhibitory response when incubated with the ovarian tumor extract. Although the exact nature of the antigenic specificities uniquely associated with common epithelial ovarian carcinomas is unknown, our data suggest that cellular immune mechanisms may be involved in the host response to cells bearing tumor-specific antigens.

McGowan and coworkers have studied peritoneal fluids and have established profiles. They found the peritoneal fluid to be very sensitive to many physiologic and pathologic gynecologic and obstetric conditions. They reported that peritoneal fluids from women with ovarian cancer had significantly higher indexes for the following biochemical parameters than did the fluids from women with benign ovarian tumors: calcium, inorganic phosphorus, urea nitrogen, uric acid, cholesterol, total protein (not albumin), total bilirubin, lactic dehydrogenase (LDH), and glutamic-oxaloacetic acid transaminase (G-OT). In normal patients the pH of the peritoneal fluid was 7.81, whereas in patients with ovarian carcinoma it was 7.43. McGowan and associates believe that these biochemical tests are affected by the amount of tumor present, but there appears to be no critical amount of disease needed, other than invasive cancer, for them to reflect change from normal and to form a biochemical pattern for ovarian cancer. Serial peritoneal fluid profiles serve to monitor the patient undergoing surgical, irradiative or chemical therapy.

In terms of function it must be emphasized that a variety of paraendocrine effects, such as hypercalcemia, hypoglycemia, and Cushing's syndrome, as well as hemolytic anemia, may rarely be related to the presence of an ovarian tumor.

Routine pelvic examination will detect few asymptomatic ovarian cancers. It is estimated that only one ovarian cancer will be found in 10,000 examinations of asymptomatic women. In addition, since tumors cannot be palpated abdominally until they reach 15 cm in size, pelvic findings are often minimal or uncertain even in patients with advanced disease. As ovarian cancer enlarges and presses against the uterus, the pelvic examination often gives a false impression of a midline mass which is mistaken for a fibroid uterus. Consideration must be given to surgery in those patients suspected of having a fibroid, but in whom the ovaries cannot be felt. Unfortunately, the ovarian cancer may be deep in the pelvis, the patient may be obese, heavily muscled, uncooperative, or aged, and the vagina may be inelastic and conical, all of which make palpation difficult, if not impossible. Detection of a truly early ovarian cancer is not possible by pelvic examination. The smallest tumor that can be detected clinically or by x-rays is usually about 1 cm^3 (1/16 in^3) in size and weighs about 1 g (1/30 oz). A tumor of this size contains at least a billion (10^9) cells and has the capacity for spreading. This information is included to highlight the difficulty of early diagnosis by clinical means.

Although pelvic findings have limited value in diagnosis, the physician must be alert to:

- A mass in the ovary
- Relative immobility due to fixation and adhesions
- Irregularity of the tumor
- Shotty consistency with increased firmness
- Tumors in the cul-de-sac described as "a handful of knuckles"
- Relative insensitivity of the mass
- Solid or semisolid consistency
- Increasing size under observation
- Bilaterality (70% in ovarian carcinoma versus 5% in benign lesions)
- Common finding of omental cake, nodular hepatomegaly, and ascites in advanced disease

The most important diagnostic procedure in any case of suspected or confirmed ovarian carcinoma is exploratory laparotomy. The indications suggested by Gusberg and Frick with additions and modifications are:

- Any mass that has appeared after the menopause, particularly an adnexal mass.
- An adnexal mass in a woman of any age that progressively enlarges beyond 5 cm while under observation.
- Appearance or persistance of an ovarian mass while the patient is on the combined contraceptive pill.
- An adnexal mass 10 cm or larger.
- A mass that cannot be definitely diagnosed as either a fibroid or a carcinoma. The pelvic mass must be considered an ovarian cancer until both ovaries are felt on palpation.
- The palpation of what is interpreted as a normal-sized ovary in the premenopausal woman represents an ovarian tumor in the postmenopausal woman.

ULTRASOUND

Ultrasound is the name given to a sound with a frequency over 20,000 cycles per second, the upper limit of the human ear. A simple explanation of the ultrasound is included for orientation purposes.

The ultrasound is basically a wave. The source of these waves is called a pulse generator, an apparatus which passes high voltage current through a crystal, causes it to vibrate at very high frequencies, and emits ultrasonic pulses at rates between 200 and 1,000 per second. These pulses are formed into a beam which is directed into the abdomen and reflected back to the crystal (transducer) whenever it meets two apposed surfaces of different density (an interface). This reflected wave or echo is converted by the transducer into electrical energy and represented on a cathode ray tube, either by a vertical deflection of a horizontal line (known as A-scanning) or by a bright spot (B-scanning). A third modality of ultrasound diagnosis involves the Doppler shift—a relative change in the frequency of a reflected echo when the wave strikes a moving object. Separate receiving and transmitting crystals are used. The receiving crystal processes frequency shifts caused by motion. The frequency differences can also be heard.

An additional technique, a gray scale of the intermediate shades between black and white, was developed to permit greater discrimination and more precise evaluation. Some have questioned the additional diagnostic value of the gray scale. Transmission imaging is an innovation which, unlike the gray scale, is still unavailable to most clinicians. Ultrasonic pulsation is passed directly through the tissues, then recorded in optical form for interpretation. The resultant soft tissue image is analagous to an x-ray in that it is isomorphic with its real-life model.

The ultrasonic examination of the pelvis employs the B-mode two- dimensional scans and the A-mode deflection patterns. The only specific preparation for examination is the drinking of four 8 oz glasses of fluid to distend the urinary bladder. The distended bladder serves as a window through which the pelvic structures are evaluated.

The normal ovaries are ordinarily not identified with certainty because of their variability in position, the superimposition of air-filled small bowel, and the difficulty of differentiating the ultrasonic pattern of ovaries from the adjacent bowel pattern.

In most instances it is possible to differentiate ovarian cysts, both malignant and benign, from solid masses. A mass separate from the uterus associated with disorganized internal echoes at normal sensitivity suggests ovarian cancer. Ascitic fluid loculations may add to confusion in evaluating suspected masses. Implants in the omentum may be interpreted as masses, especially in serial studies. It is accepted that the efficacy of preoperative evaluation of the primary mass has been adequately documented. More correlation is needed to establish the role that ultrasound will play in the diagnosis and management of the patient with disseminated ovarian carcinoma.

LAPAROSCOPY

Laparoscopy or peritoneoscopy has been found to be useful in staging suspected ovarian cancer patients and in the follow-up of these patients. It has had very limited value as a diagnostic modality in patients with ovarian cancer.

Peritoneoscopy has been employed as a tool for second-look in ovarian cancer, and has been performed in patients who have achieved clinical remission with chemotherapy. It can be summarized by saying that a positive finding with biopsy is conclusive, but a negative laparoscopy must be followed by an exploratory laparotomy before chemotherapy can be terminated. The role of laparoscopy or peritoneoscopy remains to be evaluated.

It has been reported that although patients appear at exploratory laparotomy to have disease localized to the pelvis, nearly 50% of these women will die within 5 years with recurrent tumor after what should have been curative surgical and radiotherapeutic treatment. Bagley and coworkers demonstrated the high frequency of unsuspected diaphragmatic metastases in patients with stages I and II ovarian cancer. Rosenoff and colleagues evaluated a group of patients that had been explored, staged, and then referred to the National Cancer Institute for further treatment, usually chemotherapy. Sixteen had been previously staged as I or II, but at the time of laparoscopy prior to treatment 7 (44%) were found to have metastatic disease to the diaphragm and were restaged as III.

Computerized axial tomography (CAT scan) has been a valuable tool in identifying and localizing lesions in the brain. However its value in the diagnosis of early ovarian cancer remains to be determined.

SUMMARY

Unfortunately, there is no one test or profile that helps in making an early diagnosis of ovarian cancer. The physician must have a high index of suspicion and must use any and all means including exploratory laparotomy to make the diagnosis.

Although there is hope that work being carried out in the field of immunology will provide a serologic test for early diagnosis, time will be required to bring it to fruition. Until it is possible to utilize the unusual discriminatory powers of the immunologic system, which can detect a difference of a few molecules, ovarian cancer will remain a problem that can be diagnosed only by clinical means.

Because 10% of ovarian cancers are metastatic from the bowel, breast, or thyroid, thorough work-up including a metastatic series is imperative before treatment is started.

BIBLIOGRAPHY

Abelev, G.I.: Alpha fetoprotein in oncogenesis and its association with malignant tumors. Adv. Cancer Res. 14:295, 1971.

Alexander,P.: Fetal "antigens" in cancer. Nature 235:137, 1972.

Alpert, M.E., Uriel, J., DeNechaud, B.: Alpha feto globulin in the diagnosis of human hepatoma. N. Engl. J. Med. 278:964, 1966.

Bagley, C.M., Jr., Young, R.C., Schein, P.S., et al.: Ovarian carcinoma metastatic to the diaphragm—frequently undiagnosed at laparotomy. A preliminary report. Am. J. Obstet. Gynecol. 116:397, 1973.

Bagley, C.M., Jr., Young, R.C., Canellos, G.P., et al.: Treatment of ovarian cancer: Possibilities for progress. N. Engl. J. Med. 287:856, 1972.

Baldwin, R.W.: Tumor-specific antigens associated with chemically induced tumors. Rev. Eur. Etudes Clin. Biol. 25:593, 1970.

Baldwin, R.W., Erubleton, M.J.: Demonstration by colony inhibition methods of cellular and humoral immune reactions to tumor-specific antigens associated with aminoazo-dye-induced rat hepatomas. Int. J. Cancer 7:17, 1971.

Barber, H.R.K., Graber, E.A.: Surgical aspects of ovarian tumors, in Selected Topics of Cancer Current Concepts. Symposia Specialists, Miami, 1974, p. 161.

Barber, H.R.K., Graber, E.A., Kwon, T.: Ovarian cancer. American Cancer Society, Professional Education Publication, 1975, p.2.

Barber, H.R.K. (ed.): Immunobiology for the Clinician. Wiley, New York, 1977.

Barber, H.R.K.: Surgical management of ovarian cancer. Curr. Ob-Gyn Tech. 1:6, 1975.

Coligan, J.E., Eagan, M.L., Todd, C.W.: Detection of carcinoembryonic antigen by radioimmune assay. Nat'l. Cancer Inst. Monogr. 35:427–432, 1972.

Edynak, E.M., Hirshant, Y., Old, L.J., Trempe, G.L.: Antigens of human breast cancer. Proc. Am. Assoc. Cancer Res. 12:75, 1971.

Graber, E.A.: Early diagnosis of ovarian malignancy. Clin. Obstet. Gynecol. 12:958, 1969.

Gusberg, S.B. and Frick, H.C., II: Corscaden's Gynecologic Cancer. Williams & Wilkins, Baltimore, 1970.

Haber, E.: Radioimmunoassay—Principles and Practical Applications. Little Brown, Boston, 1974.

Ioachim, H. L., Dorsett, B.H., Sabbath, M., Andersson, B., Barber, H.R.K.: Antigenic and morphologic properties of ovarian carcinoma. Gynecol. Oncol. 1:130–142, 1973.

Kobayashi, T., Osamutakantani, H.N.: Ecographic evaluation of abdominal tumor regression during antineoplastic treatment. J. Clin. Ultrasound 2:131, 1974.

Laurence, D.J.R., Munro, N.: Fetal antigens and their role in diagnosis and clinical management of human neoplasms: A review. Br. J. Cancer 26:335, 1972.

Laurora, J., Jandora, A., Skoda, Al, Zizkorska, E., Zizkorski, V.: Verhalten des Immunoglobulinspiegels im Blutserum ber Patientinsan mit Carcinoma Ovarii. Zbl. Gynaeckol. 97:540–548 1975.

Leopold, G.R., Asher, W.M.: Ultrasound in obstetrics and gynecology. Radiol. Clin. North Am. 12:127, 1974.

LoGerfo, P., Krupey, J., Hansen, H.J.: Demonstration of an antigen common to several varieties of neoplasia. N. Engl. J. Med. 283:138, 1971.

McGowan, L., Stein, D.B., Miller, W.: Cul-de-sac aspiration for diagnostic cytologic study. Am. J. Obstet. Gynecol. 96:413, 1966.

McGowan, L.: Peritoneal Fluid Profiles. Symposium on Ovarian Carcinoma. Monograph 42, National Cancer Institute Monographs, 1975, p. 75.

Melnick, H., Barber, H.R.K.: Cellular immunologic responsiveness to extracts of ovarian epithelial tumors. Gynecol. Oncol. 3:77, 1975.

Meyers, M.A.: The spread and localization of acute intraperitoneal effusions. Radiology 95:547, 1970.

Mitchison, N.A.: Immunologic approaches to cancer. Transplant. Proc. 2:92, 1970.

Rosenoff, S. H., DeVita, V. T., Jr., Hubbard, S., Young, R. C.: Peritoneoscopy in the staging and followup of ovarian cancer. Semin. Oncol. 2:223, 1975.

Rosenoff, S. H., Young, R. C., Anderson, T. et al.: Peritoneoscopy: A valuable tool for the initial staging and "second look" in ovarian carcinoma. Ann. Intern. Med. 83:37–41, 1975.

Samuels, B. I.: Usefulness of ultrasound in patients with ovarian cancer. Semin. On-col. 2:229, 1975.

Shuster, J.: Immunologic diagnosis of human cancers. Am. J. Clin. Pathol. 62:243–257, 1974.

Stolbach, L. L., Krant, M. J., Fishman, W. H.: Ectopic production of an alkaline phosphatase isoenzyme in patients with cancer. N. Engl. J. Med. 281:757, 1969.

An updated guide to diagnostic ultrasound. Contemp. Ob-Gyn 3:105, 1974

Van Nagell, J. R., Meeker, W. R., Parker, J. C., Jr., Harralson, J. D.: Carcinoem-bryonic antigen in patients with gynecologic malignancy. Cancer 35:1372, 1975.

Young, R. C., Hubbard, S. P., DeVita, V. T.: The chemotherapy of ovarian cancer. Cancer Treat. Rev. 1:99, 1974.

Zemlyn, S.: Comparison of pelvic ultrasonography and pneumography for ovarian size. Clin. Ultrasound 2:331, 1974.

9

Preoperative and Postoperative Management

Cancer of the ovary raises many challenges in the preoperative, operative, and postoperative periods. It is not only the site of origin of a variety of tumors, but also a target for metastases from many other organs, i.e., thyroid, breast, stomach, colon, and the opposite ovary. Therefore it is important to have a very thorough metastatic work-up before the exploratory laparotomy. To be forewarned is indeed to be forearmed. The diagnostic evaluation has been covered in chapter 8.

The management of ovarian cancer has come full circle since the early 1950s. At that time extended surgery was carried out, including the ultraradical surgery of pelvic exenteration. It became obvious that ovarian cancer was a surface spreader and often involved the upper abdomen with small metastases that were difficult to detect by methods then available. In spite of aggressive surgery, most patients succumbed to recurrent cancer if they survived the postoperative period.

Now, with the newer methods of management with chemotherapy, the patient has an opportunity for extended survival, particularly if the disease has been debulked. The more liberal use of hyperalimentation has permitted a more aggressive management without compromising the survival of the patient who develops a complication, especially those involving the gastrointestinal tract. This has led to an extension of the standard ovarian cancer extirpation techniques. Improvements in preoperative and postoperative care have been equally important. Even the most superior technical skill does not obviate the necessity for excellence in preoperative and postoperative management.

The patient and/or the family may ask about the particular risks involved. In the past the surgeon assumed the responsibility of explaining the risk, but in a society oriented to malpractice suits, the operative risks must be discussed. It is important for the consent form for surgical operations to have a place for writing the state, nature, and extent of the operation.

The operative risk is influenced by age, associated medical disorders (cardiovascular, respiratory, and metabolic), the familiarity of the surgeon with the natural history of the disease and the planned procedures, the experience of the anesthetist, the equipment and physical facilities necessary for the surgical procedure, the duration of the anesthesia or operation, the staff of the recovery room, and the team for managing the postoperative care of the patient.

It is important to evaluate the operative risk, and the surgeon and anesthetist must institute appropriate corrective measures in the preoperative period to establish optimal conditions before the surgical procedure. Training the patient preoperatively in the use of the IPPB method is important, particularly for patients who smoke or have any chronic lung problem. The average patient with ovarian cancer is between 40 and 60 and in general is a fairly good operative risk.

Among patients with suspected ovarian cancer the diagnostic work-up and preoperative care can be carried out simultaneously. The work-up is best accomplished at least 2 days before surgery.

It is the responsibility of the surgeon (shared with the surgical team) to evaluate the patient properly and to institute measures that prepare the patient for surgery. These measures must include a general evaluation of her physical status, as well as a detailed medical history.

The preoperative regimen should start before admission to the hospital. There should be a complete explanation of the work-up to be carried out and the anticipated surgery. It is important to reassure the patient and to prepare her psychologically. If the patient smokes, she should be advised to stop before admission to the hospital. A well-balanced diet is advised, and iron and vitamins should be prescribed.

The patient admitted to the hospital for treatment of cancer is subject to a general evaluation of her physical status. A complete history is taken, and specific answers to the following questions are included: duration of present symptoms, history of weight change, previous neoplastic disease, whether she is a twin, menstrual history, abortions, histories of pregnancies, treatment with hormones, and previous operations. The history should be carefully reviewed for sensitivity to medications and anesthetic agents. It should be determined whether the patient is taking any long-term medication that might be a factor in anesthesia, or in operative or postoperative complications. Antihypertensive drugs, diuretics, and tranquilizers are among the agents that might have such an influence.

In the routine physical examination, pelvic and rectal examination should be carefully carried out and recorded. Papanicolaou smears should be obtained, and, if feasible, smears or biopsies of the endometrium should be secured. In addition to hemoglobin, white blood count, and differential, red count and routine urinalysis should include the following blood chemistries: bleeding time, clotting time, tourniquet test, prothrombin time, prothrombin consumption time, clot retraction time, partial thromboplastin time and a platelet count. An electrocardiogram and a chest plate as well as an intravenous pyelogram are essential.

Since 10% or more of all pelvic cancers are metastatic from another organ, additional x-ray studies should be ordered as indicated and routinely included in the metastatic work-up. These studies include mammography, a gastrointestinal series, and a barium enema, as well as bone and liver scans when indicated. If barium studies are carried out, a flat plate of the abdomen should be taken before surgery to make certain that there is no residual barium in the bowel.

A patient who has cancer generally suspects the nature of her illness; or often she has been told the diagnosis, or that such a diagnosis can be ruled out. When entering the hospital she is apprehensive, regardless of appearance. A well-organized admission routine can be most reassuring. The house officer and nurse should refrain from general discussion of neoplastic disease, methods of treatment, specific diagnoses of her case, and prognosis. The terms *tumor* or *growth* should be used in relation to her condition and not the word *cancer*. On admission, medication should be prescribed to allay apprehension, to insure sleep, and to control pain.

SPECIAL PREOPERATIVE ORDERS
FOR SURGERY OF OVARIAN CANCER

For ovarian cancer surgery, the general principles of preparation for laparotomy and major pelvic surgery are followed, with the addition of the procedures listed below.

Upon return of laboratory reports, any abnormal values are rectified by appropriate measures, i.e., blood transfusions for anemia and hypoproteinemia, and indicated parenteral fluids for chloride, potassium, or sodium deficiencies. Because patients with advanced ovarian cancer are frequently debilitated and emaciated, hyperalimentation is being used more often in these patients and will be discussed later.

In debilitated patients, preoperative blood volume studies may be carried out and blood replacement ordered as needed. Ordinarily such studies are not indicated. Among patients with clinical evidence of a depleted blood volume, transfusions can be given and the patient's response monitored with serial hematocrits. A rise of 2–3% in the hematocrit after a transfusion of 500 cc of whole blood usually indicates that the blood volume deficit has been corrected.

A thorough preoperative bowel preparation is very important in patients suspected of having ovarian cancer. Although the mechanical bowel prep is the most important part, the addition of a sulfa preparation or an antibiotic has proved helpful. The bowel can be cleaned out and flattened by administration of 60 cc of 50% magnesium sulfate solution for 2 days, followed by 45 cc of castor oil on the afternoon before surgery. The question of preoperative antibiotics has not been resolved but is included in this protocol. If time permits, one of the sulfa preparations in doses up to 10 g a day for 5–7 days is given, or a short course of neomycin is instituted in a 1-g dose every hour for 6 doses on the day before surgery. The vagina is prepared with an antibiotic suppository or one of the sulfa vaginal creams for 2 or 3 days before surgery. The night before surgery, the patient takes a shower using Phisohex.

The evening before surgery an infusion of glucose and water is started with 1,000 units of heparin in the infusion. This runs through the night, during surgery, and in the postoperative period.

Preoperative medication is given 30 to 45 minutes before the patient is taken to the operating room. Although the medication and dose are selected for each patient depending on size, debilitation, and age, the average is usually 100 mg of seconal and 0.4 mg of atropine by hypodermic, or 50 mg of vistaril and 0.4 mg of atropine, or 50 mg of demerol and 0.4 mg of atropine by hypodermic.

Aggressive surgery and/or chemotherapy for the treatment of ovarian cancer has given rise to many complications. Among these are bowel fistulas and debilitation of the patient, which carried a high mortality before the use of hyperalimentation. Parenteral hyperalimentation was originally used therapeutically, but more and more it is being used prophylactically to prepare patients for their anticipated treatment or for patients who have had a weight loss of 10% or more.

Hyperalimentation is a unique form of intravenous therapy which, parenterally, provides all of the daily nutritional requirements. Parenteral hyperalimentation, or total parenteral nutrition (TPN), is the technique of providing enough calories, amino acids, and other nutrients to promote growth, weight gain, and normal healing. This technique has had a tremendous impact on the critically ill patient who faces slow starvation because of the inability to provide oral alimentation. If adequate nutrition is not available, the body will turn to itself for a source for the energy necessary to remain alive. A rapid deterioration of lean tissue, muscle, and fat ensues.

In the fasting state the body breaks down approximately 75 g of protein per day (12 g of nitrogen). Liver glycogen stores are depleted within 24 hours. The catabolism of protein to glucogenic amino acids and, finally, to glucose is responsible for the maintenance of serum glucose in starvation. The body turns to stores of lean tissue and muscle for a source of glucose, rather than to fat stores. Therefore a protein deficiency rapidly develops. As a result, secondary deficiencies develop in tissue synthesis, blood proteins, leukocytes, enzymes, hormones, and antibodies with consequent delay in healing and susceptibility to infection. The significance of supplying adequate nutrition to the seriously ill patient is quite evident. Severe injury, sepsis secondary to surgery, or other trauma may cause an increased breakdown of body protein/nitrogen of up to 50%. Thus, when hyperalimentation is considered, the daily metabolic requirements should also be calculated as 50% greater than normal.

Hyperalimentation should be used with extreme caution in patients with (1) impaired renal function, (2) hepatic insufficiency, or (3) diabetes.

The technique of catheter placement will not be discussed, nor will a detailed plan of management be described. The purpose is to emphasize the importance of hyperalimentation in managing the debilitated cancer patient.

There are typical formulas for parenteral hyperalimentation, such as the protein hydrolysate solutions and free amino acid mixtures. Electrolytes, vitamins, and minerals should be added as needed. Heparin should be added to each infusion and insulin should be given as needed.

Basic guidelines for safe intravenous feeding include daily measurement of body weight and water balance. Serum electrolytes, blood sugar, and urea nitrogen in the blood should be measured daily until they are stabilized, and then measured every 2 to 3 days. The urine sugar concentration should be measured every 6 hours. Liver and kidney function should be evaluated initially and then every 2 to 3 weeks. Periodic measurement should be made of arterial and central venous pressure, blood acidity, and dissolved gases which may be indicated in the management of patients with heart, kidney, lung, or metabolic disorders. It is a cardinal rule, however, that whenever an infection caused by a catheter is suspected, the catheter should be removed immediately and cultured. Blood cultures should also be taken.

It is important to avoid hyperosmolar, hyperglycemic, nonketotic diabetic coma. Adequate fluid intake must always be maintained and the urine carefully monitored for sugar and acetone. Insulin must be given as needed. Rapidly developing hyperglycemia syndrome may follow a too rapid infusion of glucose. The patient complains of frontal headaches followed shortly by convulsions. Insufficient insulin and hyperglycemia complications can be avoided by the prevention of hyperglycemia by not allowing the blood sugar to rise over 200 mg%.

The surgical technique is covered in chapter 16 and will not be reviewed here. Two points will be discussed briefly—the removal of a great volume of ascitic fluid and the start of oozing or bleeding during the operation. The removal of 2 or more liters of ascitic fluid may lead to an unstable vasomotor system which may result in shock. Therefore enough plasma and fluids and electrolytes should be given to correct the imbalance.

The second point concerns the diagnosis and therapy of hemorrhagic disorders that occur during surgery. Acute, unexpected bleeding during or shortly after operation in the absence of an accountable surgical source is a vexing problem which may catch the surgeon unprepared with a definite plan for management. In such an emergency there is usually little time to run a battery of time-consuming hematologic tests. The discussion that follows is based on the assumption that bleeding is not from a vessel but is related to a hemorrhagic disorder.

The plan of action suggested for the management of these patients is based upon three features: (1) clinical judgment, (2) rapid blood tests, and (3) selective therapy.

Clinical judgment is founded on a careful work-up before operation. Preexisting disorders, congenital or acquired, would presumably be exposed by a thorough history, careful physical examination, and necessary preoperative tests. When preexisting hematologic defects have been ruled out, the causes of unexpected bleeding may be narrowed down to (1) bleeding from a surgical source, (2) fibrinolysis, (3) defibrination, (4) thrombocytopenia from massive blood bank transfusions, (5) anticoagulants and their antagonists, and (6) mixed clotting problems.

Hemostasis involves an interdependence of the blood platelets, the coagulation mechanism, and the blood vessels. The least understood and least studied factor in hemostasis is that involving the blood vessels. In summary, clotting consists of platelet aggregation, then consolidation, the formation of the fibrin clot, clot retraction, and, in pathologic states, fibrinolysis. It can be assumed that blood loss sufficient to require almost constant transfusion to maintain blood pressure is attributable to a surgical cause until proved otherwise.

The circumstances before and at the time of bleeding may help to determine the cause. The onset of abnormal bleeding after massive blood transfusions is probably due to thrombocytopenia which is associated with five or more units of bank blood. A platelet count or estimation of platelet count may confirm that this is the cause of the bleeding. Bleeding that follows one transfusion may be due to a mismatch of blood and favors hemolysis and intravascular coagulation.

Rapid blood tests should be available within 10 to 15 minutes. Test tubes containing a 3.8% sodium citrate solution should be ready in the operating rooms at all times. There are five tests which can be done in all hospitals: (1) *Partial thromboplastin time* (PTT) is a sensitive test for identifying undiagnosed hemophilia, a variety of coagulation defects, and circulating anticoagulants. (2) *Rapid estimation of platelets* has helped in identifying the etiology of the bleeding. Platelet counts considerably below 100,000 may point to massive bank blood transfusions as a source of bleeding. (3) *Bleeding time* helps identify the reason for the bleeding. In patients in whom the bleeding is prolonged beyond 4 minutes, attention must be directed to a platelet abnormality or vascular hemophilia (von Willebrand's disease). Bleeding time is normal in hemophilia. (4) *Prothrombin time* that is abnormal may indicate intravascular coagulation, fibrinolysis, or liver dysfunction. (5) *Thrombin time* that is prolonged indicates overheparinization, defibrination, or fibrinolysis.

Selective treatment depends upon identification of all factors which contribute to the bleeding state. Because the emergency therapy available is rather limited, it is perhaps best to approach the diagnosis by selective treatment. In using this approach one assumes that hemophilia or other severe, lifelong bleeding disorders would probably have been diagnosed preoperatively. There are indeed very few therapeutic modalities available clinically at this time: (1) Fresh frozen plasma will replace any plasma coagulation factor deficiency, as will antihemophilic plasma. (2) Platelet concentrates (or a poor second choice of fresh whole blood) will replace platelets deficient in number or function. (3) Epsilon aminocaproic acid, used to arrest fibrinolysis, probably acts by competitive inhibition of plasminogen activators.

The triad of thrombocytopenia, hypofibrinogenemia, and lysis of a blood clot within 2 hours points to the probability of disseminated intravascular coagulation (DIC). Heparin may rapidly restore the platelet count and fibrinogen level, and thus attenuate the bleeding. After heparin has been given, the consumed clotting factors such as platelets and fibrinogen may have to be replaced in the form of plasma, platelet concentrates, or fresh blood. While the DIC is being treated, therapy for the precipitating cause (hypovolemic shock) should be carried out. In fact, DIC of short duration can be treated without heparin therapy by removing the precipitating cause. Only in profound and long-standing shock and DIC is heparin therapy necessary. Heparin should be considered an adjunct to treatment but not a panacea for the patient in hypovolemic shock who needs a massive transfusion of blood.

SPECIAL POSTOPERATIVE ORDERS
FOR SURGERY OF OVARIAN CANCER

Immediately after operation the vital signs—blood pressure, pulse, and respirations—are noted at 15-minute intervals until sensoria are fully recovered. Urine output per catheter is recorded at hourly intervals. The normal rate is about 50 ml/hour. The urine output is a simple and reliable guide for the administration of fluids.

Sedation for pain is gauged to maintain comfort and at the same time to avoid respiratory distress.

Nothing by mouth is continued until the bowel sounds are normal.

Antibiotics should be used as deemed necessary by the surgeon. Cephaloridin and gentamycin are the two usually chosen. However, in the presence of known bacteroides, cleomycin should be chosen.

Nasogastric suction should be used as needed.

The following schedule for fluids, electrolytes, and plasma should be instituted: 1,000 cc of 5% glucose and water; 1,000 cc of Ringer's lactate; 1,000 cc 5% glucose and water; 1,000 units of heparin added to each bottle. Plasma is added as needed to stabilize the blood pressure and to improve urinary output. After day 1, additional plasma, saline, and potassium are required. The losses from the nasogastric tube must be added to this baseline.

Hemoglobin and hematocrit should be recorded BID for 2 days.

Following surgery for ovarian cancer, any of the complications that are associated with major surgery may occur. However a few of the more common ones will be listed and discussed briefly. Postoperative intestinal problems are not infrequent; they include ileus, intestinal obstruction, peritonitis, and fistula formation. Postoperative infections are not unusual, particularly infections of the wound, and dehiscence is more common among these patients than among those operated on for benign disease. Thromboembolic disease and pulmonary embolization occur more frequently among cancer patients.

Ileus

Ileus is one of the most frequent complications in the postoperative period following surgery for ovarian cancer. It may vary in severity from mild distension to a full-blown picture of paralytic ileus, with its accompanying electrolyte, water, and acid-base imbalance. It is extremely important to make certain that the problem is indeed paralytic ileus and not mechanical small bowel obstruction. Although the fluid and electrolyte replacement may be the same, the definitive approach to the underlying problem is different.

Ileus is most often preceded by a diminution in urine volume. Fluids and electrolytes collect in the intestines. The abdomen becomes distended and pushes the diaphragm up. This often gives rise to an atelectasis and predisposes to respiratory acidosis. The extracellular fluid is therefore decreased, and this in turn leads to a decrease in glomerular filtration with a drop in the urinary output. The clinical picture includes the following features:

- Vomiting and distension occur on the second or third day after surgery.
- Vomiting is first mucus, then bile, and later altered blood.
- Constipation is the rule.
- The abdomen rapidly distends with gas.
- Peristalsis is absent.
- Bowel sounds are absent.
- Pain is usually absent, but if present, it is colicky.
- The patient becomes dehydrated.
- The pulse becomes rapid.
- The respiratory rate, temperature, and leukocyte count rise.
- Urinary output drops despite a good intake.
- The patient becomes toxic.
- A flat plate of the abdomen shows (1) a gas-distended loop and multiple fluid levels in the small bowel, and sometimes (2) a little gas in the cecum and pelvic colon.

Paralytic ileus must be differentiated from a mechanical obstruction. Four cardinal symptoms of mechanical intestinal obstruction are (1) Colicky abdominal pain which is intermittent, comes on suddenly, reaches a peak, then subsides. Auscultation at the time of pain reveals loud, metallic, high-pitched peristaltic rushes. This is the most important difference between obstruction and ileus; (2) Frequent and copious vomiting; (3) Distension; and (4) Obstipation.

The signs and findings that are most helpful in judging whether the patient is improving or deteriorating are (1) the pulse, (2) the respiratory rate, temperature, and white count, (3) the urine output, and (4) the follow-up flat plate of the abdomen.

Peritonitis

Peritonitis is an inflammation of the peritoneum—a condition marked by exudation of serum and by fibrin, cells, and pus in the peritoneum.

The diagnosis of the full-blown picture is easy, but early diagnosis may be elusive. The following signs and symptoms may help in the diagnosis:

- Initial stages depend upon the mode of infection.
- The temperature is elevated.
- A most important sign of pelvic peritonitis following operation is a pulse that is more rapid than would be expected from the temperature elevation.
- Once peritonitis is established, the picture is characteristic.
- Pain distribution follows the spread of infection.
- Vomiting is usual.
- Constipation is more common than diarrhea.
- The patient lies motionless and supine, most often with legs drawn up.
- The expression is anxious and the facies is drawn and gaunt.
- Abdominal muscles over the inflamed site are slightly contracted.
- In diffuse peritonitis, the whole abdomen is rigid, ligneous, and motionless. There is no movement of the abdomen with respiration.

The management of the fluid, electrolytes, and plasma imbalance will not be discussed. However the peritonitis resembles a 15–30° body burn, and the basic principles suggested by Evans for fluid and plasma protein replacement in burn cases can be adapted to the patient with peritonitis.

POSTOPERATIVE WOUND INFECTIONS

A collection of blood or serum below or above the fascia may become secondarily infected. This results from bacterial contamination from a variety of sources, but in a high percentage of cases it is the result of a break in technique.

A wound infection, particularly those forming below the fascia and behind the pubis, are characterized at first by a low temperature and slightly elevated pulse with some malaise. This progresses to a spiking fever with tenderness above the pubis but usually little induration at this point. The onset of the spiking fever usually comes later in the postoperative period than the onset associated with wound infections located above the fascia. Opening of the abscess cavity usually solves the problem. However cultures should be taken and an antibiotic regimen started. If the opening is large enough to insure good drainage, it is not necessary to insert a drain.

WOUND DEHISCENCE AND EVISCERATION

Wound dehiscence is more common in patients treated surgically for a malignancy than in those treated for a benign disease. Protein deficiency, anemia, chronic debility, vomiting, distension, malignancy, and wound infections are all contributing factors to dehiscence. The patient can usually be handled by opening the skin, irrigating the wound, and packing the area open.

Evisceration is more serious and involves the bowel outside the peritoneum and fascia. If the condition of the patient permits, the wound should be closed in the operating room with through-and-through interrupted wire or nylon sutures. Occasionally it is necessary to irrigate the wound, pack it, and strap it closed until it is possible to perform a secondary closure.

THROMBOEMBOLIC DISEASE

Thrombophlebitis is not uncommon in general gynecologic surgery and is more frequent when the operation is carried out for treatment of a malignancy. It usually develops between days 5 and 10 postoperatively. Most reports state that the phlebitis probably starts in the operating room. Thromboembolic disease may have an insidious onset with few, if any, clinical signs or symptoms until pulmonary embolization occurs. Superficial phlebitis is not dangerous and fatalities result only from deep venous thrombi.

Pulmonary embolism may be the first and only sign that thrombophlebitis is present. Other signs of phlebothrombosis and thrombophlebitis include (1) tenderness of the foot, particularly on the medial side; (2) painful dorsiflexion of the foot (Homan's sign)—a very unreliable sign and one that is difficult to evaluate; (3) an ascending stepladder pulse associated with temperature elevation and increased respiration; and (4) pain and swelling of the affected leg.

Cranley has developed phleborheography as an accurate method of diagnosing thrombophlebitis. Phleborheography, defined as the tracing of moving currents within a vein, has been considered an accurate term to designate a plethysmographic technique for diagnosing deep venous thrombosis of the lower extremity. The technique is practical and highly accurate, and it has become a standard clinical test. It is noninvasive and very accurate in diagnosing deep venous thrombosis of the lower extremity. Phleborheography can be performed by a technician in the laboratory, at the bedside, or in the office. It has taken the guesswork out of diagnosing deep vein thrombosis. Therapy consists of anticoagulation, bed rest, elevation of the extremity, and a pneumatic pad. The rationale for the use of anticoagulants is to prevent embolization, to control additional clot formation, and to interrupt the local pain and swelling.

In the past few years, prophylactic heparinization has been established as a method of treatment on many services, and it has proved most rewarding. The minidose heparin (1,000 units of heparin in 1,000 cc of infusion to run over 8 hours) is started the evening before surgery and is continued during surgery and during the first 3 or 4 postoperative days. It has been reported to be more effective by this plan of administration than if it were started in the operating room or in the immediate postoperative period.

PULMONARY EMBOLIZATION

Pulmonary embolization is a feared complication following pelvic surgery for a malignant condition. It occurs most frequently after coughing and squeezing on bed pans when the glottis closes followed by a sudden release of pressure. The embolization may be sudden and dramatic, resulting in death, or it may progress from minor symptoms. The patient may faint and have an acute pain in the chest followed by cyanosis and respiratory distress, or she may have an unexplained tachycardia for a few days with a slight elevation of temperature.

A high index of suspicion is most important in making the diagnosis. The triad of an elevated serum glutamic oxalic transaminase, bilirubin and serum lactic dehydrogenase are helpful, as is the evaluation of arterial blood gases. Lung scans have some value, but the most specific test in this diagnosis is pulmonary angiography.

SHOCK LUNG

The syndrome of life-threatening progressive pulmonary insufficiency of unknown etiology has been called shock lung. The same systemic insult may result in differing patterns of lung damage, or the same pattern of lung damage may follow varying types of systemic insult. Some of the many etiologic factors are lack of surfactant, disseminated intravascular coagulation (DIC), overtransfusion or overinfusion, heart failure, low osmolality of blood, direct lung injury, fat embolism, transfusion embolism, oxygen toxicity, damage due to a respirator, increased antidiuretic hormone, and vasospasm.

The shock lung has often been confused with such pathologic diagnoses as bronchopneumonia, patchy atelectasis, and agonal changes. In the acute state the lung grossly shows edema, congestion, hemorrhage, heaviness, and relative airlessness. The lungs are liver-like, consolidated, and markedly saturated with fluid, literally oozing fluids onto their surface. Microscopically, the same characteristics are evident with patchy atelectasis, intraalveolar edema, interalveolar edema, congestion, and hemorrhage with or without microthrombi.

The clinical picture is characterized by apprehension, tachypnea, air hunger, and sepsis, but cyanosis may not be present. Expiratory wheezes are almost pathognomonic of impending shock lung, but bronchial rales and signs of consolidation may not be present early in the disease. Three conditions that commonly lead to shock lung are systemic sepsis, massive fluid replacement, and a period of hypotension.

An x-ray of the lungs may not show any evidence of impending shock until 36 to 48 hours postoperatively. At that time characteristic "snowfield" patchy pneumonitis and pulmonary haziness may be present.

Blood gases and tidal volumes, especially serial measurements, are diagnostic and prognostic. Early in the development of shock lung the serum pO_2 ranges from 50 to 60 mmHg, and serum pCO_2 from 20 to 30 mmHg. The pH is often alkalotic. In the initial alkalotic phase the pO_2 can be maintained by increasing the inspired concentration of oxygen and by hyperventilating the patient. Later, in the untreated patient, the pO_2 declines further, but the pCO_2 rises or remains normal and the pH becomes acidotic. These measurements give an indication of both the ability of the lungs to utilize oxygen and the degree of arteriovenous shunting. When arterial pO_2 is low after the patient has inspired 100% oxygen for 30 minutes, there is a high degree of shunting and the chances for survival decrease. Prognosis is also poor when lung compliance is low and decreases progressively. In the latter instance, functional residual capacity decreases as minute volume increases.

Treatment must be aggressive and must be started early. The treatment should include maintenance of a positive and expiratory pressure (PEEP), large amounts of steroids, infusion of albumin and diuretics, administration of broad-spectrum antibiotics, restriction of fluids to levels that can be handled by a compromised cardiopulmonary system, and carefully filtration of all fluids given to decrease the chance of particles forming microemboli in the lungs. If carried out in a carefully controlled manner, these measures may greatly decrease the incidence of death from this disease.

SUMMARY

A well-planned and well-coordinated work-up may alert the physician to a diagnosis of metastatic as opposed to primary ovarian cancer. In addition, it may reveal a physiologic imbalance that could result in a high morbidity or mortality unless it is corrected. Therefore a detailed diagnostic work-up is outlined:

1. Complete history and physical examinations, including a pelvic and rectal examination
2. Careful palpation of the thyroid
3. Hemogram
4. Urinalysis
5. Blood chemistry profile
6. Serum electrolyte profile
7. AP and lateral chest x-ray
8. Electrocardiogram
9. VDRL
10. Intravenous pyelogram
11. Mammography
12. Cystoscopy
13. Proctoscopy
14. Barium enema
15. Gastrointestinal series
16. Skeletal survey
17. Lymphangiogram
18. Liver scan

19. Ultrasound
20. Prior to an exploratory laparotomy, the patient should have an examination under anesthesia and a fractional curettage. Laparoscopy or peritoneoscopy for staging the ovarian cancer is optional.

BIBLIOGRAPHY

Cranley, J. J.: Phleborheography: New noninvasive method of diagnosing deep venous thrombosis of lower extremity is highly accurate. Rhode Island Med. J. 58:111, 1975.

Cranley, J. J., Gay, A. Y., Grass, A. M., et al.: A plethysmographic technique for the diagnosis of deep venous thrombosis of the lower extremities. Surg. Gynecol. Obstet. 136:385, 1973.

Dudrick, S. J., Copeland, E. M., III, MacFayden, B. V., Jr.: Long-term parenteral nutrition. Hosp. Practice, 10:47–58, 1975.

Dudrick, S. J., Rhoads, J. E.: Total intravenous feeding. Sci. Am. 226:73, 1972.

Hull, R. L: Physiochemical considerations in intravenous hyperalimentation. Am. J. Hosp. Pharm., 31:236–243, 1975.

Kinnaird, D. W., Aldrete, A.: Preoperative care, in General Surgery. Edited by F.W. Preston, W. C. Davis. Harper & Row, Hagerstown, Maryland, chap. 12, 1975, p. 1.

Kinnaird, D.W., Aldrete, A.: Postoperative care, in General Surgery. Edited by F.W. Preston, W.C. Davis. Harper & Row, Hagerstown, Maryland, chap. 13, 1975, p. 1.

Laufman, H., Lalezari, P.: A plan for management of unexpected bleeding problems related to surgery. Pacific Med. Surg. 75:362, 1967.

Maki, D. G.: Infection control in intravenous therapy. Ann. Intern. Med. 79:867, 1973.

Miller, R. D.: Complications of massive transfusions. Anesthesiology 39:82, 1973.

Ryan, G. M., Howland, W.S.: The diagnosis and therapy of hemorrhagic disorders occurring during surgery. Surg. Digest 3:29, 1968.

10

Diagnosing and Managing the Unilateral Mass

Age is an important consideration in the management of a patient with unilateral mass. For the following discussion, I have divided patients into three age groups: birth to 20 years, 20 to 40 years, and over 40 years. Occurence during pregnancy will be considered separately.

A mass in the very young and the very old is presumed to be *abnormal*. The best management consists of a careful work-up and exploratory laparotomy. There is no time or place for observation and procastination with patients in these age groups. Management of a unilateral mass diagnosed during pregnancy or in patients between 20 and 40 may arouse controversy.

BIRTH TO AGE 20

In the newborn and the prepubertal patient, any palpable adnexal mass is suspect and a new growth must be ruled out. Although ovarian tumors account for about 1% of new growths in children under 16, they still remain the most frequent genital neoplasm of childhood and adolescence. The problems related to diagnosis are surpassed only by the problems and confusion related to therapy. It is difficult for many of those involved with patients in this group to accept the possibility of ovarian malignancy, and even more difficult for the physican to deprive a child of her reproductive potential.

Ovarian neoplasms may occur at any age in childhood or adolescence, but they tend to be most common at puberty (between 10 and 14). This fact had led to conjecture that some control mechanism may be activated or that pituitary stimulation of a latent ovarian factor may be the triggering mechanism.

The most common tumors in infants and young children are cystic teratomas (dermoids). They have been found soon after birth or later. Multiple retention cysts and luteal cysts are also occasionally seen in the newborn. If the tumors are not complicated by torsion, rupture, or infection, observation for a couple of weeks is acceptable. During this time, there should be marked regression.

Ovarian tumors in children may produce few symptoms. The symp-

125

tomatology is related to the rapidity of growth, position, and degree of malignancy, as well as to the tumor's ability to secrete hormones. The complications associated with tumors, such as twisting, rupture, infection, and hemorrhage, focus attention on them.

When symptoms occur, a general physical examination that includes the pelvic, rectal, and rectovaginal areas should be carefully carried out. It is almost universally impossible to palpate normal ovaries in children; therefore it can be assumed that a palpable ovary is abnormal. The size determines whether it can be felt abdominally or by rectoabdominal palpation. In the prepubertal girl, the ovary is an abdominal organ. It does not migrate into the pelvis until puberty.

Diagnostic procedures should include a blood count, urinalysis, chest x-ray, intravenous pyelogram, and, if indicated, x-ray studies of the gastrointestinal tract. In patients suspected of having a hormone-producing tumor, hormone assays may have some value, but x-ray studies of bone age may be even more helpful. The role of ultrasonic studies and laparoscopy in this age group remains to be clarified. Alpha-fetoprotein (AFP) and carcinoembryonic antigen levels may be significantly elevated. Elevation of AFP has been found to be associated with endodermal sinus tumor and certain embryonal carcinomas. An elevated chorionic gonadotropin titer may be present in embryonal tumors, especially when chorionic elements are found in the tumor.

The key to treatment is to be conservative. However any spread beyond the ovary demands a more aggressive approach. Treatment will be outlined by groups of tumors within a given classification. Although common epithelial ovarian tumors are rare in this age group, the physician must occasionally manage a mucinous or serous cystadenocarcinoma. If the tumor is unilateral and encapsulated, if there is negative pelvic cytology, and if the opposite ovary is negative on biopsy, unilateral salpingo-oophorectomy is acceptable therapy. With any evidence of spread of disease beyond the ovary, however, total hysterectomy, bilateral salpingo-oophorectomy, and omentectomy (if an omentum has developed) are indicated, along with the instillation of 10 mc of radioactive phosphorus (P^{32}).

Germ cell tumors vary a great deal in their response to treatment. The dysgerminoma is a highly radiosensitive tumor that occurs bilaterally in up to 10% of the patients. The treatment of choice, although controversial, is unilateral salpingo-oophorectomy and is based on the assumption that no positive cells are present in the pelvis. (The value of pelvic cytology in this tumor has not been established.) The opposite ovary must be free of tumor on biopsy as well as the paraaortic nodes. If there is spread beyond the ovary in which the tumor occurs, total hysterectomy and bilateral salpingo-oophorectomy are required. X-ray should be employed if the disease spreads to the pelvis and/or upper abdomen. The necessity for mediastinal and supraclavicular node therapy with x-ray for this age group has not been determined.

Embryonal carcinomas and extraembryonal carcinomas (endodermal sinus tumor, polyvesicular vitelline tumor, and choriocarcinoma) are highly malignant. But if unilateral and encapsulated, they are treated just as well by unilateral oophorectomy as by more radical surgery. Radiation therapy offers very little help because these tumors are relatively radioresistant. Recently, however, multiple chemotherapy has produced encouraging results; some improvement in survival rates is expected. There is controversy over whether the uterus and remaining tube and ovary should be removed before instituting triple chemotherapy. Only time will give the answer, but a conservative approach is currently recommended if there is no evidence of spread.

Gonadal stromal tumors (formerly referred to as sex-cord tumors) include tumors that have the potential to produce either an estrogenizing or masculinizing effect, although they do so in only 25% of patients. Of the female cell type, the only important malignant tumor is the granulosa cell tumor. It is usually unilateral and has late recurrence, often beyond 5 years. Typically, spread is local and recurrence is confined to the pelvis. Since the tumor has a low-grade malignancy and is seldom bilateral, unilateral oophorectomy is indicated when the tumor is encapsulated and the other ovary is normal.

Among tumors of the male cell type, the Sertoli-Leydig cell tumor (formerly called arrhenoblastoma) is the most important. If it secretes a hormone, the resulting clinical picture is defeminization followed by masculinization. When it is malignant, the natural history is similar to that of granulosa cell carcinoma, and treatment is the same for both. Once the patient has completed her family, hysterectomy and removal of the other ovary are indicated in patients who have had either a granulosa cell tumor or a Sertoli-Leydig cell tumor.

Gonadoblastoma is composed of germ cells and gonadal stromal cells in nearly equal proportion. Its malignant potential is determined by the type of germ cell present. The gonadoblastoma is usually found in the intersexual patient, and therefore the common treatment is bilateral oophorectomy.

In this age group metastatic ovarian cancer is treated as in adults. As much tumor as possible is removed, including the primary cancer.

AGE 20 TO 40

In this group, as previously noted, controversy may arise over management of an adnexal mass. A careful history is of prime importance, followed by a thorough pelvic examination to include the vaginal, rectal, and rectovaginal areas. The ideal time to examine the patient is after she has been given an enema. There are causes for the presence of an adnexal mass other than ovarian pathology. Certain diagnoses are more likely to be made at a given age; for example, diverticulitis is more common after age 40, whereas an ectopic pregnancy is more common when the patient is in her 20s. The differential diagnosis should include myomata (pedunculated); retroperitoneal tumors; pelvic-kidney, tubo-ovarian, or appendiceal abscesses; diverticultitis; adhesions; anterior sacral meningocele; ectopic pregnancy; and neoplasms of the large bowel.

The preoperative work-up must be thorough so that the primary site of a metastatic tumor is not overlooked. It should include blood counts and chemistries as well as urinalysis. Chest x-ray, intravenous pyelography, and sonography are helpful. Whether mammograms and x-rays of the intestinal tract are indicated depends on symptomatology and the age of the patient. Biologic markers such as carcinoembryonic antigen, AFP, chorionic gonadotropin titers, and lactic dehydrogenase levels have value only if they are elevated. Then they can serve to monitor response to therapy. The value of laparoscopy has not been established.

If the patient is in her 20s and the mass is cystic, smooth, and movable, it is good medical practice to reevaluate after one or two menstrual periods. A functional cyst should start to regress during this time. Some investigators have advocated the use of a combined estrogen-progesterone pill to inhibit pituitary stimulation of the ovary. If it is a functional cyst, it should promptly begin to regress. Even a short period of observation is not justified if the patient is already taking oral contraceptives.

At the time of laparotomy, management of the adnexal mass in the patient in her 20s is similar to that described for tumors in childhood. It is important to individualize treatment not only according to histogenetic classification but also according to stage of disease. In general the conservative approach is justified if the tumor is unilateral and encapsulated. Also, there should be negative cytology, the tumor should be well differentiated, and it should be a dysgerminoma or a gonadal stromal type. The patient should be of low parity or nulliparous. And there should be negative biopsy of the opposite ovary as well as negative omental or pelvic and paraaortic node biopsies.

Any evidence of spread demands maximal surgical treatment, including total hysterectomy, bilateral salpingo-oophorectomy, omentectomy, and appendectomy. Although patients between 20 and 40 become subjects of the greatest degree of controversy when an adnexal mass is found, there is no dispute over treatment if the mass is bilateral, larger than 10 cm, irregular in outline with cystic and solid areas present, or if it continues to grow under observation. Total hysterectomy, bilateral salpingo-oophorectomy, omentectomy, appendectomy, and P[32] instillation are indicated.

UNILATERAL MASS IN PREGNANCY

The adnexal mass in pregnancy is always cause for concern. Approximately 1 in 1,000 pregnancies is complicated by ovarian tumor. In pregnancy about 1 in 10 ovarian masses represents a normal cystic corpus luteum, which may get to be as large as 10 cm.

The differential diagnosis of an adnexal mass in the pregnant patient is the same as that for the nonpregnant patient in the same age group. Management of an ovarian mass depends to a certain extent on the trimester of the pregnancy and on whether torsion or hemorrhage occurs as a complication. A freely movable, encapsulated, unilateral adnexal can be observed until the patient is in the second trimester. A corpus luteum cyst will regress during this time. If the mass persists or increases in size, surgical intervention is indicated. Most ovarian tumors discovered during pregnancy are either dermoids or cystadenomas. Both can be managed by conservative therapy. However, if the mass is knobby, fixed, and/or bilateral with any signs of fluid, surgery is indicated without delay despite the trimester of pregnancy.

The incidence of malignancy in ovarian tumors diagnosed in pregnancy is variously reported between 2.5 and 5%. Fortunately, most malignancies in pregnancy are discovered at stage I because the patient seeks examination early in pregnancy. The survival rate of patients with ovarian cancer in pregnancy is the same as that of nonpregnant patients. The type of tumor and its anatomic spread determine the 5-year cure rate. Pregnancy has no effect on the tumor. Only aggressive, early exploration will save the patient. Interruption of pregnancy has no beneficial effect on the future of this disease. If the tumor is diagnosed in the third trimester, surgery can be delayed until the fetus has become viable. Delay beyond that point is not justified.

AGE 40 AND OLDER

Patients 40 years old and older compose the high-risk group because they are either perimenopausal or postmenopausal. The same diagnostic work-ups and differential diagnosis are followed as in the 20–40 age group. Metastatic cancers of the ovary are probably more common in this high-risk age group. Since chances of malignancy are higher than in the 20–40 group, there is no indication for observation, especially if the mass is larger than 5 cm and adherent, giving the impression that there are solid cystic areas.

Treatment should consist of total hysterectomy, bilateral salpingo-oophorectomy, appendectomy, omentectomy, and the instillation of P^{32}. The epithelial ovarian tumor is the most commonly encountered ovarian tumor. About 8% occur before age 40; incidence peaks at 52 to 55 years.

What is a normal-sized ovary in the premenopausal woman is an ovarian tumor in the patient who is more than 2 years postmenopausal. There is no such thing as physiologic cysts in this age group. The contrast between the premenopausal and postmenopausal ovary is striking. Whereas the normal ovary measures 3.5 × 2 × 1.5 cm., the ovary in the patient 2 or more years postmenopausal may be as small as 1.5 × 0.75 × 0.5 cm. These patients should not be followed and reevaluated; the presence or absence of a tumor must be substantiated. To wait until a solid tumor mass of up to 5 cm can be felt and then to expect a cure is an exercise in futility.

The tumors reviewed in this chapter will be discussed in greater detail in other chapters.

SUMMARY

Age is an important consideration in the management of the patient with a unilateral mass. Between birth to age 20 the germ cell tumors are the most common. Except for the embryonal and extraembryonal tumors, germ cell tumors have a respectable survival rate. Often it is possible to be conservative in the management of the ovarian tumor without compromising the survival of the patient. In the 20–40 age group a variety of ovarian tumors are encountered. Those patients at the left of the scale in the 20–30 group usually have germ cell or gonadal stromal tumors, and a conservative approach is acceptable if the findings indicate that the patient's prognosis will not be jeopardized. Those patients at the right of the scale near age 40 most often have a common epithelial tumor. The decision on management is not difficult, because a more aggressive therapy is the management chosen. The ovarian tumor in pregnancy may be followed until the end of the first trimester if it is unilateral and freely movable. However, if it is bilateral or fixed with hard knobby areas intermingled with cystic areas, the patient should be explored without a period of observation.

BIBLIOGRAPHY

Barber, H. R. K., Graber, E. A.: The PMPO syndrome (postmenopausal palpable ovary syndrome). Obstet. Gynecol. 38:921, 1971.

Barber, H. R. K., Graber, E. A.: Gynecologic tumors in childhood and adolescence. Obstet. Gynecol. Surv. 28:357, 1973.

Barber, H. R. K., Graber, E. A.: Surgical aspects of ovarian tumors, in Selected Topics of Cancer—Current Concepts. Edited by K. K. N. Charyulu, A. Sudarsanam. N.Y. Intercontinental Medical Book Corp., 1974, pp. 161–183.

Hilaris, B. S., Clark, D. G. C.: The value of postoperative intraperitoneal injection of radiocolloids in early cancer of the ovary. Am. J. Roentgenol. Radium Ther. Nucl. Med. 112:749, 1971.

Munnell, E. W.: Is conservative therapy ever justified in stage I cancer of the ovary? Am. J. Obstet. Gynecol. 103:641, 1969.

Novak, E. R., Long, J. H.: Arrhenoblastoma of the ovary. Am. J. Obstet. Gynecol. 92:1082, 1965.

Scully, R. E.: Recent progress in ovarian cancer. Hum. Pathol. 1:73, 1970.

Sjöstedt, D., Wahlen, T.: Prognosis of granulosa cell tumors. Acta. Obstet. Gynecol. Scand. 6:40, 1961.

Teilum, G.: Tumors of germinal origin. Ovarian Cancer, International Union Against Cancer Monograph Series. Vol. II, New York, Springer-Verlag, 1948, p. 58.

11

Staging of Ovarian Cancer

O varian cancer is becoming a common malignancy. It has been considered a family of malignancies arising within the ovary rather than a single entity. The ovary is complex in its embryology, histology, steroidogenesis, and potential for malignancy. It is made up of germ cells, gonadal stromal cells, and cells of the mesenchymal tissue, each with its own potential to form a tumor. Although sex is determined genetically at fertilization, the ovary passes through its early phases as an indifferent organ with parallel development that could allow it to become an ovary or a testis. Alterations or imbalances during these steps of development may provide the setting for the later cellular malfunctioning that produces endocrine imbalances as well as malignancy. The ovary is unique in that it not only gives rise to a great variety of malignancies but itself is a favorite site for metastases from many other organs.

Therapeutic statistics on ovarian cancer are of limited value if attention is not paid to the histologic type of the growth. However experience has shown that there is no clear correlation between clinical and histologic malignancy in ovarian tumors in all instances. This holds true for various types of neoplasms, but especially for epithelial tumors, granulosa cell tumors, and virilizing tumors.

In a review of the material at Lenox Hill Hospital, the conclusion reached was that staging and histologic type are both important and should be used to establish therapy. It is obvious that they are not competitive but rather complementary. The importance of grading (histologic, nuclear, and stromal) in endometrial and cervical cancers has been established and accepted. It remains for a universal grading system to be adopted for ovarian cancer. This study showed that the grade was important in predicting prognosis in the early stages of ovarian cancer but was a less reliable guide in the more advanced cancers. *In general, stage of disease has proved to be more important than histologic or nuclear grades.*

Within each stage there is a great deal of variation, making it difficult to compare results between institutions. Since there are varying degrees of malignancy in groups of a particular stage, it is important to examine tumor tissues microscopically to determine their grade or degree of malignancy according to the histologic and nuclear grade as well as the stromal reaction. *Staging is determined clinically and estimates the extent of disease and the size of the tumor, whereas histologic type and grading provide its*

131

microscopic character. It has been determined that in any stage there is considerable variation, and it is suggested that there are certain tumors more potent than others within a given stage. If these findings are accepted, *treatment should be tailored to the cancer rather than to the stage of disease.*

Unlike other gynecologic malignancies, ovarian cancer is staged at the time of exploratory laparotomy or after a complete microscopic examination of the primary specimen, and biopsies are taken from the abdominal cavity. All other gynecologic malignancies are staged before the start of therapy, and no matter what new findings are uncovered during treatment, the original and initial staging stands. This is not so with ovarian cancer.

With ovarian tumors it is desirable to have a clinical stage grouping before definitive therapy is begun. Sometimes it is impossible to come to a final diagnosis by inspection or palpation or by any other method recommended for clinical staging of carcinoma of the uterus and vagina. Therefore the Cancer Committee has recommended that the clinical staging of ovarian cancer be based on clinical examination as well as on findings at laparotomy and the microscopic findings postoperatively. In some cases of malignant tumor in the pelvis or abdomen, the condition of the patient does not permit explorative laparotomy, and the tumors cannot be clinically staged in detail. For the presentation of therapeutic results, it is necessary to have information on the number of such patients who are thought to have an ovarian malignant tumor. They should be reported in the group designated "special category."

The therapy and prognosis in ovarian cancer depend largely on the anatomic extent of the growth and on the penetration of the ovarian capsule by the tumor. Recently, subcategories have been added to stages I and II to indicate whether tumor is present on the external surface and whether the capsule had ruptured or not. In addition, in stage II a subcategory was added to include those patients with ascites or positive peritoneal washings.

The Cancer Committee of the International Federation of Gynecology and Obstetrics (FIGO) has recommended the following stage grouping for common epithelial ovarian cancer:

Stage Grouping for Primary Carcinoma of the Ovary in
Common Epithelial Ovarian Cancer

Stage I		Growth limited to the ovaries
	IA	Growth limited to *one* ovary; no ascites
		1) No tumor on the external surface; capsule intact
		2) Tumor present on the external surface and/or capsule ruptured
	IB	Growth limited to *both* ovaries; no ascites
		1) No tumor on the external surface; capsule intact
		2) Tumor present on the external surface and/or capsule(s) ruptured
	IC	Tumor either stage IA or stage IB, but

		with ascites* or positive peritoneal washings
Stage II		Growth involving one or both ovaries with pelvic extension
	IIA	Extension and/or metastases to the uterus and/or tubes
	IIB	Extension to other pelvic tissues
	IIC	Tumor either stage IIA or IIB, but with ascites* or positive peritoneal washings
Stage III		Growth involving one or both ovaries with intraperitoneal metastases outside the pelvis and/or positive retroperitoneal nodes; tumor limited to the true pelvis, with histologically proven malignant extension to small bowel or omentum
Stage IV		Growth involving one or both ovaries with distant metastases. If pleural effusion is present, there must be positive cytology to allot a case to stage IV; parenchymal liver metastases classified in stage IV
Special Category:		Unexplored cases which are thought to be ovarian carcinoma.

Stage I epithelial ovarian cancer is a disease limited to one or both ovaries. IA is limited to one ovary and IB is limited to both ovaries. Stage IC is tumor limited to one or both ovaries, but with ascites. It must be a peritoneal effusion which in the opinion of the surgeon is pathologic and/or clearly exceeds normal amounts. Patients who have cytologically positive peritoneal washings are now permitted to be classified as stage IC. Stages IA and IB are further subdivided into subgroups 1 and 2, depending on whether there is tumor on the external surface, as well as on whether the capsule is intact or ruptured. Rupture of the cyst applies to both spontaneous rupture at the time of surgery. It is obvious that rupture and ascites represents more advanced disease even within a given stage (Figure 45).

Stage II indicates growth involving one or both ovaries with pelvic extension of the tumor. Stage IIA indicates extension or metastases to the tubes and/or uterus. Stage IIB represents tumor extension to other pelvic structures, but still within the pelvis. And IIC includes those patients who have ascites as classified above or positive peritoneal washings. The change in survival between stages IIA and IIB is dramatic. It would seem that IIA may represent a geographic spread because of the proximity of the cancer to the uterus and/or tubes, whereas IIB represents a biologic spread with possibly lymphatic invasion (Figure 46).

Stage III is growth involving one or both ovaries with intraperitoneal

*Ascites is peritoneal effusion which in the opinion of the surgeon is pathologic and/or clearly exceeds normal amounts.

STAGE I : Growth Limited to the Ovaries

Ia – One ovary   Ib – Two ovaries

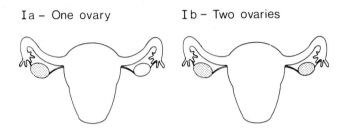

Ic – Tumor in one or both ovaries ,

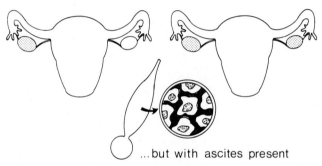

...but with ascites present

Figures 45–48. Clinical staging of common epithelial ovarian cancers. Staging is based on findings at clinical examinations and surgical exploration, as approved by the general assembly of the International Federation of Gynecology and Obstetrics.

metastases outside the pelvis and/or positive retroperitoneal nodes. Tumor is limited to the true pelvis, and there is histologically proven malignant extension to small bowel and/or omentum (Figure 47).

Stage IV indicates growth involving one or both ovaries with distant metastases. If pleural effusion is present, there must be positive cytology to designate a case as stage IV. Parenchymal liver metastases (which does not include studding or implants on the surface of the liver) are classified in stage IV (Figure 48).

The "special category" is reserved for unexplored cases which are thought to be ovarian carcinoma.

Stages I and II spell out specifically the amount of disease, but stages III and IV are not so specific. It is important for the operating surgeon to record the volume of tumor to the best of his ability, because tumor volume has an important relationship to therapy and prognosis.

Staging and detailed histology studies serve as a guide in understanding the natural history of the disease. Both are important in selecting a therapeutic regimen. Although there are many deficiences in the FIGO classification, they have focused attention on evaluating the extent of the disease. In summary, stage of disease is the most reliable guide in therapy and prognosis.

STAGE II : Growth Involving One or Both
Ovaries with Pelvic Extensions

IIa.- Extension and / or
metastases to the uterus
and / or fallopian tubes

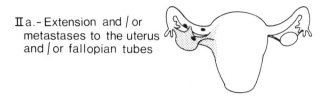

IIb.- Extension to other pelvic tissues; no ascites

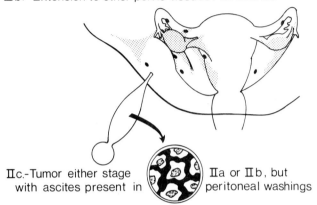

IIc.- Tumor either stage IIa or IIb, but
with ascites present in peritoneal washings

Figure 46.

STAGE III

Cross section of liver -
shows metastases
studding the surface

Histologically proven
malignant extensions to
small bowel or omentum

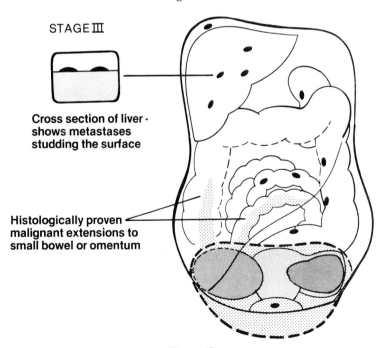

Figure 47.

135

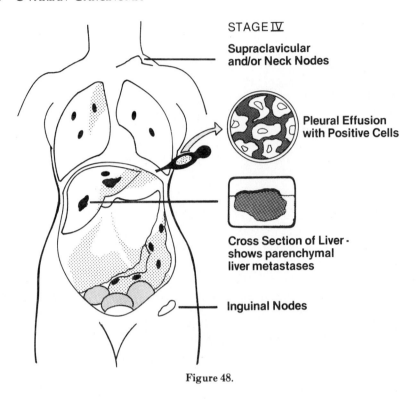

STAGE IV

Supraclavicular and/or Neck Nodes

Pleural Effusion with Positive Cells

Cross Section of Liver · shows parenchymal liver metastases

Inguinal Nodes

Figure 48.

SUMMARY

The clinical stage or anatomic extent of tumor growth at the time of diagnosis is generally considered the best indicator of prognosis. Unlike other gynecologic cancers, ovarian carcinoma is staged at the time of exploratory laparotomy or when the final histologic findings are reported. The International Federation of Gynecology and Obstetrics (FIGO) revised their 1971 classification in 1974. Although the original staging only included the common epithelial ovarian tumors, the others including germ cell and gonadal stromal are now staged according to this method. The new classification for ovarian cancer has created additional subgroups. It has been designed to explore the significance of grossly visible tumor on the external surface of the tumor and to discover whether rupture of the capsule is associated with a poorer prognosis. In stages IA and IB, rupture of the capsule or tumor on the external surface advances it to subgroup 2. Although it is important to stage the ovarian cancer, it is also important to remember that potency of tumors varies within a given stage and that treatment should be tailored to the cancer rather than to the stage of disease.

The concept of how to stage ovarian cancer is not always correctly interpreted. *It is to be restated that ovarian cancer is staged at the time of exploratory laparotomy or when the final histologic findings are reported.* Despite this, Knapp and Friedman reported on aortic lymph node metastases in early ovarian cancer and the paper is widely quoted for the incidence of aortic nodes in stage I ovarian cancer. They reported that aortic node biopsies performed in 26 patients with stage I ovarian cancer revealed 5 with metastases. The 5 patients should not have been staged as I, but rather by definition should be included as stage III ovarian cancer. The conclusion to be drawn is not that there are 19% positive aortic nodes in stage I ovarian cancer, but rather that *these patients were incorrectly staged.*

BIBLIOGRAPHY

Averette, H.E., Haskins, W.J., Dudan, R.C., Nordqvist, S.R.B.: The ovary, *in* Management of the Patient With Cancer. Edited by T.F. Nealon, Jr. Saunders, Philadelphia, 1976, p. 618.

Barber, H.R.K., Graber, E.A., Kwon, T.: Ovarian Cancer Monograph. American Cancer Society, Professional Education Publication, 1975.

Barber, H.R.K., Kwon, T.: Current status of the treatment of gynecologic cancer by site—Ovary. Cancer 38:610, 1976.

Barber, H.R.K., Sommers, S.C., Snyder, R., Kwon, T.: Histologic and nuclear grading and stromal reactions as indices for prognosis in ovarian cancer. Am. J. Obstet. Gynecol. 121:795, 1975.

Knapp, R.C., Friedman, E.A.: Aortic lymph node metastases in early ovarian cancer. Am. J. Obstet. Gynecol. 119:1013–1017, 1974.

Report presented by the Cancer Committee to the General Assembly of FIGO: New York, April 1970. Int. J. Gynecol. Obstet. 9:172, 1971.

12

Treatment of the Common Epithelial Cancers

Tumors that originate in the surface epithelium and ovarian stroma constitute 75 to 90% of primary ovarian cancers. Only about 8% of these cancers occur in women under the age of 35, but recent figures indicate that this number may be increasing. Most common epithelial cancers develop in patients between 40 and 60. In this group conservative surgery is not indicated or considered, and treatment consists of total abdominal hysterectomy, bilateral salpingo-oophorectomy, omentectomy, appendectomy, and instillation of P^{32}. Chemotherapy has been added to the protocol, as prophylaxis in stages I and II and as therapy in stages III and IV.

The treatment for common epithelial tumors will be presented by stage of disease. This will provide a framework for management, though it is impossible to assert rigid criteria for the management of each and every problem that may arise. Armed with the general principles to be outlined, the physician caring for women with ovarian cancer should be able to modify this protocol as he or she deems necessary and be in a better position to make proper decisions on the management of these patients.

The suggested management of the patient with truly invasive common epithelial cancers includes:

- Total abdominal hysterectomy
- Bilateral salpingo-oophorectomy
- Appendectomy
- Omentectomy
- Insertion of tubes and administration of P^{32} (if the disease is limited in extent)

TREATMENT PLAN BY STAGES

Stages IA, IB, and IC

Total hysterectomy, bilateral salpingo-oophorectomy, omentectomy, appendectomy, and instillation of P^{32} constitute the recommended treatment. All patients should have any free fluid aspirated before the patient is explored and, if none is present, the pelvis should be irrigated with saline and the fluid submitted for cytology according to the Papanicolaou technique. There is considerable controversy over the value of omentectomy. Occasionally, islands of tumor cells will be found in the omentum, advancing the stage from I to III. In addition, the presence of the omentum interferes with the even distribution of P^{32} and should be removed if the use of P^{32} is contemplated. Metastatic disease may be found in the opposite normal- appearing ovary. Reports in the literature indicate that approximatley 10% of patients with stage I ovarian cancer will have metastatic cancer between the liver and the diaphragm along the posterior wall of the abdominal cavity. In view of this finding, our protocol has been revised to include prophylactic chemotherapy in stage I cancer of the ovary.

Stages IIA and IIB

The treatment recommended is total hysterectomy, bilateral salpingo-oophorectomy, omentectomy, appendectomy, and P^{32} instillation. All adhesions surrounding the ovarian cancer should be biopsied to document the extent of the disease. Chemotherapy is given to all stage II cancers of the ovary.

Stage III

The surgical approach, if possible, is the same as that for stages I and II and should consist of total hysterectomy, bilateral salpingo-oophorectomy, appendectomy, and omentectomy. Total abdominal radiation is no longer employed as a definitive method of treatment. Because it is necessary to shield the kidneys and the liver, it is felt that cancer on or adjacent to these organs would not be adequately treated. Therefore these patients are selected for failure from their therapy. Chemotherapy is given in stage III cancer of the ovary.

Stage IV

The ideal management constitutes removal of as much cancer as possible, including total hysterectomy, bilateral salpingo-oophorectomy, appendectomy, and omentectomy. Chemotherapy is given as definitive therapy, and radiation is reserved for the control of disease in the supraclavicular or inguinal areas.

Although it is occasionally necessary to resect isolated segments of bowel, we do not favor exenterative or ultraradical surgery in the management of ovarian cancer because of its nature. A surface spreader, it moves swiftly over all organ surfaces and to the upper abdomen in a high percentage of cases.

We take the appendix out because it is often the site of clinically undetectable disease. Frequently we are forced to change the staging of ovarian cancer and thus its treatment by the surprise finding of tumor on appendix pathology sections.

We remove omentum primarily to establish the true extent of the disease. Contrary to the fears of some gynecologists, this has not resulted in any increased morbidity when the surgery is carried according to sound surgical principles. Unfortunately, many gynecologists do not have extensive training in upper abdominal surgery and therefore are reluctant to excise the omentum.

HOW MUCH IS TOO MUCH?

Not everyone agrees on the amount of tumor that can be excised safely. We try to remove as much as we think we can without running a risk of a gastrointestinal or genitourinary fistula. Success of subsequent chemotherapy or radiation, or both, is inversely proportional to the amount of tumor left in the abdomen after surgery. Therefore aggressive surgery is indicated, not so much because it is curative, but because it potentiates other forms of treatment. If it is true that the patient is immunized by her own tumors, this self-immunization can be more effective when the bulk of tumor has been decreased. Removal of a volume of tumor may decrease the possibility of acquired tolerance and by decreasing the number of antigen—antibody complexes reduce the chance of immunologic enhancement.

The aggressive management of ovarian cancer has evolved through a full cycle. In the early 1950s an aggressive surgical program was carried out. It was complicated by a high morbidity and an increased mortality. If the patient survived the postoperative period, the cancer recurred in spite of the debulking operation. The poor results were followed by a less radical management of the patient with ovarian cancer. Currently, the increased use of hyperalimentation has lowered the morbidity, and the improved management of the patient with chemotherapy has contributed to the control of the cancer. The philosophy at present is to be aggressive in the diagnosis and treatment of ovarian cancer.

Higher cure rates are now reported in stage I patients (up to 90%+ survival). There is a dramatic difference between the survival rates of the various stages of cancer. It is significant that there is a marked fall in survival between stages IIA and IIB. This finding is similar to those in cancer of the cervix. Although several explanations have been suggested, it would appear that stage IIA represents a geographic spread of the ovarian cancer, whereas stage IIB represents a biologic spread.

External radiation therapy has been phased out of the protocol of treatment for common epithelial cancer. This development will be discussed in chapter 21.

Chemotherapy has taken on a more significant role in the prophylaxis and therapeutic management of ovarian cancer. It is given prophylactically in stages I and II when all gross disease has been eliminated, as well as in stage III when the gross disease can be excised by an omentectomy. It is given therapeutically in stages IIB, III, and IV when gross disease has been left behind. The plan of therapy with chemotherapy is reviewed in chapter 20.

Radioactive isotopes (P^{32}) are given when all gross disease has been removed. In stages I and II as well as in a limited number of patients with stage III, the gross disease can usually be completely removed when the gross disease is limited to the omentum. P^{32} is not used in the presence of gross disease or nodules greater than 2 cm in diameter.

SUMMARY

The acceptance and use of clinical staging and histologic classification established by the World Health Organization and the International Federation of Gynecology and Obstetrics has helped compare therapeutic results among institutions around the world. It has led to a greater insight into the natural history of ovarian cancer, resulting in a more rational approach to therapy with anticipated improved results.

The philosophy of management of ovarian cancer has evolved into an aggressive surgical and chemotherapeutic attack. The use of hyperalimentation to decrease the morbidity and the judicious and more skillful use of chemotherapeutic agents to control the cancer have contributed immensely to current concepts of the management of ovarian cancer.

BIBLIOGRAPHY

Barber, H.R.K.: Ovarian cancer: Still an enigma. Dr. 1:17, 1975.

Barber, H.R.K., Kwon, T.: Current status of the treatment of gynecologic cancer—By site. Cancer 38:610, 1976.

Brady, L.W.: Radiation therapy in gynecologic cancer: Future prospects. Clin. Obstet. Gynecol. 18:125, 1975.

Buchsbaum,H.J., Keetel, W.C., Latourette, H.B.: The use of radioisotopes as adjunct therapy of localized ovarian cancer. Semin. Oncol. 2:247, 1975.

Clark, D.G.C., Hilaris, B.S., Ochra, M., Jr.: Treatment of cancer of the ovary. In the ovary. Clin. Obstet. Gynecol. 3:159–179, 1976.

Frick, H.C., II: An overall evaluation of chemotherapy for ovarian cancer. Clin. Obstet. Gynecol. 12:1003, 1969.

Fuks, Z.: External radiotherapy of ovarian cancer: Standard approaches and new frontiers. Semin. Oncol. 2:253, 1975.

Smith, J.P.: Chemotherapy in gynecologic cancer. Clin. Obstet. Gynecol. 18: 109, 1975.

Young, R.: Chemotherpy of ovarian cancer: Past and present. Semin. Oncol. 2:267, 1975.

13

Managing Ovarian Tumors of Childhood and Adolescence

The term *childhood* or *adolescent gynecologic tumor* is used to indicate any new growth (benign or malignant) that develops between birth and age 14. It implies the growth of newly formed cells derived from normal body cells or that preceding developmental cells of origin. Benign neoplasm indicates a tumor that does not itself destroy the host, whereas a malignant neoplasm, if left untreated, destroys the host.

Cancer Facts and Figures, published by the American Cancer Society in 1976, reports that cancer is second only to accidents as the cause of death among children under 15 years of age. Childhood cancer accounts for 1 of 28 deaths compared to 1 out of 6 among adults. However since 1950 death rates for all sites have declined somewhat, from more than 8 per 100,000 to 5.5. by 1973. This seems to be partly a result of the decreasing death rates for leukemia, kidney cancer, and lymphomas. The actual number of deaths has also decreased during this period.

Incidence has also decreased slightly from 1947 to 1971. If present rates continue, the number of new cases per year will be about 6,500. Deaths number about 3,000. The most common forms of childhood cancer are leukemia, brain and central nervous system cancer, lymphomas, and kidney and bone cancer. Cancer kills more children between the ages of 3 and 14 than any other disease. Leukemia accounts for about one-half of these deaths.

For all forms of cancer in children under 15, the 5-year survival rate age, adjusted for normal life expectancy, is 30%. For the 10 most frequent forms, the range is as low as 3% for some leukemias to a high of 98% for thyroid and 85% for eye tumors. In *Comprehensive Cancer Centers* the 5-year survival rate rises to 50% for children with acute lymphocytic leukemia; these results reflect aggressive treatment. More than 60% of leukemia cases in children are acute lymphocytic.

About 3% of malignancy in childhood and adolescence is related to the gynecologic system. Even the busy gynecologist, unless he specializes in pediatric gynecology, sees relatively few tumors of the genital tract in children any one year. Because the average pediatrician's exposure to pediatric gynecologic oncology is markedly limited, he should refer any case in which the diagnosis is in doubt or therapy beyond his capabilities to a qualified specialist or clinic. It must be emphasized that in some cases time is the critical factor between localized and widespread disease. Procrastinating and hoping that time will take care of the disease are fraught with great dangers for the patient; and from the physician's standpoint, they expose him not only to the disappointment, frustration, and emotional turmoil of having missed an important diagnosis, but also to the threat of a large malpractice award to his patient. If in doubt, consult!

ETIOLOGY

All tissues in the body are liable to undergo malignant change, and all cells have an inherent potential for the development of cancer. The origin may be unicentric or multicentric. All of the known carcinogenic factors that are associated with cancer in the adult, i.e., viruses, chemical factors, ionizing energy, and genetic factors are found also in the child. The theory of misplaced blastomeres may take on added significance in this age group.

NATURAL HISTORY

In dealing with the wide variety of tumors found in the female reproductive system, it is obvious that each system and indeed each tumor within a given system has a natural history that is unique unto itself. As an example, the ovary is complex in its embryology, histology, steroidogenesis, and potential for malignancy. It is made up of a variety of different types of cells, and rather than giving rise to a malignancy, it produces a family of cancers. However it can be reported that cancer originating in the reproductive system in this age group is characterized by rapid growth, early spread, and frequently a fatal outcome.

BASIC DIFFERENCES FROM ADULT PELVIC CANCER

1. The space available for tumor expansion is more limited in children.
2. The effect of therapy (especially radical surgery or irradiation) on the further development of the patient must be given greater consideration.
3. The high degree of malignancy in cancer of the young must be taken into account.
4. The most common neoplasms are a special group of ovarian tumors and a specific type of uterovaginal sarcoma, which will be elaborated on later.
5. The immunologic surveillance mechanism is very inefficient in childhood.

EMBRYOLOGY

A complete understanding of gynecologic neoplasms in children requires at least a brief review of the embryology of the female genitourinary tract. The urogenital organs include two separate sytems of organs with wholly different functions, but they are so closely related embryologically and anatomically that is is impossible to study one while ignoring the other. Although mesoderm is the major component in the development of the urogenital system, the entoderm and ectoderm also make important contributions.

The urogenital fold or mesonephric ridge is a large and important body occupying the posterior or dorsal portion of the primitive peritoneal cavity. This structure lies on each side of the midline and runs the entire length of the fetus. From this urogenital fold arise the ovaries, kidneys, Fallopian tubes, uterus, and part of the vagina. Even in the later development of the fetus, the distance between the structures is measured in millimeters. The urogenital fold serves to explain the interrelationship between these structures, as well as the possibility for congenital rests between organ systems.

The steps in normal embryologic development are outlined briefly below.

MÜLLERIAN DUCTS

The Müllerian duct (paramesonephric duct) develops as a groove in the mesonephric ridge, and by a process of folding (in front of the mesonephros and the gonadal area) it fuses in its distal portion to form the uterus, cervix, and possibly the upper part of the vagina. The female duct (Müllerian or paramesonephric duct) has an abdominal opening through the fimbriated end of the tubes. Although the mesonephric tubules and ducts degenerate, a few may remain near the ovary and are known as the epoophoron and paraoophoron. The mesonephric duct may persist as a Gartner duct and runs along the uterus, cervix, and vagina. In some instances these structures may develop cysts requiring surgery.

GONADS

The gonads appear as a swelling on the medial surface of the urogenital fold close to the mesonephros and mesonephric duct and run parallel to it. The gonad is relatively short, so that the mesonephros extends beyond it at both ends. The ovary and the testis have a similar embryonic origin, and up to a certain point they cannot be distinguished from each other. The coelomic epithelium covering the gonad is thickened to form the germinal epithelium. The sex cords grow into the mesenchyme from the coelomic epithelium. Oogonia probably come from the entoderm of the yolk sac and migrate by ameboid movement via the gut mesentery to the ovary. These cells, called primordial germ cells, develop into ova, each surrounded by a group of follicular cells to form a primary follicle.

KIDNEYS

The three kidneys arise from the mesonephric area in succession: the pronephros, the mesonephros (Wolffian body), and the metanephros—the permanent kidney. The metanephros has a double origin. The ureter, pelvis, calyces, and collecting tubules arise grom an outgrowing of the Wolffian duct, whereas the secreting parts of the tubules are formed directly from the posterior end of the intermediate cell mass.

ADRENAL (SUPRARENAL) GLAND

Although the adrenal gland is not a part of the urogenital system, its proximity, overlapping function, and propensity for producing aberrant rests in the reproductive system proper make it appropriate to include a brief outline here.

The adrenal gland is formed by a combination of mesodermal elements which develop into the cortex, and an ectodermal portion which forms the medulla. Mesothelial cells located between the root of the mesentery and the developing gonad begin to proliferate during the fifth week of development and penetrate the underlying mesenchyme. Here they differentiate into formation of the fetal or primitive cortex. Shortly thereafter a second wave of cells from the mesothelium penetrates the mesenchyma and forms the definitive cortex of the gland. During the time that the cortex is developing, cells originating in the sympathetic system (ectoderm) invade its medial aspect and become arranged in cords and clusters forming the medulla.

PROGRESSION OF GENITOURINARY EMBRYOLOGIC DEVELOPMENT

1. Genetic sex (time of fertilization)
   A. Determined by sperm
      1) Each ovum contains one X chromosome.
      2) Approximately half of all spermatozoa contain an X chromosome and the other half a Y chromosome.
2. Undifferentiated gonad (1–6 weeks)
   A. Undifferentiated ("sexless") gonads come into existence when primordial germ cells migrate into primitive gonadal folds.
3. Differentiation of the gonad (seventh week)
   A. A still unidentified factor (evocator) stimulates the primitive gonad to develop in a direction corresponding to the genetic sex, and, depending upon which sex predominates, an ovary or testis develops. In the male the Wolffian system becomes dominant in the development of the genital system, and the Müllerian system atrophies. In the female the opposite occurs. Any upset in this mechanism causes variations with mixtures.
      1) The cortex basically forms an ovary.
      2) The medulla basically forms a testis.
4. Development of the internal genital system (8–12 weeks)
   A. Müllerian ducts originate from the lateral aspect of the urogenital fold.
   B. Wolffian ducts originate from the mesonephros.

    C.   Jost showed that castration of the embryo before any sexual development has begun results in development of the female internal and external genital system.

5. Development of the external genital system (13 weeks to birth)

    A.   Differentiation of external genitalia involves changes in the urogenital sinus and genital tubercle, the anlage of which are already present in the fifth week.

6. Birth to puberty

    A.   There is little change until puberty, when the reproductive system matures toward the adult form.

OVARIAN NEOPLASMS: ORIGINS AND CONCEPTS

From the time when the ovary differentiates as a modified portion of coelomic epithelium after the menopause, it is a constantly changing organ. The primitive germ cells migrate in the dorsal mesentery from the primitve hind gut to the genital ridges, and from these cells the primordial follicles are stimulated to grow. The stroma of the ovary arises from the same cells as do the follicle cells, and no new germ cells are formed after the early postnatal period.

The ovary is made up of germ cells, cells of the sex cord, and cells from the mesenchymal tissue, each with its own potential to form a tumor. It is generally agreed that at least 10% of all ovarian neoplasms in children are malignant and that the germ cell tumors make up the greatest number. Papillary serous and mucinous cystadenocarcinomas are relatively rare in childhood. The most common benign tumor in childhood and adolescence is the cystic teratoma, or dermoid, which makes up approximately 30% of all ovarian tumors in this age group.

A major conceptual advance in cancer research was achieved when it was established that cancers do arouse a specific immune response in the organism within which they appear. In fact, antigenic differences represent the first known qualitative distinctions between cancer cells and their normal counterparts. Following Gold's work on the carcinoembryonic antigen (CEA), a great number of different tumors have been subjected to immunologic study. Although the CEA is related to endodermal structures, a carcinoembryonic-like antigen has been found in many other systems. Closely related to the endodermal carcinoembryonic antigen, it may come from the same chromosomal group. Lawrence reported that plasma CEA levels were elevated in 7 of 20 ovarian cancer patients (35%), whereas none of 4 patients with a benign tumor showed an elevation. Presenting one case to support his hypotheses, Ballas reported that teratoid neoplasms containing a significant vitelline component are most likely to give rise to alpha fetoprotein in the serum. The significance of these studies in relation to diagnostic technique is yet to be proved, but so far the findings appear promising.

Ectopic production of human chorionic gonadotropin by neoplasms has received a great deal of attention. Teratocarcinomas containing chorionic elements, as well as choriocarcinomas of the ovary, give positive results. Currently, the β-subunit component of human chorionic gonadotropin, a specific test for gonadotropins produced by the placenta, is being evaluated. Studies suggest a positive human chorionic gonadotropin titer in 30 to 40% of adenocarcinomas of the ovary, and a much higher incidence in embryonal cancers.

Most tumors are now classified according to histogenesis, behavior, and functional attributes. Recent advances in finding tumor-specific antigens on the tumor surfaces may promote a new field in diagnostic pathology which would provide answers to etiology as well as predict behavior patterns and prognosis. Furthermore, such techniques offer promise as a means of monitoring the effects of treatment.

TUMORS OF THE OVARY

Among the common epithelial cancers, about 8% occur under the age of 35, and of this number very few occur among the pediatric and adolescent groups. The ovarian cancers that are found in childhood almost always arise from the germ cell or sex cord (mesenchymomas or gonadal stromal) cells. The malignant germ cell tumors are generally encountered in childhood or among young adults. However malignant changes (2% of cystic adult teratomas) are encountered in dermoid cysts.

When ovarian cancer is diagnosed, the question of management is raised, and rightfully so in view of the young age of the patient. To help formulate a plan of therapy, each tumor type in the germ cell and sex cord groups will be reviewed individually. The tumor types are classified below. According to the FIGO classification, only the tumors of epithelial and stromal origin are usually discussed. However in childhood the germ cell tumors are more commonly encountered and the sex cord tumors less so. Therefore the classification has been modified to emphasize this difference.

CLASSIFICATION OF OVARIAN NEOPLASMS

1. Tumors of epithelial and stromal origin
    A. Serous
    B. Mucinous
    C. Endometrioid
    D. Clear cell (mesonephric)
2. Germ cell tumors
    A. Dysgerminoma
    B. Tumors in teratoma group
        1) Extraembryonal forms
            a) Endodermal sinus tumor (mesoblastoma vitellium, yolk sac carcinoma, extra-embryonic membrane tumor)
            b) Choriocarcinoma
        2) Embryonal teratomas, solid and cystic

       3) Adult teratomas
          a) Solid
          b) Cystic (dermoid cyst)
             (i)   Benign
             (ii)   With malignant change
       4) Struma ovarii
       5) Carcinoid
    C.   Mixed forms of the above
3. Gonadoblastoma
    A.   With germinoma
    B.   Without germinoma
4. Gonadal stromal tumors (sex cord mesenchymal tumors)
    A.   Female cell types
       1) Granulosa cell tumor
       2) Thecoma-fibroma type
    B.   Male cell types
       1) Sertoli-Leydig cell tumor (arrhenoblastoma, androblastoma)
       2) Sertoli cell tumor (androblastoma tubulare)
       3) Hilus (Leydig) cell tumor
    C.   Mixed cell types (gynandroblastoma)
    D.   Indeterminate cell types
5. Tumors not specific for ovary
    A.   Lymphoma
    B.   Burkitt's lymphoma
6. Miscellaneous
    A..   Sarcomas
    B.   Fibromas
7. Metastatic tumors
    A.   Krukenberg
    B.   Choriocarcinoma

The stage grouping for primary common epithelial cancer is presented in chapter 11. Although FIGO's clinical staging of ovarian cancer was designed to include only the common epithelial ovarian tumors, it has been used as a guide to judge the extent of disease for germ cell tumors and gonadal stromal tumors.

Wollner and coworkers proposed a new grouping to define the extent of disease. They considered the new approach more useful in planning therapy; it is also applicable to the extent and location of disease found at the time of disease recurrence, which is the time when most of these patients are seen for the first time at the Comprehensive Cancer Centers. The grouping is presented in Table 1.

In the Wollner study, grouping or staging of the extent of disease at the time of diagnosis seemed to contribute little to determining the patient's prognosis. If, however, some means of indicating the extent of disease must

Table 1.   Proposed Grouping for Malignant Ovarian Tumors in Childhood

Group	Extent of disease
I	Disease limited to one ovary. Negative peritoneal washing.
II	Disease limited to one ovary and ipsilateral paraaortic nodes. Bilateral primary ovarian tumors without pelvic extension, with or without paraaortic node involvement. Negative peritoneal washing.
III	Disease spread to pelvis, mesenteric and paraaortic nodes, abdominal wall, peritoneum, diaphragm, liver, and other organs in the peritoneal cavity.
IV	Distant metastases (lungs, bone, brain, peripheral nodes).

be utilized for documentation or future comparative studies, Wollner believes that this new grouping system is better able to chart the course of these tumors in children.

It has been shown that there is no correlation between clincial and histologic malignancy in ovarian tumors. This holds true for various types of neoplasms, but especially for epithelial tumors, granulosa cell tumors, and virilizing tumors. The committee recommended that cases of germ cell tumors, hormone-producing neoplasms, and metastatic carcinomas should be excluded from therapeutic statistics on ovarian epithelial tumors. However, a clinical plan for staging ovarian cancer does focus attention for carefully evaluating the extent of all ovarian cancers.

There are five primary points that should be emphasized concerning ovarian tumors in childhood: (1) The ovary is the most common site of new growths involving the gynecologic organs appearing in childhood. (2) The ovary in a child is essentially an abdominal organ, and tumors are abdominal rather than pelvic. (3) Ovarian tumors in childhood are especially susceptible to torsion because of a longer ovarian suspensory ligament. (4) About 1 in 10 ovarian neoplasms are malignant; therefore, the odds are generally good that the tumor is benign. Panic is not justified, but judicious concern is indicated. (5) The evolution of ovarian tumors in children is more rapid because of contracted spacial relationships. Large tumors produce relatively greater pressure symptoms and dyspnea. Cachexia and ascites are increased.

Incidence

Ovarian tumors comprise about 1% of all new growths in children who are less than 16 years of age. However they are the most frequent genital neoplasm in childhood and adolescence. The problem of diagnosis is surpassed only by the confusion related to therapy. It is difficult to accept psychologically the possibility of ovarian malignancy in this age group, and even more difficult for the physician to deprive a child of her reproductive potential. In general, although certain ovarian tumors are more common in children, almost any tumor found in the adult may also be found in the child.

Age

Analysis of age distribution shows that although ovarian neoplasms may occur at any age in childhood or adolescence, they tend to be most frequent at puberty, between the ages of 10 and 14. This fact permits the conjecture that some control mechanism is released or that pituitary stimulation of some latent factor in the ovary is the triggering mechanism.

The most common tumors in infants and young children are cystic teratomas (dermoid tumors) and teratosarcoma. These may be found soon after birth or later. Multiple retention cysts and giant follicle cysts have also been described at birth. Occasionally theca lutein and corpus luteum cysts are found in neonates. In adolescents the most frequent tumors, in their order of frequency, are cystic teratoma, mucinous cystadenoma, serous cystadenoma, corpus luteum cysts, paraovarian cysts, and endometrioma. To this list we can add the more infrequent embryonal teratoma, granulosa cell tumors, dysgerminoma, endodermal sinus tumor, and carcinoma.

Diagnosis

Symptoms and Signs. Ovarian new growth in children may produce minimal symptoms in its early state of development. The degree of symptomatology and the physical finding signs relate directly to the rapidity of growth, position, degree of malignancy, potential to produce hormones, and possible accidents associated with these neoplasms (torsion, rupture, hemorrhage, infection, etc. in children). Since ovarian tumors are frequently abdominal and have their embryologic origin from the level of T10, it is not surprising that abdominal pain and abdominal tumors are common. Pain may be related to the relatively small pelvic and abdominal cavity which causes the new growth to stretch the peritoneum and produce pressure on adjacent organs. Rectal examination often reveals that the pelvis is free of tumor, but a negative rectal examination does not rule out an ovarian neoplasm because frequently it presents only as an abdominal mass during childhood.

The hormone-producing tumor, although rare, produces the clinical picture related to the type of hormone being secreted.

The clinical history should be carefully assessed for symptoms not related to the abdominal contents, such as persistent and unexplained headaches for possible space-occupying lesions in the brain, pain in the back related to specific vertebral bodies, symptoms related to the extremities or control of sphincters, and cough, chest pains, or bone pain.

Physical Findings. A general physical examination including pelvic and rectal examination should be carried out. In most instances it is impossible to palpate normal ovaries in children. Therefore it can be assumed that if an ovary is enlarged on palpation, it is abnormal. The size determines whether it can be felt abdominally or by rectoabdominal palpation.

Diagnostic Procedures. Baseline blood counts should be determined, and urinalysis and blood chemistry studies should be performed. A flat plate of the abdomen may help determine whether a dermoid cyst is present. Intravenous pyelograms and x-ray studies of the gastrointestinal tract are indicated if time permits. In those patients suspected of having a hormone- producing tumor, x-ray studies of bone age may be helpful. A hormone assay profile sometimes documents the type of tumor. Pneumoperitoneum has been used to outline small tumors, and ultrasonic methods have recently been introduced. The role of laparoscopy in the study of abdominal and pelvic problems in this age group remains to be clarified. Levels of alpha fetoprotein and carcinoembryonic antigen should be determined for follow-up of tumor activity and regression. Urinary levels of chorionic and pituitary gonadotropins should be measured and, if abnormal, may serve as baselines for evaluation of therapy.

Special studies include scans of the brain (with 99m Tc pertechnetate), soft tissue gallium (with 67 Ga citrate form) and liver (with 99m Tc sulfur colloid) as well as lymphangiography.

Differential Diagnosis.   The clinical picture and physical findings usually point to the diagnosis. However the differential diagnosis should include appendiceal abscess, intussusception, obstruction, salpingitis, hematometra, and pyelonephritis.

Origin

Tumors of the ovary in childhood and adolescence may be derived from any of a number of cellular elements: coelomic epithelium or its derivatives (mesotheliomas), including serous, mucinous, endometrioid, and clear-cell tumors: and gonadal stromal tumors, including granulosa cell, thecal cell, Sertoli-Leydig, Sertoli, and germ cell tumors (dysgerminomas and embryonal teratomas).

COMMON EPITHELIAL TUMORS

Ninety percent of the ovarian tumors in the adults originate in the ovarian surface epithelium and stroma. In premenarchal girls, about 90% of ovarian tumors are of germ cell origin. On the other hand, in patients between 13 and 20, 40% of ovarian neoplasms are of nongerminal origin. Tumors of epithelial origin include the serous and mucinous types. No endometrioid tumors have been reported in this age group. However, after puberty, serous and mucinous tumors may occasionally be diagnosed.

Primary epithelial tumors occur in the postpubertal period; almost all are unilateral and most are on the right. The malignancy rate, 7.5%, is less than that among older patients. Most investigators believe that these tumors arise from invagination of the surface coelomic epithelium of the ovary or its derivatives. Because these tumors occur almost exclusively after puberty, the question of hormonal stimulation has been raised, but no correlation has been established.

Therapy must be tailored to the patient's needs and to the extent of the disease. A frozen section is carried out to determine whether the tumor is benign or malignant. Benign disease is treated by extirpation of the tumor, leaving as much normal ovary as possible. If the tumor is malignant, the most important considerations in therapy and prognosis are the *stage* and *grade* of the neoplasm. A malignancy that has spread beyond the ovary should receive radical extirpative therapy including total hysterectomy, bilateral salpingo-oophorectomy, omentectomy (the omentum is usually very small in the child), appendectomy, and the instillation of radioactive P^{32}.

If there is any doubt about the type of tumor or whether a malignancy is present, and if the tumor has an intact capsule and is freely moveable, it is better to do a salpingo-oophorectomy on the side of the tumor. If the tumor proves to be highly malignant on permanent section examination, the abdomen may be opened and the remaining reproductive organs excised if this appears to be the best course.

X-Ray therapy has been practically phased out in the treatment of common epithelial tumors. Chemotherapy (with single alkylating agent) has been chosen as the treatment for the common epithelial ovarian cancers. In certain low-grade malignancies the previously performed treatment may be considered sufficient to insure a cure. Borderline or potentially malignant (low-grade) tumors are relatively benign; their 5-year survival rate is between 90 and 95%.

GERM CELL TUMORS

Germ cell tumors are almost always found in children or adolescents. A knowledge of the natural history of these tumors can be used as a guide in avoiding undertreating or overtreating these patients.

Teilum has reported the scheme shown in Figure 49 to illustrate the histogenesis and interrelationship of ovarian and testicular tumors of germ cell origin. In this classification Teilum reports that the term *embryonal carcinoma* is restricted to tumors composed of undifferentiated neoplastic embryonal cells representing the undifferentiated forms of extraembryonic as well as embryonic types. This relationship is demonstrated in Figure 49.

Dysgerminoma (Germinomas)

Dysgerminomas are ovarian tumors of an embryonal type resembling the sexually undifferentiated germ cells of the early gonad. Hughesdon reported that the origin of this tumor, composed of germ cells and undifferentiated stromal cells, is problably linked to the continuing proliferation of unencapsulated germ cells and to the associated stimulation of the surrounding stromal or ovarian mesenchymal cells.

Certain patients with these tumors show subnormal gonadal development and coincidental abnormal secondary sex characteristics (pseudohermaphroditism); the ambiguous sex status is not reversed after removal of the tumor.

Dysgerminoma is characteristically smooth or lobulated and surrounded by a dense capsule. It has a doughy or rubbery consistency and may vary in size from a few centimeters in diameter to a mass large enough to fill the pelvis and abdomen.

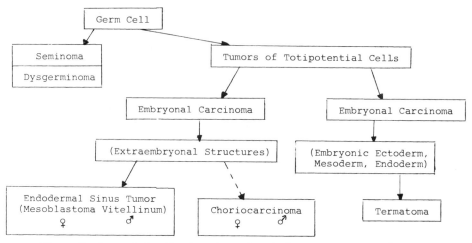

Figure 49. Interrelationship of ovarian and testicular tumors of germ cell origin.

Histologically, the tumor is characterized by large round cells with dark-stained nuclei, and by stroma that divide the tumor into nests of cells. The septa are heavily infiltrated with lymphocytes and symplasmic giant cells. These lymphocytes may be associated with a cell-mediated immunity, which perhaps explains the good prognosis (70 to 90% survival at 5 years) with pure dysgerminoma. The survival rate in bilateral ovarian involvement ranges from 5 to 12%.

The germinomas have the same nuclear sex as their host (sex chromatin-positive in the dysgerminomas of the female; sex chromatin negative in the male seminomas). Presumably these neoplasms are derived from diploid germ cells prior to haploid reduction division.

In the broad controversy about the treatment of dysgerminoma, most disagreement is related to incorrect diagnosis. It is important to distinguish pure germinomas (dysgerminoma) from those intermingled with teratoid elements. The latter may be of widely varying types, such as endodermal sinus tissue, embryonal forms of cancer (Schiller's mesonephroma), or choriocarcinoma (dysgerminoma with choriocarcinoma elements) that may produce a positive pregnancy test. Pure dysgerminomas are not associated with hormone activity. However the diagnostic problem here is that with hemagglutination inhibition tests, and even with radioimmunoassay, HCG (human chorionic gonadotropin) cross-reacts with LH (luteinizing hormone). A newly developed test for the β-subunit of human chorionic gonadotropin uses an antiserum that can differentiate between tumor LH and HCG. Incidentally, some mixed dysgerminomas also produce human placental lactogen (HPL).

Although dysgerminomas are highly radiosensitive, tumors possessing other teratoid elements (e.g., endodermal sinus and choriocarcinoma) are relatively insensitive to radiation therapy and are particularly deadly. Thus an accurate histologic diagnosis is crucial.

In the pediatric and adolescent group the question is raised, and right-fully so, about the type of treatment to be followed. The cure rate for unilateral pure germinoma ranges between 80 and 90%, even greater than the general cure rate previously cited. On the other hand, if the tumor is bilateral or shows local extension, the chance of 5-year cure drops to 20—30%.

Ascites or the discovery of a mixed teratoma or choriocarcinoma element within the tumor, or rupture through the capsule, are prognostic of a poor outcome. When the neoplasm is unilateral, encapsulated, and free, it should be treated by unilateral oophorectomy with wedge biopsy of the opposite ovary; microscopic metastases are infrequently found. This recommendation is based both on reports in the literature and on personal experience.

There are three possible methods of therapy: unilateral oophorectomy; unilateral oophorectomy followed by radiation therapy; and excision of the uterus, tubes, and ovaries with or without postoperative x-ray therapy. The experience at many tumor centers indicates that a conservative operation yields about the same 5-year survival rate as do the more radical procedures; the recurrence rate, however, is higher following the more conservative opera-tion. Fortunately, these recurrent tumors are highly sensitive to radiation therapy, and an appreciable number can be cured. Dr. Hans Kottmeier of the Radiumhemmet at the Karolinska Institute suggests that, in addition to unilateral oophorectomy, the opposite ovary should be shielded and radiation therapy directed to the side from which the ovary was removed as well as to the paraaortic area. But since the 5-year survival rate in these patients does not differ from that in those treated by unilateral oophorectomy without x-ray therapy, we do not recommend this procedure.

At the time of exploration the paraaortic area should be carefully explored and biopsies taken of any enlarged nodes. This is an important part of management, since dysgerminoma, like seminoma, metastasizes to the retroperitoneal paraaortic nodes. Although there are no data to support our view, we do not recommend the use of radioactive substances such as P^{32} following unilateral oophorectomy.

When disease invades pelvic structures outside the reproductive tract or cannot be encompassed by conservative surgery because of spread outside the pelvis, a more radical approach is indicated: The uterus, tubes, ovaries, omentum, and appendix should be removed, and radiation therapy to the pelvis and paraaortic areas should be instituted. Neither pelvic nor paraaor-tic lymphadenectomy is performed for dysgerminoma; this tumor drains to the mid or upper abdomen, and these cases can best be treated with irradia-tion. If spread is within the abdomen, total abdominal irradiation is in-dicated, even though radiation injury may result in tissues such as bone (retardation of growth at the epiphyseal line, bone necrosis, and, perhaps as a late effect, osteogenic sarcoma). When metastatic disease is found, the pa-tient is fighting for survival; therefore, aggressive radiation therapy is justified and acceptable.

The greatest incidence of recurrence, 25 to 40% falls within the first 3 years after the initial therapy. The patient should be seen every 3 or 4 months during this period. Any change is highly suspect, and rather than a long period of observation, early exploratory laparotomy with biopsy is recommended along with plans for additional therapy if indicated.

The role of the second-look operation merits some discussion, particularly in the pediatric and adolescent patient. If the mass was greater than 15 cm in diameter at the time of the original operation, if the pathology report indicated a triad of anaplasia, medullary structure, and numerous mitoses, and if residual tumor is left, routine postoperative x-ray is indicated. If no residual tumor is palpable after completion of therapy, abdominal exploration is indicated at 8 months. Our experience suggests that 6 months is too early to detect early growth, and that 12 months is too late to treat a recurrence adequately. At the time of the second look, any recurrent or residual tumor is removed in toto. As a general rule, however, a second look is useless with a palpable tumor. Dr. Howard Jones of the Johns Hopkins Hospital states that these tumors exhibit the troublesome clinical and pathologic phenomena of very late recurrence in the opposite ovary. Therefore it is prudent to remove the intact ovary after the patient's reproductive destiny has been fulfilled.

Teratoma Group

Five basic types comprise this category of germ cell tumors. The first is the extraembryonal form, of which there are two subtypes: endodermal sinus tumor and choriocarcinoma.

Endodermal Sinus Tumors. These tumors are known by many names, such as membrane tumor, embryonal carcinoma, yolk-sac carcinoma, extraembryonic (endomesodermal) membrane tumor, mesonephroma ovarii (Schiller), and endodermal sinuses of Duval, or Teilum's tumor. This mesometanephric rest tumor was so designated to cover both Müllerian and mesonephric origins, but this term is no longer used. On the basis of his research, Scully believes that this tumor has a Müllerian origin. Although the tubular structures resemble renal tubules and the masses of clear cell suggest renal carcinoma (hypernephroma) and Growitz tumor, neither term is now accepted and all have been included as endodermal sinus tumors.

Endodermal sinus tumors are highly malignant neoplasms characterized by an overgrowth of extraembryonic mesoblast associated with yolk-sac endoderm. They have been interpreted by Teilum as recapitulating a yolk-sac structure. The microscopic picture is similar to that found in the placenta of a rat. These tumors may contain a great number of blastocyst-like yolk-sac (endoblast) vesicles and are referred to as polyembryonic, whereas the polyvesicular vitelline tumor has a typical histologic pattern occasionally found as a predominant characteristic of vitelline tumors in the ovary.

The endodermal sinus tumor and its related group occur in young patients and are not sensitive to radiation. Cure rates following conservative surgery do not differ from those following radical surgery. Only an occasional 5-year survival is reported, and these tumors whose incidence is less than 1% of all ovarian cancers, are almost 100% fatal within 5 years.

Some reports indicate tumor response following triple therapy with methotrexate, dactinomycin, and chlorambucil. Although the dosages must be calculated for each individual according to age, weight, and general health, certain guidelines can be stated: Initially, 5 mg of methotrexate daily and 10 mg of chlorambucil daily are given simultaneously. Both agents are administered orally. This regimen is continued for 16 to 25 days. In addition, 0.5 mg (500 μg) of dactinomycin is given intravenously daily for 5 days, starting on the third, 12th, and 21st days after methotrexate and chlorambucil therapy is initiated. A repeat course, started 2 weeks after completion of the initial treatment if blood count and chemistries are normal, consists of 5 mg of methotrexate and 10 mg of chlorambucil given orally as a single dose daily for 5 days, with 0.5 mg (500 μg) of dactinomycin begun intravenously on the third day and repeated daily for 5 days. Subsequent repeat courses are given 2 to 3 weeks after completion of the previous course—provided that blood count and chemistry values remain within normal limits—and repeated at 2- to 3-week intervals until there is no evidence of disease. An alternate plan which is simpler and appears to be equally effective is a 5-day regimen which includes 200 mg cytoxan, 0.5 mg actinomycin D, 1 mg vincristine, and 50 mg adriamycin on day 1; on days 2, 3, 4, and 5 only cytoxan and actinomycin D are given. All drugs are given intravenously. The patient is carefully monitored by daily blood counts and blood chemistries. The E.K.G. is checked before adriamycin is given and is stopped if there is any change in the rhythm or voltage. The toal dose of adriamycin never exceeds 450 mg/m^2.

Exploratory laparotomy and biopsy to confirm eradication of the tumor may be indicated before therapy is stopped. Blood counts and blood chemistries should be done at least every 2 weeks during treatment, and a bone marrow biopsy is indicated at the start of treatment as well as every 4 to 6 weeks during treatment.

Choriocarcinoma. In children, choriocarcinoma is an extremely rare, highly malignant tumor composed of trophoblasts. Although it is placed in the broad category with extraembryonic germ cell tumors, it may arise from a teratoma, from an ovarian cancer, or as a metastasis from a primary teratoma originating elsewhere. Postpubertal ovarian choriocarcinoma is more likely to be associated with an ovarian preganancy than it is to be a primary germ cell tumor.

The gross picture of choriocarcinoma, identical to that in an adult, is characterized by extensive hemorrhage, ulceration, and necrosis which convert it into a brittle, spongy, friable, red mass. The tumor may attain huge proportions and has a propensity for invading the blood vessels.

Histologically, this tumor is characterized by columns or alveoli of trophoblastic cells with nests of Langhans' cells enveloped by syncyiotrophoblast. The cell masses are usually separated by spaces filled with clotted blood. Extensive necrosis often makes tumor diagnosis difficult.

Choriocarcinoma may be associated with rapidly developing sexual precocity. In part, this syndrome is triggered by ovarian estrogen production induced by chorionic gonadotropin elaborated by the tumor. The titers of estrogen and chorionic gonadotropins, which may be markedly elevated, will drop when the tumor is entirely removed and will rise if the tumor recurs.

Tumor growth is rapid, filling the pelvis and abdomen and becoming fixed to surrounding tissue, with early metastases, particularly to the lungs. The child becomes rapidly cachectic. If the tumor is discovered early, the uninvolved ovary may be markedly enlarged with multiple cysts of both the follicular and lutein types as well as a pseudodecidual reaction.

As stated above, the tumor is not radiosensitive. Radical excision has no advantage over conservative surgery if the neoplasm is unilateral and encapsulated. However, if the neoplasm has spread outside the ovary, total hysterectomy, bilateral salpingo-oophorectomy, appendectomy, and omentectomy should be carried out. The role of radioactive phosphorus has not been established, but the isotope will control ascites if there is not a large volume of tumor. Although these tumors have not responded as well to chemotherapy as those arising from an intrauterine pregnancy, some success has been achieved with a 3- or 4-day regimen outlined above.

Embryonal Teratoma.   The second tumor type in the teratoma group is the embryonal teratoma. In premenarchal girls the most frequent germ cell tumors (90%) are either dysgerminoma or embryonal teratoma; the remainder are mixed germ cell neoplasms. Embryonal, i.e., immature, teratomas are usually solid but may also contain small cystic areas that rarely take the form of a single large cyst. Their degree of malignancy can be determined only by microscopic examination, but these tumors are rarely benign and most are highly malignant and rapidly fatal. They contain a mixture of embryonal and mature tissue derived from all three embryonic layers, whereas the solid, adult teratoma (discussed below) is composed of adult, i.e. mature, tissue from all three layers. Survival is directly related to the pathology rather than to the mode of therapy.

The embryonal teratoma has a poor prognosis, with less than 5% of patients surviving 5 years, whereas the solid, adult teratoma is benign. However the cystic adult teratoma has a 2% malignancy rate. The degree of maturity or lack of it is best judged by histologic examination and provides a more logical basis for nomenclature than does the gross appearance.

According to Teilum, the term *embryonal carcinoma* should be restricted to tumors composed of undifferentiated neoplastic cells. Embryonal teratomas often show histologic evidence of other types of germ cell tumors. Consequently, some investigators have used the terms *malignant embryonal teratoma* and *embryonal carcinoma* interchangeably, and the result has been some confusion. The prognosis in embryonal carcinoma depends on the predominant type of cell present; malignant neural tissue or malignant struma ovarii has a much better prognosis than does a tumor containing choriocarcinoma or endodermal sinus components, for example. Other combinations are melanoepithelioma, adenocarcinoma, spindle-cell sarcoma, fibrosarcoma, rhabdosarcoma, chondrosarcoma, and osteogenic sarcoma.

In approximately 10% of patients, involvement is bilateral. When the tumor is unilateral and encapsulated, radical surgery has shown no advantage over unilateral oophorectomy. However, if the tumor has spread, excision of the uterus, tubes, ovaries, appendix, and omentum is advocated. Unfortunately, the extent of the surgical procedure has little effect on the outcome; practically all patients with tumor spread die within 14 months. These tumors are radioresistant, and there is insufficient positive data to support the use of prophylactic chemotherapy. But data do support treating recurrence with a regimen of 3 or 4 drugs like that outlined above for endodermal sinus tumors.

Adult Teratoma. The third basic type of teratoma is the adult, i.e. mature, teratoma or the cystic teratoma (dermoid cyst). More than one-third of ovarian tumors in children are benign cystic teratomas, which are composed of all three germinal layers, although epithelial structures predominate.

Nuclear sex chromatin in ovarian teratomas uniformly shows a female pattern, and XX sex chromosomes have been confirmed by chromosome studies. Nuclear sex chromatin also suggests that these cells are diploid rather than haploid. Interestingly, a significant portion of teratomas in the male have shown the sex chromatin pattern of females; this discrepancy may be explained by the fact that teratomas in males are derived from haploid germ cells by autofertilization or fusion of adjacent haploid cells. The result would be a diploid with either XX or XY chromosomes. The same process in the female could result only in XX diploid cells. Because some teratomas in the male have shown a mosaic pattern with sex chromatin-positive and sex chromatin-negative cells, it has been suggested that their origin may be multicentric rather than from a single germ cell.

The cystic (dermoid) teratoma reveals a round, doughy, nontender, smooth, heavy, mobile mass more likely to be present in older children than in the very young. In small children the mass is usually above the true pelvis, and x-ray studies of the abdomen will demonstrate teeth or calcification in about 40% of the cases.

Microscopic examination may reveal all types of mature ectoderm, mesoderm, and endodermal elements. It is not uncommon to find gastrointestinal mucosa, stratified squamous epithelium, hair follicles, sebaceous glands, cartilage, and nerve and respiratory tract elements. Giant cells and pseudoxanthoma cells are often seen. Occasionally, an overgrowth of thyroid tissue may result in a functioning struma ovarii.

The first sign may be a mass in the abdomen, although often it is a complication from the cyst—twisting, hemorrhage, rupture, infection, or malignancy—that brings the patient to the physician's office.

Although 2% of all dermoids are complicated by malignancy, the incidence of malignancy among children is lower. In adults the malignant change is usually confined to one ovary, and squamous carcinoma within the cyst carries a much higher survival rate than do the other forms of malignancy—sarcoma, carcinoids, and adenocarcinoma. No comparable studies have been reported for children.

Torsion of the cyst occurs in about 16% of reported cases; 1.3% are said to rupture spontaneously, producing a clinical picture suggesting chronic granulomatous peritonitis, tuberculosis, or carcinomatosis. These possibilities should be ruled out by biopsies and frozen section studies.

When a dermoid cyst is suspected, the pelvis should be well walled off by laparotomy pads at surgery. If spillage occurs, a thorough saline wash should be carried out to prevent the chemical peritonitis that may result from the oily component of the cyst fluid. Dermoid cyst is best managed by dissecting the cyst from the ovary with preservation of the ovary, although occasionally the ovary will be damaged beyond salvage from torsion, hemorrhage, or infection; unilateral oophorectomy is then indicated. Since the bilaterality rate ranges from 5 to 12% wedge biopsy should be carried out on the opposite ovary.

Struma Ovarii.   The fourth type of teratoma is the struma ovarii, a dermoid tumor with thyroid tissue as its main or sole teratoid element. Few of these tumors prove to be malignant. About 10% of the patients with these tumors show evidence of thyrotoxicosis.

Carcinoid Tumors.   Carcinoid tumors (argentaffinomas) of the ovary, the last category of teratoma, may arise in the wall of a dermoid cyst, either from intestinal or bronchial epithelium, and occasionally they metastasize. The syndrome resulting from this tumor includes intermittent flushing, cyanosis, diarrhea, and asthmatic attacks. The clinical manifestations are attributed to production of excessive quantities of 5-hydroxytryptamine (serotonin) by the argentaffin cells of the tumor. Argentaffin granules can be identified with silver nitrate stain. Although dermoid cysts in children may contain thyroid or argenaffinoma tissue, they rarely grow large enough to cause the typical symptoms.

Gonadoblastoma

This third major ovarian tumor type is found in patients with Turner's syndrome, pure gonadal dysgenesis, mixed gonadal dysgenesis, male hermaphroditism, or true hermaphroditism. Bilateral involvement occurs in about one-third of the patients. The coincidence of gonadoblastoma mixed with choricarcinoma is 1 in 75 cases.

Composed of a mixture of germ cells (dysgerminoma) and sex cord cells (granulosa-Sertoli), the tumor had previously been reported only in intersex individuals and was called *dysgenetic gonadoma.* In most cases in which sex chromatic studies have been done, the nuclear pattern has been negative in the patient (46XY) or has shown a sex chromosome mosaicism (XO/XY).

Most patients with a gonadoblastoma are intersexual with a phenotype female habitus, amenorrhea, and perhaps virilization.

Grossly, the tumor ranges from a solid mass of gray-to-cream-colored fleshy tissue resembling a dysgerminoma to a firm, fibrous mass. A characteristic feature is calcification, which may be evident on x-ray examination of the pelvis. Microscopic examination reveals masses of large germ cells which wrap themselves around immature granulosa-like cells. Between the nests of these cells are large numbers of others, suggestive of Leydig cells.

The malignant potential of pure gonadoblastoma has not been established. Some investigators consider it an in situ carcinoma because its germ cells commonly progress to invasive germinoma. However the possibility of malignant behavior may well depend on the mixture of gonadoblastoma with other germ cell elements, such as dysgerminoma or endodermal sinus tumor. Because these patients often reveal eunuchoidal features, sterility, or signs of Turner's syndrome, and because the tumor has a potential for malignancy, removal of both gonads is indicated. In fact, late recurrence in the remaining gonad mandates bilateral extirpation. All streaks should be removed as well.

Estrogen and progesterone should be prescribed for these girls when they reach the age of puberty. The prognosis after removal of these tumors is usually good. Neither recurrence nor metastasis has been reported after removal. However, if the tumor is extensive or only partially removed, subsequent difficulty may ensue.

Gonadal Stromal Tumors (Sex Cord Mesenchymal Tumors)

This fourth major tumor group is composed of neoplasms derived from ovarian mesenchyme. There are three basic categories: (1)gonadal stroma tumors of the female cell type (granulosa and granulosa-thecoma tumors); (2)the male cell type (Sertoli-Leydig cell tumors, i.e., arrhenoblastoma or adrenoblastoma), Sertoli, and hilus (Leydig) cell tumors; and (3)mixed cell types (gynandroblastoma). Tumors in this group are not as common as the germ cell tumors, nor are they as malignant. The first subcategory includes granulosa cell tumors, which in childhood are infrequent. Although approximately 100 have been reported in children, only 3 have proved to be malignant. From 5 to 10% of the tumors occur before the patient reaches the age of puberty and may feminize an occasional patient. For example, they may produce a feminine habitus, maturation of the genitalia, and enlargement of the breasts, but with scant pubic hair. Vaginal bleeding may occur.

Although precocious puberty is usual constitutional and only rarely results from an ovarian tumor, it must be remembered that it may also result from gonadotropin production (by tumors such as teratoma and choriocarcinoma) which in turn triggers estrogen production. Also, precocious heterosexual puberty may result from masculinizing tumors such as Sertoli-Leydig cell tumors or lipoid cell tumors. Of 225 cases of female sexual precocity reported in the literature, 6 were due to ovarian tumors.

Usually the diagnosis is made after an abdominal or pelvic mass is discovered. Exploratory laparotomy shows that the tumor is rounded or lobulated with a smooth surface. A thin capsule covers the tumor, and the bulk is either solid or marked with numerous cystic spaces which may be filled with clotted blood. If these cysts rupture, acute abdomen may result from hemoperitoneum. These cysts are bilateral in about 5% of patients.

Treatment for the unilateral encapsulated tumor is unilateral oophorectomy with wedge resection of the opposite ovary. For extension beyond the ovary to pelvic structures, hysterectomy and bilateral salpingo-oophorectomy should be carried out, followed by postoperative x-ray therapy. The tumor carries a good prognosis, depending upon its degree of anaplasia and the stage of the disease. The malignancy rate, about 25% in adults, is much lower in children, ranging from 3 to 6%.

Malignant granulosa cell tumors have the capacity to produce estrogens from androstenedione, dehydroepiandrosterone, progesterone, and test-osterone. Recurrences are usually local, and distant metastases are rare. Recurrences often take many years to develop, although they may occur at any time. The histologic appearance of a tumor of this group offers no index to its final behavior. If the tumor is primarily a thecoma, its potential for malignancy is less than 1%. It can be classified as malignant only if there is metastasis.

These tumors are sensitive to x-ray, which should be employed for widespread or recurrent disease. Classifying these tumors separately into granulosa cell and theca cell groups has recently been abandoned because most tumors are mixtures and both cell types have identical origins. Some researchers disagree with this concept, stating that pure granulosa cell tumors tend to be more malignant, either initially or after many years, whereas granulosa cell/theca cell mixtures or thecomas are more benign.

It is important to follow children with these tumors for life. Vaginal cytology in the premenarchal child will reveal increasing estrogen stimulation if recurrence is developing. Late recurrence is a well-documented characteristic of granulosa cell tumors. The remaining ovary should be removed after childbearing is completed.

The term *Sertoli-Leydig cell tumor* is used instead of the more familiar *arrhenoblastoma* because many of these tumors are nonfunctioning or have estrogenic physiologic effects rather than masculinizing tendencies. The more immature the tumor cells, the greater their potential for producing hormones.

Tumors with a predominance of functioning Sertoli cells may have the effect of a feminizing neoplasm. However, if the Leydig cells are predominant and functional, the patient is first defeminized (atrophy of breasts, loss of female contour, amenorrhea), then masculinized (hirsutism, hypertrophy of clitoris, voice changes). Androgens suppress normal ovarian function and cause the signs of virilization, and it is a high level of testosterone that mediates the masculinization resulting from this tumor.

The tumor usually affects women of childbearing age and is very rare in childhood. Malignant behavior, seen in 3 to 20% of patients, is usually manifested by intraabdominal spread rather than by distant metastasis. The tumor is bilateral in 5% of the patients. The plan of management outlined for the granulosa cell tumor can be applied to this tumor, and a wedge resection of the opposite ovary is indicated if unilateral oophorectomy is elected.

Signs and symptoms regress after tumor excision; however the patient may be left with permanent hirsutism and voice changes. Since these tumors have a history of late recurrence, the question is raised about the validity of reexploration after the patient has completed her reproductive life. Some clinicians suggest that hysterectomy with oophorectomy be carried out. Unfortunately, this question cannot be resolved at this time.

Whenever a child develops virilization, virilizing adrenal tumors must be kept in mind; they are not uncommon in young girls. The key test here is dexamethasone suppression challenge.

Included among the gonadal stromal tumors is a mixed type, *gynandroblastoma*. Gynandroblastoma should contain typical aggregates of granulosa cell with Call-Exner bodies and hollow tubules of Leydig cells containing crystalloids of Reinke. There are no reports of this tumor in childhood, but there is no reason to believe that it would differ in behavior from granulosa cell or Sertoli-Leydig cell tumors, depending on which group of cells predominates. Malignancy of gynandroblastoma is undocumented.

Nonspecific Ovarian Tumors

The ovary may be involved as part of disseminated Hodgkin's disease. Although these tumors are usually found almost exclusively among the adult population, ovarian involvement has been reported in children suffering from Burkitt's tumor. It is interesting that the first virus to be suspected of causing a human cancer was isolated as a result of epidemiologic observations made in populations of tropical Africa, particularly in those with Burkitt's tumor. The particular distribution of the tumor from the geographic and ecologic standpoint, as well as its age distribution, typical of an infectious disease, has led to the suspicion that Burkitt's tumor may be caused by an infectious agent. A concerted effort has in fact resulted in isolation of a virus (EB virus) from Burkitt's tumor cells. Cytoxan is very effective in treating these tumors, but a large tumor causing symptoms should be excised.

Miscellaneous Tumors

This category includes *fibroma* and *sarcoma*. Ovarian fibromas are more common in adults than in children; these tumors are benign and should be removed when their size makes the diagnosis obvious or complications cause symptoms.

On the other hand, ovarian sarcomas occur more frequently in children than in adults. Grossly, these tumors are solid, lobulated, or soft growths that rapidly fill the abdomen. The cut surfaces of the cellular sarcomas are soft and fleshy, whereas the more fibrous ones are firm and somewhat granular when sectioned. Azoury and Woodruff, reporting on 47 primary sarcomas of the ovary, noted that the most common symptoms were abdominal pain and swelling.

Regardless of the types of therapy employed, survival is poor. In patients with unilateral encapsulated disease, unilateral oophorectomy is as efficacious as more radical surgery. The most common type of sarcoma in this age group is teratoid (90%), and the tumor is undifferentiated; the prognosis is uniformly poor.

Metastatic Cancer

The final major tumor type that can affect the ovary in children is metastatic cancer. Metastatic ovarian tumor must be considered whenever a primary malignancy of any other pelvic structure or abdominal organ, or of the thyroid gland, is found. The diagnosis can be made only with a high index of suspicion. Involved ovaries are usually smooth, firm, and freely movable, and involvement is bilateral in approximately 55% of the patients. Twenty percent of involved ovaries are of normal size, although many have a bizarre histologic pattern. The main lesion will reflect the characteristics of the primary tumor.

Krükenberg tumor, for example, usually arises in the gastrointestinal tract and metastasizes to the ovary, although this tumor may occur primarily in the ovary as well. Probably arising in germinal epithelium having Müllerian potentialities, it is often bilateral and typically solid, and the ovary retains its normal shape. A few cases have been reported in children. Krükenberg tumors are characterized histologically by large, swollen, signet-ring-like cells that lie in clumps within areas of mucoid degeneration, and these are scattered through an edematous stoma-like matrix. Only tumors meeting these criteria should be so designated. Ovarian metastases should be removed whenever feasible.

SUMMARY

Some additional comments must be made about ovarian cancer in children.There are certain characteristics that distinguish the picture from that in adults:

- Limited space for tumor expansion
- A high degree of virulence in cancer
- A less effective immunologic response
- The possibility that therapy may affect future physical and emotional development

Thus the picture is usually one of rapid progression once the tumor has expanded beyond its original site. In dealing with advanced cancer, the physician must strike a balance between doing too little and too much. Therapy should be aimed at relieving symptoms with palliative measures to keep the patient comfortable for as long as possible. This approach should include surgery for relief of intestinal obstruction, drainage of abscesses, or repair of fistulas. If liver, bone marrow, and kidney functions are adequate, chemotherapy may be valuable in selected cases, and, when indicated, judicious use of irradiation is helpful.

Ovarian tumors in children trigger excessive emotionalism in the child, in her parents, and in her physician. Parents may first tend to deny the threat to their child's life. If a diagnosis of cancer is made, they tend to become utterly panic-stricken and seem to lose the ability to think clearly. The physician must be a pillar of strength in this situation and assume broad responsibilities. He must guide the parents and soothe the child. But above all else, he must control his own feelings of pity and avoid projecting himself into the picture as a surrogate parent, lest emotion cloud clinical decisions.

In dealing with ovarian tumors in children, the gynecologist must use the same principles of assessing operability as those used for adults. This approach offers the maximum opportunity for successful treatment. The ancient medical philosophy of not inflicting harm if one cannot achieve good is especially applicable to children with ovarian cancer. It is better for a child to die at home in the loving care of her parents than alone in a cold, forbidding hospital room.

However the greatest tranquilizer for all concerned is to emphasize that most ovarian tumors in children are nonmalignant. In all likelihood the child can be hospitalized and cured in a few short days. These young patients heal quickly and recuperate at a remarkably rapid rate; most can be sent home in 4 or 5 days. Even for malignant tumors that are encapsulated and free of adjacent tissue, cure rates are very high, depending, of course, on the type of tumor. This positive philosophy should pervade our discussions whenever ovarian tumors in children are evaluated.

BIBLIOGRAPHY

Averette, H.E., Hoskins, W.J., Dudan, R.C., Nordqvist, S.R.B.: The ovary, *in* Management of the Patient with Cancer. Edited by T.F. Nealon, Jr. Saunders, Philadelphia, 1976, p.618.

Azoury, R.S., Woodruff, J.D.: Primary ovarian sarcoma: Report of 47 cases from the Emil Novak ovarian tumor registry. Obstet. Gynecol. 37:920, 1971.

Ballas, M.: Yolk sac carcinoma of the ovary with alpha fetoprotein in serum and ascitic fluid demonstrated by immuno-osmophoresis. Am. J. Clin. Pathol. 57:511, 1972.

Barber, H.R.K.: A guide to ovarian tumors in children. Consultant 15:83, 1975.

Barber, H.R.K., Graber, E.A.: Gynecological tumors in childhood and adolescence. Obstet. Gynecol. Surv. 28:369, 1973.

Barber, H.R.K., Graber, E.A.: Managing ovarian tumors of childhood and adolescence. Contemp. Ob/Gyn 3:123, 1974.

Boles, E.T., Hardacre, J.M., Newton, W.A.: Ovarian tumors and cysts in children. Arch. Surg. 83:112, 1961.

Brownstein, G.D., Vaitukaitis, J.L., Carbone, P.P., et al.: Ectopic production of human chorionic gonadotropin. Ann. Intern. Med. 78:39, 1973.

Butt, J.A.: Ovarian tumors in children. Obstet. Gynecol. 69:833, 1955.

Devi, N.S.: Mesodermal mixed tumors of the female generative tract. Presented at the 6th International Congress on Obstetrics and Gynecology, New York, 1970.

Gold, P., Freedman, S.O.: Demonstration of tumor-specific antigens in human colonic carcinoma by immunological tolerance and absorption technique. J. Exp. Med. 121:439, 1965.

Heald, F.O., McCraig, J., Ming, P-M.L.: Ovarian tumors in adolescents: Types and presenting feature. Clin. Pediatr. Phila. 6:401, 1967.

Hughesdon, P.E.: Structure, origin and histological relations of dysgerminoma. J. Obstet. Gynecol. Br. Commonw. 66:566, 1959.

Huffman, J.W.: Gynecology of Childhood and Adolescence. Saunders, Philadelphia, 1968, p.286.

Kaufman, R.H., Gardner, H.L.: Benign mesodermal tumors. Clin. Obstet. Gynecol. 8:953, 1961.

Knox, J.M., Freeman, R.G.: Epidermal tumors. Clin. Obstet. Gynecol. 8:925, 1965.

Lawrence, D.J.R., Neville, M.A.: Fetal antigens and their role in the diagnosis and clinical management of human neoplasms: A review. Br. J. Cancer 26:335, 1972.

Luisi, A.: Metastatic ovarian tumors, in Ovarian Cancer, International Union Against Cancer Monograph Series. Vol. II Springer-Verlag, Berlin, 1968, p.87.

Miller, O.J.: Sex chromosome abnormality. Am. J. Obstet. Gynecol. 90:1078, 1964.

Moore, J.G., Schifrin, B.S., Erez, S.: Ovarian tumors in childhood and adolescence. Am. J. Obstet. Gynecol. 99:913, 1967.

Morris, J., McLean, O., Scully, R.E.: Endocrine Pathology of the Ovary. Mosby, St. Louis, 1969, pp.65—95.

Parson, L., Sommers, S.C. (Eds.): Gynecology. Saunders, Philadelphia, 1963.

Pepus, M., Hutchison, J.B., Ruffolo, E.H., et al.: Ovarian neoplasm and sexual precocity. Obstet. Gynecol. 29:828, 1967.

Radman, H.M., Koman, W.: Ovarian tumors in children. Am. J. Obstet. Gynecol. 79:989, 1960.

Scheelhaus, H.F., Trujillo, J.M., Rutledge, F.N., et al.: Germ cell tumors associated with XY gonadal dysgenesis. Am. J. Obstet. Gynecol. 109:1197, 1971.

Scully, R.E.: Recent progress in ovarian cancer. Hum. Pathol. 1:73, 1970.

Scully, R.E.: Sex cord-mesenchyme tumors, in Ovarian Cancer, International Union Against Cancer Monograph Series. Vol. II. Springer-Verlag, Berlin, 1968, p.40.

Southam, A.L.: Disorder of menstruation in adolescents. Clin. Obstet. Gynecol. 9:779, 1966.

Taylor, E.S.: Editorial comment: Virilizing adrenal tumors. Obstet. Gynecol. Surv. 23:981, 1968.

Teilum, G.: Tumors of germinal origin, in Ovarian Cancer International Union Against Cancer Monograph Series. Vol. II. Springer-Verlag, Berlin, 1948, p.58.

Wallach, E.E.: Female isosexual pseudoprecocious puberty. Clin. Obstet. Gynecol. 11:795, 1968.

Wollner, N., Exelby, P., Woodruff, J.M., Cham, W.C., Murphy, M.L., Lewis, J.L., Jr.: Malignant ovarian tumors in childhood. Cancer 37:1953, 1976.

14

Ovarian Cancer Complicating Pregnancy

The incidence of ovarian cancer has doubled in the United States in the last 30 years. Unfortunately, early cases are as difficult as ever to diagnose clinically, but the obstetrician has one great advantage—the patient presents herself for pelvic examination. With a high index of suspicion, the diagnosis can be made earlier. If the disease is diagnosed in stage I, the chance of a 5-year survival is between 60 and 90%; but once it spreads outside the ovary and involves adjacent organs, the 5-year survival falls to 10 to 25%.

Cancer of the ovary complicating pregnancy occurs very rarely, and the incidence usually given is 1 in 18,000 deliveries. It should be remembered that these figures include abortions. The malignancy rate of ovarian tumors in pregnancy is 2 to 5% lower than 18 to 21% listed for the nonpregnant patient. The signs and symptoms are not basically different from those in the nonpregnant state. If the patient is seen in the first trimester, the ovarian tumor can be detected with some degree of success. The diagnosis may at times be quite fortuitous. The patient presents herself during the first trimester of pregnancy with an enlarged uterus plus an adnexal mass. This should immediately arouse suspicion, and from then on, observation and evaluation over a short period should permit the physician to pursue a given course with vigor and decision. The physician should suspect any mass in the adnexal area that is immobile and fixed with adhesions, irregular and shotty, fixed in the cul-de-sac, and increases in firmness and size, especially if it is bilateral. An abdomen that grows larger than would be expected for the time of pregnancy should alert one immediately.

Although some advocate diagnostic culdoscopy or laparoscopy, use of these techniques is very questionable and may increase the complication rate. Direct inspection is indicated but it should be done with great care to avoid the risk of trauma to the tumor and possible rupture and extension or damage to other organs that might be adherent. Finally, frozen section and total removal is the therapy of choice.

There really is not much difference between a 1-inch incision for laparoscopy and a 5- to 6-inch incision which permits thorough evaluation of

167

the tumor, thorough inspection of all the other abdominal viscera, and removal of affected organs. Diagnostic work-up should include a Papanicolaou smear, proctosigmoidoscopy, pelvic and rectovaginal examination, and a careful search for extrapelvic metastasis. If there is an omental cake, hepatomegaly, or gross ascites, the outlook for long survival is grim. Only about 8% of patients with ascites live 5 years. The toll of cancer will be lowered only if physicians begin to suspect cancer in every enlarged ovary that persists.

It is rare to make a diagnosis in either the second or third trimester, however, unless a high degree of suspicion is carried over from the first trimester. Unless the tumor becomes incarcerated or fixed in the cul-de-sac, it usually rises up into the abdomen and is difficult to identify. Any shotty, fixed tumor that is bilateral is highly suspect and deserves exploration without delay. If a cyst or tumor which is 5 cm or less, unilateral, smooth, and freely movable is detected in the first trimester, it should begin to regress in the second trimester. If it does not, laparotomy is indicated by the 16th week of pregnancy if it is 5 cm or larger. Laparotomy is indicated at the first visit if the cyst is 10 cm or larger or if it is fixed and nodular.

The presenting symptom may be a complication of ovarian tumor, such as torsion, rupture, hemorrhage, or infection. This may be accompanied by acute abdominal pain with vomiting and possible shock. Surgical intervention is indicated immediately. In other instances the cysts or tumor should be removed to eliminate the need for cesarean section, to remove the danger of the complications listed above, and to eliminate the danger of malignancy. Cesarean section can then be reserved for the usual obstetric indications.

THERAPY OF OVARIAN CANCER IN PREGNANCY

If the surgeon finds an ovarian tumor, cyst, or malignancy during abdominal exploration, his first obligation is to stage the disease, to collect peritoneal fluid for cytologic and cell block examination, and to remove the lesion for immediate frozen section for definitive diagnosis and documentation. This procedure is followed by whatever further surgery is indicated, depending upon the type of tumor, its histologic grading, and the degree of anatomic spread. Biopsies of omentum, peritoneum, or any other intraabdominal area where one suspects tumors are indicated. The information may prove helpful in selecting the appropriate therapy and in future follow-up examinations and studies.

Papillary serous cystadenocarcinoma is the most common type of ovarian malignancy and is probably an advanced stage of a benign serous cystadenoma. If it is contained so that papillary processes are within an intact capsule, the prognosis is reasonably good. Once there is an extension through the capsule with papillation on the exterior of the tumor, extension to the surrounding organs appears promptly with a great diminution of 5-year survival. General abdominal carcinomatosis soon follows with death. The treatment is total hysterectomy, bilateral salpingo-oophorectomy, appendectomy, omentectomy, P^{32} (if no gross disease is left) and chemotherapy. Therapy must be tailored to the patient and the extent of disease. If there is any doubt about the type of tumor or whether a malignancy is present, if the tumor has an intact capsule and is freely movable, especially in a patient under 30, it is better to do a salpingo-oophorectomy on the side of the tumor. The pelvis should be aspirated prior to the excision and sent for a cell block. If the tumor proves to be highly malignant or the cell block is positive, the abdomen may be opened and the remaining reproductive organs excised as outlined above, if that appears to be the best course. In certain low-grade malignancies the previously performed treatment may be considered sufficient to insure a cure.

Papillary mucinous cystadenocarcinoma is the next most common type of ovarian cancer. About 1 in 4 is bilateral. The clinical picture and operative findings again depend on whether the issue is contained in an intact capsule. The spread of this tumor is fortunately slower than the spread of the papillary serous variety, so the prognosis is better. Treatment is the same as that for serous cystadenocarcinoma.

Solid Adenocarcinoma

Is a common epithelial ovarian carcinoma with the same cells as those found in papillary serous or mucinous carcinoma of the ovary. These tumors are solid, highly undifferentiated, and have a greater potential to spread and metastasize. They are bilateral in more than 50% of the patients and the prognosis is extremely poor. Treatment is similar to that outlined above.

Dysgerminoma

In the young group of patients, dysgerminoma is not as aggressively malignant. Pure dysgerminoma has a surprisingly high 5-year survival rate. If the tumor is unilateral and still encapsulated, unilateral oophorectomy may be carried out if the remaining ovary is negative on biopsy, the peritoneal fluid is negative and if external, common, and paraaortic nodes are negative as well. Dysgerminoma in the patient over 35 and surely in the one over 40 years should undergo more aggressive attack. If the tumor is bilateral or if the capsule is perforated, bilateral salpingo-oophorectomy, hysterectomy, omentectomy, appendectomy, and postoperative x-ray therapy must be carried out in any age group.

Other germ cell tumors, both extraembryonal and embryonic carcinomas, are highly malignant. The treatment is generally excision of the uterus, tubes, ovaries, appendix, and omentum. Multiple chemotherapy agents given at monthly intervals up to 2 years have increased the salvage rate of this generally lethal group of malignancies. As a group these tumors are relatively radioresistant.

The gonadal stromal tumors (granulosa cell, Sertoli-Leydig) are rarely associated with pregnancy. However, if they are unilateral and encapsulated, with a negative opposite ovary on biopsy, negative cytology, and no evidence of spread, unilateral salpingo-oophorectomy is usually adequate therapy. If there is any evidence of spread or if the tumor is bilateral, it should be managed as outlined above. These tumors are characterized by local, late recurrence and are very radiosensitive.

Sarcoma of the ovary, either primary or metastatic, is highly malignant and spreads quickly by local invasion and blood vessel and lymphatic extension. It is usually found before the childbearing age. The prompt therapy should be complete removal of the pelvic gynecologic organs. Multiple chemotherapeutic agents should be given over an extended period of time.

Metastatic carcinoma of the ovaries from the uterus, breasts, thyroid, stomach, or colon may occur, although it is extremely rare. There is confusion over whether all or merely certain secondary cancers are properly but eponymically designated as "Krukenberg tumors." The signet-ring cell type of carcinoma described by Krukenberg is most often metastatic to the ovary from the stomach. The ultimate prognosis is poor, but removal of the uterus, ovary, and tubes may permanently control the pelvic manifestations of the problem. Bilateral tumors are the rule. Of course, removal of the original focus of the disease probably will not result in cure at this late date, but at least adequate palliation might be accomplished. Some Krukenberg tumors in pregnancy may be hormonally active. Reports of androgenicity as well as estrogen secretion effecting even the fetus can be found in the literature.

It should be noted that the ovaries at term in pregnancy are resting ovaries and are comparatively small. They often have shaggy, eosinophilic, wispy material on their surfaces which is decidua. *Any enlargement of the ovaries in a term pregnancy should be suspect,* and it is in the best interest of the patient for the operating surgeon to take biopsies and frozen sections as a guide to an indicated additional therapy.

Nonmalignant ovarian tumors may be encountered in pregnancy. After they are diagnosed as benign, the question of their management is raised. A brief discussion is included to serve as a guide to management.

Therapy for Nonmalignant Ovarian Tumors

There are eight basic principles of therapy for this group of tumors.

1. If the tumor is cystic, less than 6–8 cm in diameter, and steadily diminishes in size as the pregnancy continues, it can be observed. Operation is not indicated unless there is torsion or rupture. If the tumor becomes enlarged, however, operative intervention is mandatory. When cystic tumors do not regress, the ideal time for operation is in the early part of the second trimester (12–14 weeks). By this time the corpus luteum of pregnancy is no longer important in maintaining the pregnancy. In most instances, after the 60th day of pregnancy, removal of the corpus luteum will not materially affect the outcome. If the tumor is benign on frozen section, the cyst should be resected, and as much of the normal portion of the ovary as possible should be left.

2. Solid or suspicious tumors should be removed at once regardless of the trimester of pregnancy. With evidence of torsion, hemorrhage, or necrosis, prompt surgery is mandatory.

3. The uterus should be handled as little and as carefully as possible in the early months. Excessive manipulation contributes to an increased abortion rate. Although some advise prophylactic progesterone therapy postoperatively, it is generally unnecessary. The results do not justify the means.

4. After the 18th week it may be more difficult to remove a tumor because of the enlarged uterus. It can be done, but there are more technical problems. Also, the closer the patient is to term, the greater is the stress on the healing abdominal wound by the enlarging uterus with possible weakening and herniation. The earlier the surgery is done, the greater is the time remaining for proper healing.

5. In the last trimester of pregnancy the main problem is a known or unsuspected tumor blocking delivery. The fetal and maternal complications make operation mandatory. If the diagnosis is made before the onset of labor, surgical intervention is indicated about 1 week before the anticipated delivery date, or if this is unreliable, in early labor. The operation consists of low flap cesarean section, and either ovarian resection or oophorectomy.

If the exit of the child is not blocked and the tumor lies above the inlet, the child should be delivered vaginally and the tumor removed abdominally as soon as the patient's condition permits. This usually is within the first 48 hours postpartum. During the interval between delivery and operation, one must watch for acute torsion because, as mentioned previously, torsion in the puerperium is a very likely complication.

6. A tumor above the inlet and evidence of pain, tenderness, or peritoneal reaction while the patient is in labor probably indicates torsion or rupture. Prompt surgery is indicated. Cesarean section plus oophorectomy is the surgery of choice.

7. If a tumor blocking the pelvis is first diagnosed when the patient is in advanced labor and fully dilated, the abdomen can be opened, the tumor dislodged, and the baby delivered vaginally by an assistant. The tumor is then removed, and the abdomen closed. This maneuver is quite spectacular, but most obstetricians will not see one case of this type in a lifetime. It is really an indictment of the patient's medical care. At the very least, the diagnosis should have been made in early labor.

8. If the tumor is diagnosed during the puerperium, operation within 48 hours is indicated. With torsion, immediate surgery is mandatory.

SUMMARY

The problem of ovarian cancer in pregnancy is quite simple. Be aware of the condition, have a high index of suspicion, make the diagnosis early, and tailor the treatment to the needs of the patient and the extent of the disease. One of the main reasons for difficulty is that the patient resists abdominal exploration during pregnancy because she fears abortion or possible damage to her fetus. She should be assured that this is not a valid argument against operation. The potential danger to the mother far exceeds the imagined danger to the child. The extra time spent gaining the patient's confidence, a consultation when necessary to reinforce one's advice, and a steadfast stand on the necessity of operation are important. Most of the tumors seen with ovarian tumors are sins of omission, rather than commission. If the patient will not follow the advice of her physician, he must remove himself from the case and relieve himself of the responsiblity of future difficulty. The mortality from ovarian cancer will never be lowered with the present state of our diagnostic armamentarium unless the tumor is attacked early and completely.

If the surgeon finds an ovarian malignancy during the abdominal exploration, his first obligation is to stage the disease, to collect peritoneal fluid for cell block diagnosis, and to remove the lesion for immediate frozen section for definitive diagnosis and documentation. This procedure is followed by whatever further surgery is indicated, depending upon the type of tumor, its histologic grading, and the degree of anatomic spread. Biopsies of omentum, peritoneum, or any other intraabdominal area where one suspects tumors are indicated.

If the tumor is unilateral, well encapsulated, shows no anatomic evidence of spread, and is reported as one of those listed with a comparatively low degree of malignancy, and if the peritoneal fluid shows no malignant cells, it is permissible to do a unilateral oophorectomy and to permit the pregnancy to continue. The other ovary, however, should be split and biopsied to insure its freedom from disease. This procedure is permissible with a histologically low-grade mucinous cystadenocarcinoma, dysgerminoma, granulosa-thecal cell tumors, arrhenoblastoma, gynandroblastoma, and possibly with a low-grade papillary tumor when it is doubtful whether it is a cystadenoma or a cystadenocarcinoma. The patient is then delivered from below at term. Six weeks after delivery of the child, the patient is re-explored and a total hysterectomy and bilateral salpingo-oophorectomy are done. If the patient wishes to take a calculated risk, she can be carefully observed while another pregnancy is permitted and surgery follows the next delivery. If, on the other hand, the tumor is beyond stage IA, or if the cancer is any other than those enumerated, the therapy must be immediate total hysterectomy, bilateral salpingo-oophorectomy, and omentectomy when indicated. Implantation of polyethylene tubes for postoperative instillation of radioactive chromic phosphate is our usual routine. Chemotherapy is instituted promptly. If the entire tumor cannot be removed, the pregnancy should still be terminated, as much tumor as possible should be removed surgically, and chemotherapy should be instituted as soon as feasible. The pregnancy is secondary.

The responsibility of the physician is to treat primarily the mother. If the baby can be saved, it is an added dividend. Before undertaking surgery in a patient with possible ovarian cancer in pregnancy, it is mandatory that the problem be completely disclosed to the patient and that informed consent be given to allow the surgeon to proceed in any manner deemed necessary.

In most reported series, about one-third of the cases are stage III or IV at surgery. One must be prepared for this contingency. The most aggressive in terms of early spread are the solid adenocarcinomas and serous cystadenocarcinomas.

The survival of pregnant patients with ovarian cancer is no different from survival in the nonpregnant group. The type of tumor and its anatomic spread determine the 5-year cure rate. Pregnancy has no effect on the tumor. Only aggressive early exploration will save the patient. Interruption of pregnancy has no beneficial effect on the future course of this disease.

With metastatic disease of the ovary from the stomach, colon, liver, or breast, the decision on therapy must be made on an individual basis. Certainly nobody would quarrel with a decision to "shoot the works" and clean out the entire pelvis. In certain instances the expectant parents, being aware of the poor prognosis in the mother, may elect to have the baby for whatever joy it may bring to the remaining time of the mother's life and to the father in the future. Under these circumstances, delivery from below (if there is no tumor blocking the pelvic canal) followed by pelvic surgery after the birth of the child might well be the more compassionate procedure. Cesarean section is performed if indicated for obstetrical reasons, and the uterus and tumor are removed at this time.

The basic principles of cancer of the ovary in pregnancy can be summarized as follows:

- It occurs in one out of 18,000 pregnancies including abortions.
- The malignancy rate of ovarian tumors complicating pregnancy is 2 to 5%, in contrast to an 18 to 20% malignancy rate in the nonpregnant state.
- The signs and symptoms are not basically different from those of the nonpregnant state.
- Usually an adnexal mass is found at the time of the first antepartum visit.
  —If it regresses on follow-up, the diagnosis is functional cyst.
  —If it is 5 cm or larger and persists, laparotomy is indicated at about 16 weeks.
  —If it is hard, knobby, fixed, or bilateral, surgery is indicated without a period of observation.
- Rarely is the ovarian tumor bilateral.
- The presenting symptom may be a complication of the ovarian tumor, such as torsion, rupture, hemorrhage, or infection. There may be sudden acute abdominal pain with vomiting and possibly shock.

The management depends upon the findings, but a general plan can be described:

- Treat the cancer as it would be treated in a nonpregnant patient.
- If it is a low-grade malignancy confined to one ovary, unilateral oophorectomy and bisection of the opposite ovary are recommended. When the peritoneal cavity is opened, prior to exploration, the abdomen and pelvis should be aspirated for cytologic examination. The pregnancy is allowed to go to term.
- If the ovarian cancer has extended byond the ovary from which it arose, total hysterectomy, bilateral salpingo-oophorectomy, omentectomy, ap-

pendectomy, and the instillation of P^{32} and postoperative chemotherapy are recommended.

- At all cesarean sections, routine inspection of the tubes and ovaries is mandatory.

BIBLIOGRAPHY

Barber, H.R.K.: Gynecologic cancer complicating pregnancy, *in* Gynecologic Oncology. Excerpta Medica, Amsterdam, 1970, pp. 283–288.

Barber, H.R.K.: Editorial comment, *in* Surgical Disease in Pregnancy. Edited by H.R.K. Barber, E.A. Graber. Saunders, Philadelphia, 1974.

Barber, H.R.K., Brunschwig, A.: Gynecologic cancer complicating pregnancy. Am. J. Obstet. Gynecol. 85:156, 1963.

Barber, H.R.K., Graber, E.A.: Surgical aspects of ovarian tumors, *in* Selected Topics of Cancer—Current Concepts. Symposia Specialists, Miami, 1974.

Betson, J.R., Golden, M.L.: Primary carcinoma of the ovary coexisting with pregnancy. Obstet. Gynecol. 12:589, 1958.

Betson, J.R., Golden, M.L.: Cancer and pregnancy. Am. J. Obstet. Gynecol. 81:718, 1961.

Breecher, N.A., Butterly, B.W., Fortune, D.W., Macafee, C.J.: Ovarian tumors in pregnancy. Aust. N.Z. J. Obstet. Gynecol. 11:208, 1971.

Creasman, W.T., Rutledge, F., Smith, J.C.: Carcinoma of the ovary associated with pregnancy. Obstet. Gynecol. 38:111, 1971.

Fox, L.P., Stamm, W.J.: Krukenberg tumor complicating pregnancy. Am. J. Obstet. Gynecol. 92:702, 1965.

Frymire, L.J.: Arrhenoblastoma with two subsequent pregnancies. Obstet. Gynecol. 17:248, 1961.

Graber, E.A.: Ovarian tumors in pregnancy, *in* Surgical Disease in Pregnancy. Edited by H.R.K. Barber, E.A. Graber. Saunders, Philadelphia, 1974, pp. 428–437.

Green, W.L., Jones, E.H.: Coexistent pseudomucinous cystadenocarcinoma and pregnancy. Obstet. Gynecol. 13:349, 1959.

Greene, G.G., Smith, A.E., McClelland, T.: A malignant granulosa cell tumor associated with pregnancy. Am. J. Obstet. Gynecol. 60: 686, 1956.

Jubb, E.D.: Primary ovarian carcinoma in pregnancy. J. Obstet. Gynecol. 85:345, 1963.

Lawrence, W.D., Larson, P.N., Hange, E.T.: Primary Krukenberg tumor of the ovary in pregnancy. Obstet. Gynecol. 10:84, 1957.

McGowan, L.: Cancer in pregnancy. American Lecture Series. Thomas, Springfield, 1967.

Phelan, J.T.: Cancer and pregnancy. N.Y. State J. Med. 68: 3011, 1968.

Smith, A.H., Ward, S.V.: Dysgerminoma in pregnancy. Obstet. Gynecol. 28:502, 1966.

Spadoni, L.R., Lindberg, M.C., Mottet, N.K., Herrman, W.L.: Virilization coexisting with Krukenberg tumor during pregnancy. Am. J. Obstet. Gynecol. 92:981, 1965.

Taylor, E.S.: Ovarian tumors in pregnancy. Obstet. Gynecol. Surv. 27: 43, 1972.

Tweeddale, D.N., Dockerty, M.B., Pratt, J.H., Hranilovich, G.T.: Pregnancy with recurrent granulosa cell tumor. Am. J. Obstet. Gynecol. 70:1039, 1955.

15

The Postmenopausal Palpable Ovary Syndrome (PMPO)

The time has come to reevaluate our clinical approach to ovarian pathology. Although cancer of the cervix is still the most prevalent cancer of the female reproductive system, ovarian cancer has become the leading killer of women who die from gynecologic malignancy. With the present state of diagnostic development, diagnosis of an ovarian tumor is a matter of chance rather than a scientific method. By the time it is diagnosed, ovarian cancer in more than 50% of the patients has spread beyond the ovary. The hard fact remains that a pelvic mass found during a pelvic examination is the only practical and consistent clinical method availabe to us to detect an ovarian tumor. Certain functional or dysontogenetic tumors with hormone activity are the exception. However there are only a few such tumors compared to the number of epithelial tumors, which compose the main group of killers.

We euphemistically state that women are protected if they have a pelvic examination every 6 months. However it has been reported that the chance of detecting an ovarian neoplasm during routine pelvic examination in an asymptomatic woman is 1 in 10,000.

The insidious onset of ovarian cancer needs no elaboration. Many competent gynecologists have had the devastating experience of finding widespread disease in a patient who had a negative pelvic examination 6 months before. Pelvic examination itself has many limitations because of the difficulties inherent in evaluating the pelvic contents in the presence of obesity, a long conical inelastic vagina with contracted fornices, vaginal atrophy, or lack of cooperation from an apprehensive or defensive patient. Among patients who survive, it is merely serendipitous that she was seen at a particular time when the tumor was still localized and could be removed intact. In many, the tumor is found accidentally or incidentally. By the time a patient complains of a mass, abdominal enlargement, or pain, the tumor has usually involved the surrounding organs with disease or adhesions; indeed, in a high percentage of such patients, the regional lymph nodes are already affected. It follows that since it is not usually possible to diagnose ovarian

175

cancer in its early stages, it is not possible to treat it with any predictable degree of certainty for cure.

It is an accepted axiom that the ovary may be too old to function but never too old to form tumors. Since the peak incidence of ovarian cancer is between the ages of 40 to 60, especially careful evaluation (combined with constant suspicion) should be carried out in this high-risk group.

One diagnostic sign of early cancer in the ovary of postmenopausal patients has proved to be both valuable and consistent in our hands. It is simply that the palpation of what is interpreted as a *normal-sized ovary in the premenopausal woman represents an ovarian tumor in the postmenopausal woman.* This suggestion may appear to be insignificant in terms of the total problem, but it has been my experience that all such palpable findings proved to be a new growth; they were not all necessarily malignant, but none were functional or dysfunctional. It is my opinion that the postmenopausal palpable ovary is a most significant finding, and I hope that this observation will alert the gynecologist to its importance.

The designation *postmenopausal palpable ovary syndrome* is a misnomer, and it is unfortunate that a more descriptive term had not been chosen. *It does not mean that anything that is palpated in the adnexa is abnormal.* Every gynecologist has been able to feel an ovary that measures 2 cm in a very thin, relaxed patient with an elastic and distensible vagina. It is to be reemphasized that the PMPO syndrome is simply that the palpation of what is interpreted as a normal sized ovary in the premenopausal woman represents an ovarian tumor in the postmenopausal woman. Figure 50 represents the normal ovary, the ovary in early menopause, and then in late menopause, drawn to scale. The drawing shows a dramatic difference in size between the normal premenopausal ovary and the ovary in the late menopausal period.

Several points can be enumerated to support this thesis. There is no such thing as physiologic enlargement of the postmenopausal ovary. Physiologic cysts can only arise from the nonrupture of a Graffian follicle (follicle cysts) or from cystic degeneration of a corpus luteum (lutein cysts). There are no follicle or lutein cysts in a postmenopausal ovary, simply because there are no follicles or corpora lutea.

The contrast between the premenopausal and postmenopausal ovary is striking. Whereas the normal ovary measures 3.5 x 2 x 1.5 cm, the menopausal ovary tends to atrophy and shrink when the Graffian follicles and ova disappear. The tunica albuginea becomes very dense and causes the surface of the ovary to become scarred and shrunken. The cortex is marked with increased thinning as well as numerous corpora fibrosa and corpora albuginea with areas of dense fibrosis and hyalinization. The ovary shows varying degrees of avascularity. Eventually the ovary becomes an inert residue that consists of connective tissue, and it clings to the posterior leaf of the broad ligament. Its pink color becomes pure white. It shrinks to 2 x 1.5 x 0.5 cm, and in some it may be as small as 1.5 x 0.75 x 0.5 cm (Figure 50). Its wrinkled surface resembles the gyri and sulci of the cerebrum. At this point it

Normal ovary
Premenopausal
3.5 x 2 x 1.5 cm

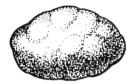

Early menopause
(1 - 2 years)
2 x 1.5 x 0.5 cm

Late menopause
(2 - 5 years)
1.5 x 0.75 x 0.5 cm

Figure 50.   Relative sizes of premenopausal, menopausal, and late menopausal ovaries.

cannot be palpated. The postmenopausal palpable ovary (PMPO) is not a normal ovary for this stage of life.

Traditionally, a woman who is amenorrheic is clinically considered menopausal. However, chemically and anatomically, the changes described above occur over a period of time. Although they are quite rapid, it takes approximately 3 to 5 years for the terminal picture to be achieved. The conclusion must then be drawn that if an ovary is palpated 3 to 5 years after the clinical menopause, it is a pathologic ovary until proved otherwise, regardless of its size in centimeters. It is our recommendation that the patient (without delay for observation) should have the benefit of an expedited examination under anesthesia and, if the previous impression is verified, she should undergo laparotomy. A careful abdominal exploration followed by total hysterectomy and bilateral oophorectomy should be the treatment chosen. Although splitting and biopsing the ovary may be justified in detecting early cancer in the premenopausal patient, the ovaries should be removed without biopsy in the postmenopausal group.

SUMMARY

On the basis of the Third National Cancer Survey data, about 1.4% or 1 of every 70 newborn girls will develop cancer of the ovary during her life. Cancers of the ovary account for roughly 5% of all cancers in women, according to both the State of Connecticut and the Third National Cancer Survey.

The age-specific incidence rates for ovarian cancer rise steadily up to age 80, then they drop off slightly in the older ages. The greatest number of cases is found in age groups 50–54 through 55–59 years. The mean age was 62.3

while the median age was 59.0. The trends in age-standardized death rates for major sites show that the rate for the ovary is increasing.

The observed median survival times by age are 1.4 years for all ages, 5.4 years for those under 45, 1.8 years for those aged 45 to 54, 1.3 years for those 55 to 64, 0.9 years for those aged 65 to 74, and 0.8 years for those aged 95 and older.

If we are to save more women and diminish the mortality rate from ovarian cancer, we must become more liberal in our indications for operation. We suggest that the palpation of what appears to be a normal-sized ovary in a patient who is 3 to 5 years postmenopausal is indicative of an ovarian tumor and should be investigated promptly. These patients should not be followed and reevaluated, but rather subjected to proof of the presence or absence of an ovarian tumor. To wait until one feels a solid tumor mass of up to 5 cm and then to expect a cure is an exercise in fancy and futility.

John Gardner said, "We are all faced with wonderful opportunities brilliantly disguised as insoluble problems." Ovarian cancer is not insoluble. Perhaps, by adding a small segment at a time, the total picture will emerge to the benefit of our patient. Remember the PMPO syndrome!

BIBLIOGRAPHY

Barber, H.R.K., Graber, E.A.: The PMPO syndrome (postmenopausal palpable ovary syndrome). Obstet. Gynecol. 38.921, 1971.

End Results in Cancer. Report No. 4 U.S. Department of Health, Education, and Welfare. Public Health Service, National Institutes of Health, Bethesda, Maryland, 1972, p. 113.

Kistner, R.W.: Gynecology, Principles and Practice. Second edition. Year Book Publishers, Chicago, 1971.

Silverberg, E.: Gynecologic cancer. Statistical and epidemiological information. American Cancer Society, Professional Education Publication, 1975.

16

Technique for the Surgical Treatment of Cancer of the Ovary

Surgical excision of ovarian cancer should be approached with a planned, methodical technique. The goal in ovarian cancer surgery is to excise as much tumor as possible and at the same time avoid the possibility of hemorrhage. Granted that ovarian cancer may be a surprising finding, these early, well-encapsulated ovarian cancers can be managed without difficulty. However 60 to 80% of all ovarian cancers present in stages III and IV. Proper surgery for ovarian cancer patients then requires relatively sophisticated techniques, not always available in every hospital. Add to this the requirements for chemotherapy, radiation, accurate pathology, and the fluid and electrolyte management that almost invariably follows abdominal surgery, and it is not hard to make a case for a large medical center as the optimum place for ovarian cancer care. The extensive dissection required to adequately debulk the disease will often compromise the patient to the extent that hyperalimentation is needed. With this disease, we must assume the worst and be ready for any emergency or complication.

The gynecologic oncologist has come full cycle from a very radical surgical attack to a conservative approach, back to a super-aggressive surgical attack. Why has this come about? In the late 1940s and early 1950s, after carrying out a radical surgical operation, oncologists did not have enough knowledge of chemotherapy to control the residual disease; thus recurrence or continued growth of persistent disease was usual. In addition, the management of these patients was difficult postoperatively because of the fluid and electrolyte imbalances as well as the problems of metabolism and proper nutrition. With the improved knowledge of fluids and electrolytes as well as the increased use of hyperalimentation, many of these problems have been overcome.

TECHNIQUE

To cut down on the possibility of hemorrhage or to hold blood loss to a minimum, a very methodical and planned approach should be used in operating on patients with ovarian cancer. The abdomen must be opened by a vertical incision that extends beyond the upper limits of the mass. Unless this is properly carried out it will be impossible to stage accurately the amount of ovarian cancer present. In addition, a small incision such as a Pfannenstiel may compromise the necessary exposure which may result in a well encapsulated cancer, thus converting it from a lesser stage to a stage with spill compromising the chance for cure. In many instances a Pfannenstiel incision selects patients for therapeutic failure. It is the height of professional integrity to choose an incision that extends beyond the upper limits of the gross disease and allows adequate and easy exploration, providing the optimum chance to remove the tumor intact (Figure 51). Morally, professionally, and medico-legally, the Pfannenstiel incision is to be condemned in the management of an ovarian tumor.

When the abdomen is opened, any fluid present is collected for cytology and, in the absence of fluid, about 50 ml of saline should be instilled into the pelvis and then aspirated for cytologic examination. The abdomen and pelvis should be carefully and thoroughly evaluated to determine the extent of disease. If tissue is readily available for easy biopsy, a frozen section diagnosis is desirable to document the site and type of primary lesion. It is especially important to evaluate the area on the posterior abdominal wall between the liver and the diaphragm. Cancer has been found here in stage I cancer of the ovary in about 10 to 15% of cases.

When one has determined the extent of disease, it is desirable to incise the posterior peritoneum lateral to and just above the pelvic brim, as carried out at the start of a radical hysterectomy (Figures 52 and 53). This approach exposes the infundibular ligament and by clamping it decreases the blood loss that occurs when ovarian cancer is excised. This procedure permits identifica-

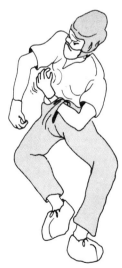

Figure 51. The Pfannenstiel and low transverse incision has no place in the management of ovarian cancer. Denis Cavanagh says it is like scratching your axilla through your fly.

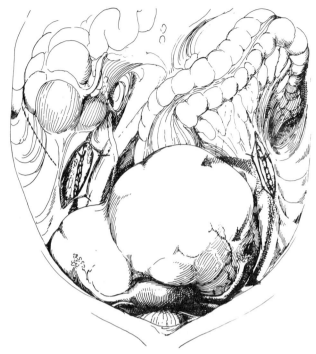

Figure 52. On opening the peritoneal cavity, it is most important to identify all landmarks. The cecum will be mobilized on the right and the sigmoid on the left for identification of the ureter and high ligation of the infundibulopelvic ligament. The drawing shows the ureter in relation to all of the vessels in the infundibulopelvic ligament. [Reprinted from *Current Ob/Gyn Techniques.* Copyright © Surgical Communications, Inc. All rights reserved.]

tion of the ureter, which can be isolated and left attached to the medial peritoneal flap. The ovarian vessels running in the infundibular ligament can be isolated, clamped, cut, tied, and doubly ligated in toto. As soon as a similar procedure is carried out on the opposite side, a considerable amount of blood is diverted from the ovarian cancer.

With the ureter protected from injury, it is possible by blunt and sharp dissection to incise the peritoneum down to the round ligament and, after it is clamped and ligated, to continue the incision of the peritoneum lateral to the bladder. If the bladder flap of peritoneum is involved with cancer, the incision in the peritoneum should be continued to the pubis (Figure 54). The lateral side of the peritoneum over the bladder can be elevated and dissected by a sharp and blunt dissection from the bladder, which is then left denuded. The flap of peritoneum is dissected off the dome of the bladder and left attached to the lower uterine segment and is removed as an en bloc dissection with the uterus. Posteriorly, with the ureter under direct vision, the peritoneum medial to the ureter is incised down over the rectum. This frees up the cul-de-sac from the bowel and leaves it attached to the back part of the uterus (Figure 55). The entire specimen can be removed as the hysterectomy is carried out.

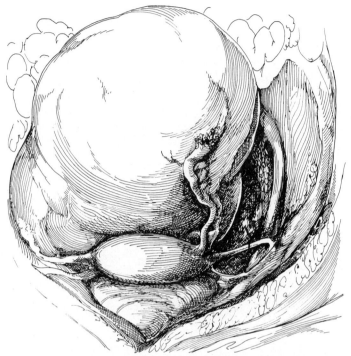

Figure 53.   The round ligament, the uterus, and the large pelvic mass. [Reprinted from *Current Ob/Gyn Techniques.* Copyright © Surgical Communications, Inc. All rights reserved.]

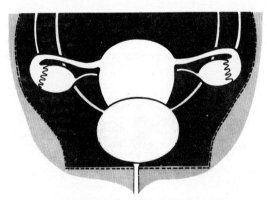

Figure 54.   The shaded area represents the extent of the peritoneum removed in a radical operation for a fixed ovarian tumor. Front view.

With this technique it is possible to remove a large bulk of cancer without an inordinate blood loss. If the tumor involves the rectum and constitutes the only place where macroscopic disease would be left behind, a decision must be made on whether the bowel should be resected to encompass disease. When this is accomplished, the omentum should be removed at the level of the transverse colon. It is important to use suture ligatures to protect against

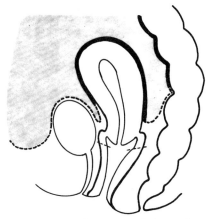

Figure 55. The shaded area represents the extent of the peritoneum removed in a radical operation for a fixed ovarian tumor. Side view.

possible postoperative bleeding. Because the appendix is often involved in the tumor mass, and because it is the site of metastases, its removal is recommended.

P^{32} tubes are placed into the abdomen through trocars, which are pushed through the abdominal wall from inside the abdomen to the skin in each lower quadrant (Figure 56). The trocars are directed lateral to the epigastric vessels. Small baby-feeding tubes with extra holes cut in them are then threaded into the trocar, and the trocar is withdrawn into the pelvic cavity with the tube. The ends of the tubes remain sealed so that when the P^{32} is instilled it has a watering-can effect (Figure 57). The trocar is removed and the tube is placed along the lateral gutter as high as the diaphragm on the right side and to the liver on the left side. The tubes are sutured into place with black silk sutures. One suture is placed in the opening made by the trocar and left long so that it can be tied in place when the P^{32} tube is removed following instillation of the radioactive phosphorus. Phosphorus is instilled within 24 to 48 hours after the completion of the surgery.

The abdomen and pelvis are carefully washed with saline, and the peritoneum is closed with a running chromic #1 suture, which is interrupted at the halfway mark; another similar suture is used to complete the closure. The abdomen is closed without drains. It is important to close the peritoneum carefully so that there will be no leakage from the instillation of the radioactive material. The fascia is closed with #1 chromic interrupted and running sutures. Approximately six to eight nylon retention sutures are used also. The retention sutures are placed through the skin and fascia about 1 cm from the incision and continue to the opposite side, where they secure just the edge of fascia. They continue under the fascia on the opposite side to about 1 cm from the incision, where they are brought through the fascia and skin. When these sutures are tied in place they close the subcutaneous spaces and give good support. Black silk sutures are used to close the skin. A dry

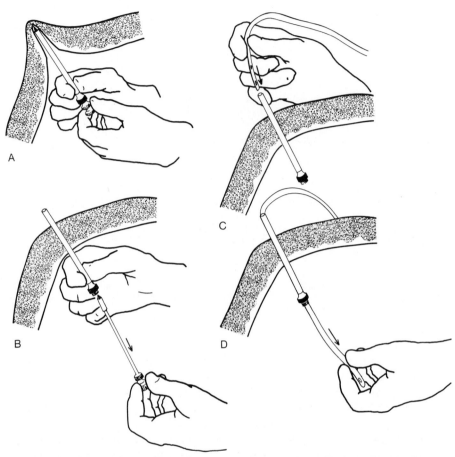

Figure 56. (*A*) Before inserting the tubes for postoperative P^{32} instillation, a trochar is inserted through the abdominal wall from inside the abdomen by raising the skin just above the inguinal ligament. (*B*) The trochar is now through the abdominal wall and the stylet is being removed. (*C*) A small catheter—a baby feeding tube—is being threaded through the trochar. (*D*) Threading the catheter is now advanced. After this, the trochar will be removed.

sterile dressing is placed on the incision. The tubes are taped to the abdomen and the opening made by the trocar is covered with dry sterile dressings.

How Much Is Too Much?

We don't all agree on the amount of tumor that can be excised safely. I try to remove as much as I think I can without risking a gastrointestinal or genitourinary fistula. The success of subsequent chemotherapy or radiation or both, is inversely proportional to the amount of tumor left in the abdomen after surgery. Therefore aggressive surgery is indicated not so much because it is curative, but because it potentiates other forms of treatment. If it is true that the patient is immunized by her own tumors a point is reached where there is acquired tolerance or excess antigen may stimulate a great number of

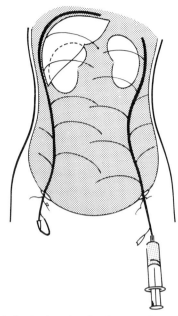

Figure 57.   Cutting multiple holes in the tubes but leaving the ends sealed results in a watering can or sprinkler effect when P^{32} solution is instilled.

antibodies which may form complexes around the tumor. These blocking factors result in a immunologic enhancement which protect the tumor from attack by killer lymphocytes. Therefore, the patient's immune response is improved when the volume of tumor has been decreased.

SUMMARY

Surgical excision should be approached with a planned, methodical technique. The ideal incision is vertical, extending above the limits of the bulk of the cancer and permitting easy exploration. The abdomen and pelvis should be aspirated before the patient is explored. No attempt should be made to excise the tumor mass until the infundibular ligaments are clamped, cut, suture ligated, and doubly secured with a free tie. Attacking the tumor before these steps are taken often results in a hemorrhage that curtails any possibility to debulk or remove the cancer. As much tumor should be removed as is possible without an inordinate morbidity and mortality and without running a risk of a gastrointestinal or genitourinary fistula.

BIBLIOGRAPHY

Barber, H.R.K.: Surgical aspects of ovarian tumors, *in* Selected Topics of Cancer—Current Concepts. Symposia Specialists, Miami, Florida, 1974, p. 161.

Barber, H.R.K.: Ovarian cancer: Still an enigma. Dr. 1:17, 1975.

Barber, H.R.K.: Surgical management of ovarian cancer. Curr. Ob-Gyn Tech. 1:6, 1975.

Barber, H.R.K., Brunschwig, A.: Pelvic exenteration for locally advanced and recurrent ovarian cancer. Review of 22 cases. Surgery 58:935, 1965.

Brunschwig, A.: Attempted palliation by radical surgery in pelvic and abdominal carcinomatosis primarily in the ovaries. Clin. Obstet. Gynecol. 4:875, 1961.

Griffiths, C.T.: Surgical resection of tumor bulk in the primary treatment of ovarian cancer. Natl. Cancer Inst. Monogr. 42:101–104, 1975.

Hudson, C.N., Chir, M.: Surgical treatment of ovarian cancer. Gynecol. Oncol. 1:370–378, 1973.

Symmonds, R.E.: Some surgical aspects of gynecologic cancer. Cancer 36:649–660, 1975.

17

Surgical Treatment of Recurrent Cancer of the Ovary

With the increased use of a radical surgical attack on cancer of the cervix in the 1940s, the same approach was attempted when recurrent ovarian cancer was present. There were ten indications for a radical surgical attack.

1. The tumor was confined to the pelvis.
2. The tumor was surgically resectable.
3. The patient was young enough and in good enough condition to withstand an extensive surgical procedure.
4. All other forms of therapy had been exhausted and there was no other modality of treatment left to offer.
5. The duration of symptoms and extent of disease as determined by clinical and biopsy examination indicated that metastases out of the pelvis are unlikely.
6. The responsible surgeon and his team had to be acquainted with the anatomy and have the technical skill and background to perform the extensive surgery.
7. A thorough knowledge of the natural history of disease was essential.
8. An in-depth knowledge of preoperative and postoperative care was important.
9. An ability to anticipate fluid and electrolyte problems and to correct them in their early stages was necessary.
10. One physician had to manage the patient, and although he could consult freely, it was his responsibility to give painstaking attention to the most minimal details.

The early attempts at a radical surgical approach to ovarian cancer were not too rewarding. In many instances it was possible to remove the macroscopic disease but without a proper knowledge of chemotherapy and the appropriate drugs, recurrent cancer usually appeared within a year. In addition, having undergone extensive resections such as small bowel resection, colectomy, retroperitoneal node dissections, gastrectomy, and removal of large bulky tumors, the patient often experienced fatal metabolic imbalances. Hyperalimentation has changed much of this scenario, and it is now possible to carry these patients in a good nutritional status for long periods of time. Surgery has now come full circle, and with improved chemotherapy and hyperalimentation surgeons are once again becoming surgically aggressive in managing recurrent ovarian cancer.

Cancer of the ovary is characterized by its wide dissemination over peritoneal surfaces of the pelvis, upper abdomen, and omentum, and by the frequent involvement of both ovaries, either as spread from the one primarily involved or as bilateral primary growths. The tendency for rapid extension to the upper abdomen, on theoretical grounds, contraindicates radical surgery. Unlike cervical cancer, ovarian cancer is a surface spreader, while cancer of the cervix infiltrates structures. Obstruction usually is not caused by an absolute occlusion at one point, but by a carcinomatous ileus which results from malignant cell infiltration of the bowel wall and prevents peristalsis.

NONEXENTERATIVE RADICAL SURGERY

Brunschwig carried out extensive resections, short of pelvic exenteration, on 65 patients. He pointed out that many patients with far-advanced cancer of the ovary—who have often been treated in some fashion or another on one or more occasions—present the clinician with a most frustrating problem. Usually such patients have only a short time to live, and immediate relief of symptoms as they evolve is all that is possible. Ironically enough, many of these patients may still appear to be in fair or even good general condition.

Most of the patients exhibited ascites, which in the advanced stage of the disease recurs after previous paracentesis. The large volume of tumor makes it as difficult to control the ascites with radioactive substances, external x-ray therapy, or even chemotherapy. If they do produce a favorable response, it is short-lived in the presence of bulky disease. Debulking the disease usually makes the patient more comfortable, if it can be accomplished without producing inordinate morbidity and mortality. Currently it provides an opportunity to get a second response from chemotherapy and from combinations of chemotherapy and immunotherapy.

There were 65 patients in the heterogenous series reported by Brunschwig. The surgical mortality, defined as death within 30 days of operation, consisted of 7 patients, an incidence of 11%. Three of the postoperative deaths were those of patients who of necessity received very radical upper abdominal excisional procedures involving partial hepatectomy, partial gastrectomy, and partial pancreatectomy. Excluding these, the mortality rate was 4 in 62 patients, a 6% incidence.

Among the survivors in this series, 3 lived 8 to 9 years and 1 lived 10 years free of disease; 1 died of uremia after 5 years, and 8 lived almost a year to 1 year and 5 months. In the 3 surviving 8 to 9 years, the 1 living 10 years, and the 1 surviving more than 5 years, the disease, although recurrent after previous treatment, had metastasized only locally and was macroscopically entirely resectable. The fact that the involvement was localized, however, was not appreciated until laparotomy had been performed.

Obviously, judgment must be exercised in performing radical excisional surgery in these patients. Patients should not be subjected to operation if they are debilitated or elderly individuals with cancer that has spread beyond the abdomen, or with advanced disease which is not causing, at the moment, particularly acute and distressing symptoms. Resection is considered only when symptoms (gastrointestinal disturbances) are severe enough to warrant attempted relief at the cost of the discomforts and risks of an operation.

In the absence of very emphatic contraindications, laparotomy is indicated in selected patients of the type described, because there is always the possibility that the recurrence and/or metastases are localized and macroscopically entirely resectable. With an increased knowledge of chemotherapy and hyperalimentation, there is new hope for salvaging many of these patients after their tumor is debulked.

EXENTERATIVE SURGERY FOR OVARIAN CANCER

In some instances the growths and their local extensions appear to be limited to the pelvic structures, and when there is peritoneal involvement of the pelvis, pelvic colon, and bladder, and/or when the cancer has actually penetrated more deeply into these structures, the question of pelvic exenteration arises as a method of dealing with the situation.

The tendency of such neoplasms toward relatively widespread extension, manifested simultaneously in the pelvis and in the upper abdomen, would, on theoretical grounds, contraindicate these radical procedures. However, since little documentation for the possible palliative effects of incomplete operations on these patients has been recorded, except perhaps for an occasional instance, pelvic exenterations were carried out in a number of cases to ascertain whether they should be more frequently attempted for ovarian cancer, at the moment limited to the pelvis. Twenty-two cases of advanced ovarian cancer, 21 previously treated by surgery and/or irradiation, and 1 a fresh case in which the growth macroscopically was confined to the pelvis, were treated by pelvic exenteration.

Fourteen patients were operated upon 5 or more years previously, including the single fresh case. Total pelvic exenteration was performed on 13, and 1 underwent an anterior pelvic exenteration (excision of bladder, vagina, uterus, adnexae, lower ureters, etc., with preservation of the rectum).

Although the series is small, the 5-year survival rate is 7% among those operated upon between September 1947 and the end of 1958. The single long survivor died of uremia without evidence of recurrent cancer 71 months after operation.

In the postoperative course of these patients, there was a high incidence of complications. Eight of the 11 survivors of the operation required secondary operations, mostly for intestinal fistulas and/or intestinal obstruction. All of these had had previous radiation therapy as well as conservative surgical procedures, and this may account for the incidence of complications.

In 4 of the 11 operative survivors, carcinomatosis was probably the immediate cause of death, the survival period averaging 10 months (7 to 13 months). Others had cancer present at the time of death, except for the 5-year survivor who died of uremia without cancer present. Among the remaining 7, the immediate causes of death were intestinal fistula in 1, intestinal obstruction in 2, uremia in 1, hemorrhage in 2, and cachexia in 1.

Eight patients were operated upon during the years from 1958 through 1962. Six had total and 2 anterior pelvic exenterations. One patient is living and clinically well 27 months after operation, while 6 others all had carcinoma present at the time of death.

The overall surgical mortality, i.e., death within 30 days of operation regardless of cause, was 22.7%. This result contrasts with an overall surgical mortality of 15.2% for 576 total and anterior pelvic exenterations done between 1947 and 1961 for cancer of the cervix.

The eventual course of cancer of the ovary is notoriously unpredictable. Patients without treatment may survive for periods of many months or several years. In the series reviewed above, the average length of time from the first symptom or previous treatment to pelvic exenteration was 42 months or 3.5 years. The extremes were 6 months to 20 years; there was one exception, a single patient not previously treated but whose symptoms began 6 months previously.

The average survival after exenteration, excluding the single survivor for 71 months who died of uremia and the 5 surgical deaths as well as the patient still clinically well at 27 months, was almost 13 months.

It would appear that, in the presence of advanced cancer of the ovary previously treated by conservative surgery and/or irradiation, the indications for pelvic exenteration may be questioned even though the disease appears still confined to the pelvis. The reason for this statement is that usually, when the question of this procedure is posed, the surgeon is operating in the presence of a recurrent or persistent lesion already treated for some months or years previously, and the lesion itself is known to have a marked tendency to widespread metastases to the upper abdomen.

The patients dealt with here were all very unfavorable candidates for any radical procedure by virtue of the situations presented, and these experiences can hardly serve as a basis for firm conclusions on the question of whether or not pelvic exenterations are justified for advanced ovarian cancer even when apparently limited to the pelvis. Certainly, further experiences are necessary before a categoric rejection of the operation is to be recommended. The case of the single long-time survivor (71 months), who eventually died elsewhere of uremia, would suggest that some patients, although admittedly very few, can be salvaged.

The question may be raised as to why, on the basis of the poor 1947 to 1957 results, further surgical procedures were advised and carried out. The answer is that the symptoms were severe enough to warrant an attempt at relief and that there is at least a ray of hope, when by clinical history and knowledge of the situation in these patients the alternative was certain rapid demise. The authors have yet to witness such patients "dying in peace"—a favorite axiom of the proponents of conservative treatment when faced by patients in advanced stages of cancer. Obviously the patients operated upon above were selected. Most of these seen with recurrent or advanced widespread cancer of the ovary were not subjected to pelvic exenteration. Patients were operated upon only if their neoplasms were macroscopically confined to the pelvis and macroscopically completely excisable.

All patients operated on by pelvic exenteration were selected by nature, as evidenced by the fact that all survived from more than 1 year to 13 years from the initial therapy to the diagnosis of recurrence. As stated above, those patients were operated upon only if their neoplasms were macroscopically confined to the pelvis and macroscopically completely excisable. In general, ovarian cancer does not lend itself to excision by pelvic exenteration because of its spread to the upper abdomen. However the series of pelvic exenterations did not include any endometrioid tumors. These tumors have a lesser tendency to be bilateral and also spread less to the upper abdomen than do the other ovarian tumors. In highly selected cases endometrioid ovarian cancer may be controlled by pelvic exenteration. In summary, it can be stated that the natural history of cancer of the cervix permits a radical surgical attack by pelvic exenteration, *while ovarian cancers lend themselves to an exenteration only if they do not have their usual method of spread and, therefore, violate their natural history.*

Indications for Removal of the Bulk of Tumor

1. Psychologic effect
2. To improve response to —
    X-Ray therapy
    Anticancer drugs
3. To reverse—
    Immunosuppression
    Acquired tolerance
    Immunologic enhancement
    Immunoselection
    Antigenic modulation

If a patient goes to the operating room with a large abdomen and returns with the same mass, obviously she knows that nothing could be done. Therefore it is important to try to reduce the tumor mass.

The volume of tumor is important in considering patients for therapy. Radiation therapists feel strongly that nodules over 2 cm do not respond in a predictable manner to therapy because the middle of the nodule contains anoxic cells that respond poorly to radiation therapy. These cells recover and grow. Radiation therapy is not my choice for the treatment of ovarian cancer. The anticancer drugs reduce a constant percentage of tumor cells that are in cycle. For example, the same dose will kill 99% of 100,000 leukemia cells or

99% of 100 cells, whichever number of leukemia cells is present. Therefore 1,000,000 cells can be reduced to 10,000, and 10,000 reduced to 100, and 100 to 10 or less, and then 10 cells to zero. It is obvious why a reduced volume of tumor is important in attempting to achieve a cure.

The immune response fails for many reasons. It is important to reverse some of the factors that inhibit a good immune response. The tumor itself is *immunosuppressant.* Removing a bulk of tumor overcomes a great deal of immunosuppression. This allows the host's own immune response to function more efficiently. *Acquired immunologic tolerance* may occur if a large amount of antigen is released by large tumors, which would thus overwhelm the host's immunologic response. Following the removal of such a large tumor mass, the hosts exhibit resistance to the reimplantations of their own tumor cells, suggesting that the intrinsic failure of the immune response was not the cause of the original lack of immune reaction. Rather, the temporary paralysis observed was due to the fact that the system was unable to cope with too big a challenge.

Immunologic enhancement results from enhancing or blocking antibodies present in the serum. This is a humoral response. These antibodies block the antigenic sites on the surface of the tumor and prevent the killer lymphocytes from attacking the tumor. Removal of a bulk of the tumor removes a great number of these antibodies that have formed complexes on the surface of the tumor. This argument has been advanced to show that a tumor is destroyed by cell-mediated mechanism rather than a humoral mechanism.

Immunoselection suggests that cells within a tumor are presumed to be descendants of a single transformed cell. Thus the bulk of the cells have the same antigen. However, through mutation some develop more antigen and attract a greater number of specific antibodies. They are then eliminated while the cells with few antigens continue to grow. The tumor therefore grows relatively slowly at first and often appears to be restrained, but then it progressively acquires more autonomy and greater invasive properties.

Antigen modulation occurs when an antibody is formed and present, causing the cell to cease synthesizing tumor antigens. This renders an immunologic reaction against tumor cells ineffective. Immunoselection and antigen modulation have not been documented in humans.

SUMMARY

The new orientation in the management of ovarian cancer is to be aggressive. Radical surgery exclusive of pelvic exenteration has proved to be of value in debulking a volume of disease. When this has been accomplished, additional therapy is better able to control the disease. There is only a very limited place for pelvic exenteration in the management of ovarian cancer. Ovarian cancer lends itself to an exenteration only if it does not have its usual method of spread and therefore violates its natural history.

The increased use of hyperalimentation and the improved methods of chemotherapy have expanded the indications for an aggressive surgical attack. The immune response of the host fails for many reasons. Because the tumor itself is immunosuppressant, removing it or debulking it allows the host's own immune response to function more efficiently. The tumor produces antigens which stimulate antibody formation. A great volume of tumor may produce an antigen-antibody complex which acts as a blocking agent on the surface of the cell. Removing a volume of tumor decreases the production of antigens and cuts down on the formation of blocking complexes. The killer lymphocytes are then better able to attack the tumor.

BIBLIOGRAPHY

Barber, H.R.K.: Relative prognostic significance of preoperative and operative findings in pelvic exenteration. Surg. Clin. North Am. 49:431, 1969.

Barber, H.R.K., Brunschwig, A.: Pelvic exenteration for locally advanced and recurrent ovarian cancer. Review of 22 cases. Surgery 58:935, 1965.

Barber, H.R.K., Graber, E.A.: Surgical aspects of ovarian tumors, in Selected Topics of Cancer—Current Concepts. Symposia Specialists, Miami, 1974, pp. 161–183.

Barber, H.R.K., Kwon, T.; Current status of the treatment of gynecologic cancer by site—Ovary. Cancer 38:610, 1976.

Brunschwig, A.: Attempted palliation by radical surgery in pelvic and abdominal carcinomatosis primarily in the ovaries. Clin. Obstet. Gynecol. 4:875, 1961.

Griffiths, C.T.: Surgical resection of tumor bulk in the primary treatment of ovarian cancer. Natl. Cancer Inst. Monogr. 42:101–104, 1975.

Hudson, C.N., Chir, M.: Surgical treatment of ovarian cancer. Gynecol. Oncol. 1:370–378, 1973.

Symmonds, R.E.: Some surgical aspects of gynecologic cancer. Cancer 36:649–660, 1975.

Tobias, J.S., Griffiths, C.T.: Management of ovarian cancer. Current concepts and future prospects. N. Engl. J. Med. 294:818, 1976.

18

Second Look Operation

Early diagnosis in ovarian cancer is a matter of chance rather than a scientific method. The same frustration confounds any attempt at detecting early recurrence of disease. Currently, laparoscopic examination and laparotomy are the only means available that have a predictable rate of accuracy. Periodic gynecologic examinations have not been helpful. Cul-de-sac aspiration, cytology, and serum enzyme studies have limited application in the initial diagnosis and have offered very little as methods for monitoring the progress of these patients. Sonography is currently being evaluated but has not been helpful in following these patients. There is no accumulated data available on the new scanners such as computerized axial tomography (CAT).

The second look concept has many interpretations. The one followed in this chapter relates to patients who have had known disease that could not be adequately removed at the time of surgery, but in whom the tumor regressed after additional therapy so that there was no longer any evidence of disease. The other group of patients in whom a second look has been employed consists of those from whom all the disease was removed at the time of the original operation, and to whom prophylactic chemotherapy was then given for a period ranging from 18 months to 2 years. At this time, in order to judge whether treatment can be stopped in the absence of any palpable disease, an exploratory laparotomy with multiple biopsies is carried out. If disease is palpable or detectable by any means prior to surgery, it is not a second look procedure but a planned type of therapy, hopefully to excise all the tumor or to relieve a complication such as an obstruction, fistula, or abscess.

The second look operation has become an established part of the protocol of many centers for patients with common epithelial or nonepithelial ovarian cancers who have received radiation therapy, chemotherapy, or a combination of treatments. Recently, *C. parvum* has been added to the therapy regimens in a limited number of centers. Following therapy for 1 or 2 years without evidence of palpable disease, the patient is reexplored to see if the disease has been controlled. A few centers are doing laparoscopy evaluations at stated intervals to follow the response of treatment in their patients. Evidence of disease is a positive response, but inability to demonstrate disease does not mean that disease is not present, and laparotomy is then indicated to evaluate accurately the response to treatment.

The most important question concerning the second look operation is whether it is possible to offer the patient a second chance for cure if disease is present. An attempt will be made to answer this question from personal experience and a review of the literature.

The second look operation was popularized, if not introduced, by Wangenstein, for patients who had cancers arising in the stomach and colon and who had a response to treatment and were asymptomatic at the time of the second look operation. About half of these patients were found to have disease present and only 9% were salvaged by this operation. Park, Corscaden, Kottmeier, Rutledge, and Burns and Smith have carried out second look procedures. None of their patients had a dramatic response in the presence of residual or recurrent tumor, despite a change in their therapeutic regimen.

The second look operation gave the surgeon the opportunity (1) to explore the patient and remove all of the residual tumor or to reduce the tumor mass and improve the patient's chances with a new regimen of treatment; (2) to outline the site of the tumor and to determine the status of the residual tumor; and (3) to program a plan of therapy for the patient. It is obvious that patients with stage I or II disease in whom all disease has been removed and chemotherapy is given prophylactically will have fewer recurrences than patients in stages III and IV treated therapeutically for residual disease after initial treatment.

It is difficult to interpret the reports in the literature based on the natural history of common epithelial ovarian cancer. The results from initial therapy for invasive epithelial ovarian cancer range from a 15% to a 35% 5-year survival. Therefore from 85 to 65% (based on a survival of 15 to 35%) should present with recurrence after initial therapy. Having treated those patients with a recurrence after a second look operation, the physician faces the question of whether additional treatment has anything to offer.

Tepper reported a series of 17 patients with advanced cancer who had exploratory laparotomy, 3000 rads of radiation therapy, thio-tepa, and second look surgery. His results were that 10 of the 17 patients were dead in less than 2 years because of pelvic and abdominal recurrences. Seven survived over 3 years (41%) 4 with repeated courses of chemotherapy and/or irradiation for recurrence. The average survival time of the whole group from the time of diagnosis was 29 months and 20 months without a recurrence, and for stage III it was 30 months and 23 months without a recurrence. Three patients were free of disease at 48, 67, and 77 months. One was stage IIB and 2 were stage III. The respective histologic types of these 3 patients were papillary serous cystadenocarcinoma, mucinous carcinoma, and granulosa cell carcinoma. The survival of the patients who underwent removal of the tumor was 39 months, versus 20 months in those with gross residual tumors.

Wallach, Kabakow, and Blinick performed a second look operation 10 times in 240 patients with advanced carcinoma of the ovary treated initially by surgery and postoperative chemotherapy with triethylenethiophosphoramide. Following second look operation, survival ranged from 8 months to 100 months. The patient who survived 100 months continued living with a palpable tumor. Therefore 8 of 10 patients died and 1 was living following the second look procedure. Wallach and coworkers report that the second look operation should be performed for patients with retained ovaries and complete clinical regression of tumor after administration of chemotherapy, and for selected patients in whom interval treatment permits surgical clearance of tumor. They conclude that the new drugs may create an expanded role for second look operation.

Rutledge lists several reasons for reexploration: (1) The patient may have had a sufficient amount of the drug. (2) The tumor may become more localized and possibly resectable for the first time. (3) The benefit from the drug may be exhausted and it may be time to switch to another drug. (4) The mass may now be suitable for irradiation. (5) It may be suspected that the mass that has served as a guide to the drug action is not cancer, as was originally presumed.

Smith reports that about 1 in 8 of the patients treated at M.D. Anderson Hospital with melphalan have had a second look operation. Among 103 patients who had a second look operation, 65% survived an additional 2 years and 34% survived 5 years. Twenty-three patients were found to have no cancer by multiple biopsies and cytologic studies, and chemotherapy was stopped. Five of these patients developed recurrent cancer; however 4 had received only four cycles of chemotherapy before surgery and the fifth patient probably had inadequate sampling at the time of the second look operation. The patient developed distant metastases several months after surgery. Fourteen of 103 patients who had a second look operation and were found to have cancer at the time of their surgery are presently alive 2 to 10 years after surgery without evidence of disease. Thirteen of these patients had all or almost all of their cancer removed at their second look operation and were either continued on chemotherapy or given irradiation. Those receiving radiation had a survival rate of only 14% after second look operation, but 30% of those given chemotherapy survived for 5 years.

The survival rate for patients who had a second look operation was proportional to the number of cycles of chemotherapy they received before surgery. Among patients who received four or fewer cycles of chemotherapy before the second look operation, 2 of 23 (9%) survived 5 years, whereas among those receiving five to nine courses, 6 of 19 (32%) and those receiving 10 or more courses, 8 of 10 (80%) survived 5 years. All of the patients who received more than 12 cycles of chemotherapy before the second look operation were alive and well. Only patients from whom it was possible to remove all or almost all of the remaining cancer were benefited by a second look operation. Therefore an aggressive approach is indicated at the time of surgery.

It is difficult to answer the initial question about the value of a second look operation. If it is possible to control and/or reduce the tumor volume so that all or almost all of the remaining cancer can be removed, the procedure has value. However in most instances this is not possible. The greatest contribution of second look operation may be demonstrated if the new drugs (adriamycin, cis-platinum, and hexamethylmelamine) give a predictable response after the present first line of drugs fail. Currently the second look operation serves its greatest purpose in the decision on whether anticancer therapy can be safely stopped. It must be carried out with great caution after radiation therapy or radioactive gold instillation. The complication rate is increased considerably over that following treatment with anticancer drugs.

SUMMARY

The contribution made by the second look operation has given rise to a great deal of controversy. One of the problems has been the lack of a firm definition. The definition chosen for this chapter relates to the apparent regression of disease left at laparotomy but controlled by additional therapy, or to the evaluation of the patient who has no apparent disease after surgery but has been on chemotherapy for 2 years and is clinically free of disease. Currently, the most important use of the second look operation is in the decision on whether to stop anticancer therapy. If the new drugs such as adriamycin, cis-platinum, and hexamethylmelamine prove to have value after the first line drugs (alkylating agents) fail, there will be an additional indication for a second look procedure. If disease is palpable or detectable by any means prior to surgery, the operation cannot be literally called a second look procedure. It is a planned procedure carried out to excise known tumor or to relieve a complication.

BIBLIOGRAPHY

Arhelger, S.W., Jenson, C.B., Wangensteen, O.H.: Experience with the "second look" procedure in the management of cancer of the colon and rectum. Lancet 77:412, 1957.

Mackman, S., Curreri, A.R., Ansfield, F.J.: Second look operation for colon carcinoma after fluorouracil therapy. Arch. Surg. 100:527, 1970.

Perez, C.A., Olson, J.: Preoperative vs. postoperative irradiation: Comparison in experimental animal tumor system. Am. J. Roentgenol. Radium Ther. Nuc. Med. 108:396, 1970.

Rutledge, F., Burns, B.C.: Chemotherapy for advanced ovarian cancer. Am. J. Obstet. Gynecol. 107:691, 1970.

Smith, J.P.: Chemotherapy in gynecologic cancer. Clin. Obstet. Gynecol. 18:109, 1975.

Tepper, E., San Filippo, L.J., Gray, J., Romney, S.: Second look surgery after radiation therapy for advanced stages of cancer of the ovary. Am. J. Roentgenol. Radium Ther. Nucl. Med. 112:755, 1971.

Wallach, R.C., Kabakow, B., Blinick, G.: Current status of the second look operation in ovarian carcinoma. Natl. Cancer Inst. Monogr. 42:105, 1974.

Wallach, R.C., Kabakow, B., Jerez, E., Blinick, G.: The importance of second look surgical procedures in the staging and treatment of ovarian carcinoma. Semin. Oncol. 2:243, 1975.

19

The Role of Radioactive Isotopes in the Management of Ovarian Cancer

A working knowledge of the physics of radioactive isotopes is important in the management of clinical problems. A few definitions and a superficial review of basic principles will be reviewed. An *isotope* is a chemical element having the same atomic number as another (i.e., the same number of nuclear protons) but with a different atomic mass (i.e., a different number of nuclear neutrons). A *radionuclide* is an atomic nucleus that will decay spontaneously into some other radioactive nuclear species, accompanied by the liberation of energy. *Bremsstrahlung (Brems rays)* is a name applied whenever high-speed electrons, regardless of their source, are abruptly slowed down, and their energy is converted to electromagnetic radiation. If the energy is large enough, the electromagnetic radiation is in the x-ray region. High energy β-particles, passing close to atomic nuclei, undergo deceleration and also give rise to Brems radiation.

All matter is made up of chemical substances which can be divided into two kinds, elements and compounds. An *element* is a distinct kind of matter that cannot be decomposed into two or more simpler kinds of matter. A *compound* is formed when two or more elements combine chemically to produce a more complex type of matter. *Atoms* are the smallest particles of an element that can exist without losing the chemical properties of the element. *Molecules* are the smallest particles of a compound that can exist without losing the chemical properties of the compound.

The atom is an electrical structure with three basic units—the proton, the neutron and the electron. This concept is adequate for an understanding of most phenomena in radiological physics.

The simplest atom is the element hydrogen. It consists of a central nucleus comprising one proton around which one electron moves in a shell or orbit. The proton is a heavy particle carrying a positive charge, and the electron is a very much lighter particle with a negative charge of exactly equal magnitude (but of opposite sign) to that of the proton. Therefore almost all of the mass of the atom is in the nucleus, and the positive charge of the nucleus is balanced by the negative charge of the electron to make the atom as a whole electrically neutral (Figure 58).

The next simplest atom is the element helium. Its nucleus comprises two protons and two neutrons and there are two orbital electrons moving around the nucleus. A *neutron* is a particle with a mass approximately equal to that of a proton but with no electrical charge. The nucleus of the helium atom therefore has a positive charge of 2 units (because there are two protons) and a mass of approximately 4 units. Also, the two positive charges of the nucleus are balanced by the two negatively charged electrons around the nucleus.

Every element has a mass number and an atomic number (Z). The *atomic number* of an element is the number of protons in the nucleus of an atom of that element; this number is equal to the number of electrons around the nucleus. The *mass number* of an atom is the total number of protons and neutrons in the nucleus. It gives a measure of the mass of the nucleus. Protons and neutrons are known collectively as *nucleons* because they are found in the nucleus. The atomic number is written to the left and below the symbol for the element. For sulfur it is $_{16}S$. The atomic mass is written above and to the right, e.g., S^{32}. Atomic mass and number may also be designated by placing the mass above the atomic number, e.g., $^{32}/_{16}$.

The radioactive isotopes now referred to as radionuclides occur as natural or artificial radionuclides. Most radioisotopes remain permanently unchanged. However some isotopes, especially the very heavy ones (which have many more neutrons than protons), are unstable. Their nuclei undergo a process of spontaneous readjustment or transformation with partial disintegration so that they change into isotopes of other elements. In this process they emit ionizing radiation, and this emission of radiation accompanying nuclear transformations is called radioactivity.

Naturally occurring radioactivity is found mostly in a few heavy elements, e.g., radium. However it is now possible to produce artificial

Fundamental Building Blocks
of an Atomic Nucleus

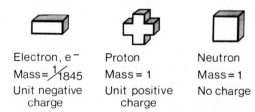

Electron, e^-	Proton	Neutron
Mass $= 1/1845$	Mass $= 1$	Mass $= 1$
Unit negative charge	Unit positive charge	No charge

Figure 58. The massive central portion of the atom consists of two major components: positively charged protons and uncharged neutrons. The mass of the protons and that of the neutrons is nearly the same. The number of protons in any atom determines and is designated by the atomic number (Z); the atomic mass (A) is the number of protons and neutrons in the nucleus. The electron has a mass of only 1/1845 of the mass of the proton. It has a negative charge of equal magnitude to that of the proton.

radioactive isotopes of all the chemical elements by subjecting them to bombardment by neutrons in the nuclear reactor or atomic furnace where atomic energy is produced.

These radiations, whether from natural or artificial radioisotopes, are of three kinds, named after the first three letters of the Greek alphabet—alpha rays (or particles), beta rays (or particles), and gamma rays (electromagnetic energy).

Alpha particles are streams of high-speed helium nuclei (two protons and two neutrons packed tightly together) that have been ejected from radioactive substances.

Beta rays are streams of fast-moving electrons (particles) ejected from radioactive substances with velocities that may be as high as 0.98 of the velocity of light. In soft tissues beta rays can travel distances ranging from small fractions of a millimeter up to about 1 centimeter, producing ionization in their path.

Gamma rays come from radioactive substances. When they are produced by electrical machines we call them x-rays. They differ fundamentally from alpha and beta radiations, in that they are not particles but waves of the same type as light and radiowaves but with different properties because of their very much shorter wave length.

Where does the beta particle arise? The beta particle is an electron. Since there are no electrons in the nucleus, how can a beta particle be emitted when the nucleus undergoes a process of spontaneous readjustment or transformation? The answer is that the beta particle comes from a neutron in the nucleus. Neutrons change into a proton and an electron, and the electron is then ejected from the nucleus. Emission of this electron or beta particle from the nucleus (beta decay) does not change the mass number (the total number of particles in the nucleus), but it does increase the atomic number by one: $_{15}P^{32} \longrightarrow {}_{16}S^{32} + 1B^0$. To complete the picture, isotopes were found which emitted positively charged electrons or positrons. Where do the positrons come from? The answer is that a positron is ejected: $_{25}Mn^{52} \longrightarrow {}_{24}Cr^{52} + 1B^0$. Again the atomic mass remains the same, but since the proton is changed to a neutron there is loss of the proton and the atomic number decreases by one (Figure 59).

Any adjunct therapy must be directed to the areas involved by ovarian cancer. This type of cancer spreads over the surface of organs and structures rather than infiltrating them early, as so many other cancers do. Ovarian cancer involves the right diaphragm as well as the paraaortic nodes in a high percentage of the patients studied. As much as 80% of the lymphatic drainage of the peritoneum is to the right thoracic trunk by way of the diaphragmatic lymphatics and the retrosternal nodes. In stage I ovarian cancer with an encapsulated unilateral cancer and without evidence of tumor elsewhere, on careful examination about 10 to 15% are found to have metastases to the right diaphragm. Meyer injected radioactive material into the peritoneal cavity in human beings and monitored its course. Ascent up the left paracolic gutter was found to be blocked by the left phrenicocolic liga-

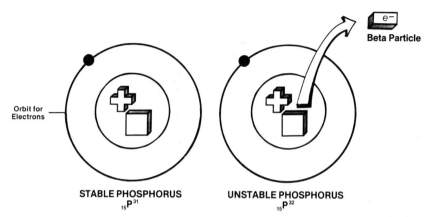

Figure 59. Beta rays are high-speed electrons that are ejected from the nucleus at speeds approaching the velocity of light rays.

ment. Virtually all of the flow was found to progress to the right subhepatic and subphrenic spaces.

Radionuclides instilled into the peritoneal cavity covered the serosal surfaces and the omentum, as well as being taken up by retroperitoneal nodes. In 1945 Muller first used radionuclides clinically in the management of ovarian cancer. Radioactive zinc (^{63}Zn) was first produced with the cyclotron in 1945 and used to control malignant effusions. Radioactive gold (^{198}Au) was introduced in 1947. Other isotopes such as radioactive phosphate (^{32}P) and yttrium (^{90}Y) have been introduced. Currently only two radionuclides, gold and phosphate, are being used. Their characteristics are recorded as shown in Table 1. It often comes as a surprise that radioactive phosphate is more expensive than radioactive gold. The explanation is that neutrons produced by the fission of uranium 235 can be used to convert natural elements into artificial radioactive isotopes by so-called neutron capture. This is the preferred way to produce radioactive cobalt 60, gold 198, iridium 192, and many other radioisotopes used in medicine. ^{32}P, which is widely used in radiation therapy, cannot be produced in this simple way because it requires an intermediate step: First, sulfur (^{32}S) is converted by neutron capture to ^{33}S. ^{33}S then decays to ^{32}P, which then must be chemically separated from the sulfur (Figure 60).

Currently, the radionuclides gold and phosphate are most often used. Several important observations have been made following the instillation of these radionuclides:

1. Malignant effusions can be controlled in up to 80% of patients.
2. Little or no control of malignant effusions has been observed in patients with residual bulk disease.
3. Prophylactically, the instillation of radioactive substances has been found to improve survival results, especially in stage I ovarian cancer.
4. In the presence of multiple adhesions, the instillation of radionuclides is followed by a complication rate that offsets the benefit received.

	Gold ^{198}AU	Chromic Phosphate $CrP^{32}O^4$
Physical characteristics	Colloid	Suspension
Particle size (micra)	0.003–0.0007	0.5–1.5
Emission (%)	Beta 90 Gamma, 10	Beta 100
Energy (Kv)	1700	960
Maximum energy	0.97 Mev Beta 0.411 Mev Gamma	1.7 Mev
Maximum path in tissue (mm)	4	4–6
Half-life (days)	2.7	14.3
Dose (mCi)	100 to 150	10–15
Cost	$64	$250
Side effect	Up to 30 including nausea, vomiting, ileus, temperature elevation, and pain at the site of instillation. Late dense adhesions and bowel necrosis.	Rare
Radiation precautions	Yes, for at least 6.5 days	None

Stable Phosphorus , Unstable Phosphorus and Stable Sulfur

$$_{15}P^{32} \longrightarrow {}_{16}S^{32} + {}^{-1}\beta^{0} \qquad\qquad _{15}P^{32} \xrightarrow{\ \beta\ } {}_{16}S^{32}$$

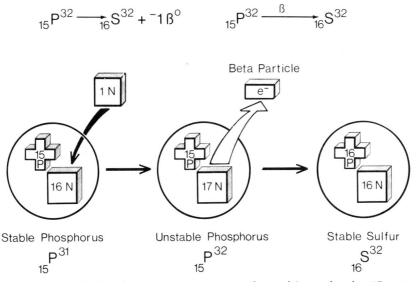

Beta Particle

Stable Phosphorus $_{15}P^{31}$	Unstable Phosphorus $_{15}P^{32}$	Stable Sulfur $_{16}S^{32}$

Figure 60. When stable phosphorus captures a neutron, the resulting nucleus has 17 neutrons, its energy has been raised to a higher level, and it is heavier by the addition of 1 mass unit. The atom is still phosphorus, for as yet there has been no change in the number of protons. For this unstable phosphorus atom, phosphorus 32, to return to a stable state, it must eliminate one of its 17 neutrons. This is accomplished by converting one into a proton with the formation of an electron e^-. The electron is ejected from the nucleus as a beta particle.

5. In patients who have had external radiation therapy, the instillation of radionuclides increases the complication rate, especially of the gastrointestinal tract.

The author has had limited experience with radioactive gold but considerable experience with radioactive phosphate. The reasons for selecting radiophosphorus was a direct result of the increased complications from the radioactive gold. Although the initial complications were minor, they included nausea, vomiting, temperature elevation, and pain. It was the delayed complication rate that was disturbing. The adhesions which followed the instillation of radiactive gold were very dense. In addition, the serosa of the bowel was thickened and fibrosed, and the intestine often lost its pink color and looked white. There were some late complications of bowel necrosis and fistula. Among patients treated by radioactive gold who required laparotomy for any reason, the complication rate, particularly of the gastrointestinal tract, was prohibitive. However radioactive gold is employed as an adjunct therapy and will be discussed.

Currently Keetel and Buchsbaum have accumulated the largest experience with radioactive gold as an adjunct therapy of localized ovarian cancer. In addition to the beta ray which makes up 90% of the colloid, the gold also gives off a gamma ray. The usual dose of radiogold is 150 mCi instilled into the peritoneal cavity. It has been calculated that the serosa receives 4,000 rads, the omentum 6,000 rads, and the retroperitoneal nodes and mesenteric lymph nodes 7,000 rads (maximum up to 10,000 to 30,000 rads). Spilling of activity into the reticuloendothelial system of the liver and spleen accounted for 130 rads and 250 rads respectively, while the kidney received 30 rads. Approximately 750 rads of diffuse penetrating gamma radiation has been reported. Keetel found the ultramicroscopic gold particles are picked up by the peritoneal macrophages and fixed to serosal surfaces. In addition, cells floating in the peritoneal cavity are subjected to a lethal dose of radiation.

The technique used for radioactive gold instillation into the peritoneal cavity was the same as that employed to instill radioactive phosphorus. This technique will be described in detail, but first the technique employed by Buchsbaum and Keetel will be described as reported by them. The technique is carried out as follows:

The patient is asked to void and is then sedated with intramuscular diazepam. The abdomen is prepared with providine-iodine and draped. The abdominal wall is infiltrated with a local anesthetic, and a long polyethylene catheter is introduced into the peritoneal cavity over a trocar needle. A puncture site is selected which is away from previous scars. After the needle is withdrawn, the catheter is attached to the infusion system. One infusion bottle contains a radiopaque contrast material in normal saline; the other bottle contains normal saline which is used to flush the gold into the peritoneal cavity. A three-way stopcock controls the flow of liquid.

The catheter is fixed to the abdominal wall and approximately 400 ml of saline with radiopaque medium is introduced into the peritoneal cavity. The distribution of the contrast material is monitored under fluoroscopy. Careful monitoring is necessary to insure that the catheter tip is in the peritoneal cavity and not in the abdominal wall or in the bowel lumen. When contrast material is seen above the liver and in the pelvis films are taken. Only after adequate distribution has been documented is the radioactive gold (150 mCi) introduced into the peritoneal cavity. An additional 600 ml of saline is instilled to create a hydroperitoneum.

The catheter is then removed, the puncture site sutured, and a collodion dressing applied. In the past, we had the patient change positions frequently to aid in the distribution of the isotope. We now use an electrocircular bed which allows the patient's position to be changed in a controlled fashion for the first four hours. The patient is kept in the supine position, head down, and head up, and in the prone position, head down, head up, for 15 minutes each. After four hours she is taken off the bed and housed in a controlled environment for the required $6\frac{1}{2}$ days.

The radionuclide ^{32}P is instilled after treatment of stages I and II ovarian cancer and in stage III when there is no disease left in place (when disease is limited to the omentum or only small scattered metastases are present). If the patient has had bowel pathology, marked adhesions, or evidences of infection, it is in the best interest of the patient to withhold the instillation of the ^{32}P.

The technique employed for the instillation of ^{32}P is now described. The only equipment necessary in the operating room is a trocar and a small catheter (a baby-feeding tube) which is threaded through the trocar. Just before the abdomen is closed, the trocar is taken from inside the abdominal incision and brought out in both the right and left lower quadrants. The trocar is passed above the external iliac artery and vein lateral to the psoas muscle to avoid injuring any vessel. Lateral to the epigastric vessels it is pushed through the peritoneum lateral to the rectus muscle and out through the skin. The trocar emerges above the inguinal ligament. The stylet of the trocar is removed and the small catheter (a baby-feeding tube) is threaded through the trocar and pulled into the abdomen. The trocar is pulled back into the abdominal cavity and removed. Some small extra holes are cut in the catheter but the tip is left sealed. This causes a "watering-can" effect when the ^{32}P is instilled through the tube. The tube is placed high in the abdomen. On the right side it is placed above the liver and on the left side is brought high into the abdomen. The skin around the catheter is then stiched in a fashion that resembles the lacing of an old-fashioned ankle-high shoe. The final stitch is left long so that it can be tied after the radioactive substance has been instilled and the tube pulled out. This assures that there will be no leakage of the radioactive material from the abdominal cavity. The tubes are slowly withdrawn during the process of the ^{32}P instillation.

In the early part of the study, radiopaque material was instilled into the peritoneal cavity to study the distribution. By observing the criteria established and reported above it was found that the distribution was excellent. Covington and Hilaris utilized ^{32}P scans for intracavitary distribution studies. Since ^{32}P is a pure beta emitter, the question is raised about its use as a screening agent. Bremsstrahlung x-ray (with energies from 1.7 MeV to 0) is produced when electrons are slowed down passing by a positively charged nucleus of tissue atoms. Scans are produced by the Bremsstrahlung x-ray. When intracavitary doses (5–20 mCi) of ^{32}P chromic phosphate are used, enough Bremsstrahlung x-ray (about 1% of the total energy) is produced to make good scans, even in large patients. Covington and Hilaris reported that this fact was not appreciated in the past, and probably accounts for the lack of use of ^{32}P scans for intracavitary distribution studies. The previous disappointing and poor results of ^{32}P as a scanning agent for the detection of tumors were attributable to the very small amount of isotope used (usually less than 0.5 mCi); this amount simply did not give off enough Bremsstrahlung x-ray to produce a diagnostic scan. The findings at Lenox Hill Hospital from our studies agreed with those of Covington and Hilaris. The distribution was generally very good when omentectomy was added to the hysterectomy and bilateral salpingo-oophorectomy.

It is difficult to compare series from the literature. However our results in stage I ovarian cancer was approximately 90% when surgery plus ^{32}P was the treatment. In other series some form of radiation therapy was used in conjunction with radioisotopes. The combined use of ^{32}P and external x-ray therapy added to our complication rate, and the combination was discontinued. Clark and associates reported a 92.8% and Moore and Langley a 90% 5-year survival in patients treated with radioisotopes for stage I ovarian cancer.

SUMMARY

The role of radioactive isotopes in the management of ovarian cancer has not been completely accepted. The use of radionuclides in the management of patients with common epithelial ovarian cancer is controversial. Each physician charged with the responsibility of treating patients with ovarian cancer must make his own judgment on whether to include it in his protocol of therapy. We feel that it has been beneficial in stage I cancers of the ovary. Although it has been employed in stages II and III where gross disease has been removed, the results in survival are not as dramatic as those reported for stage I.

The origin of the beta rays and the characteristics of gold 198 and phosphate 32 are discussed. It is included as a review for those physicians using radionuclides.

BIBLIOGRAPHY

Aure, J.C., Hoeg, K., Kolstad, P.: Radioactive colloidal gold in the treatment of ovarian carcinoma. Acta Radiol. (Ther.) 10:399, 1971.

Bagely, C.M., Jr., Young, R.C., Schein, P.S., et al.: Ovarian carcinoma metastatic to the diaphragm—Frequently undiagnosed at laparotomy: A preliminary report. Am. J. Obstet. Gynecol. 116:397, 1973.

Buschsbaum, H.J., Keetel, W.C., Lataurette, H.B.: The use of radiosotope as ajdunct therapy of localized ovarian cancer. Semin. Oncol. 2:247, 1975.

Clark, D.G.C., Hilaris, B., Ochoa, M.: Treatment of cancer of the ovary. Clin. Obstet. Gynecol. 3:150, 1976.

Clark, D.G.C., Hilaris, B., Roussis, C., et al.: The role of radiation therapy (including isotopes) in the treatment of cancer of the ovary (results of 614 patients treated at Memorial Hospital, New York). Prog. Clin. Cancer 5:227, 1973.

Covington, E., Hilaris, B.: ^{32}P scans for intracavitary studies. Am. J. Roentgenol. Radium Ther. Nucl. Med. 118:895, 1973.

Decker, D.G., Webb, M.J., Holbrook, M.A.: Radiogold treatment of epithelial cancer of ovary: Late results. Am. J. Obstet. Gynecol. 115:751, 1973.

Feldman, G.B., Knapp, R.C.: Lymphatic drainage of the peritoneal cavity and its significance in ovarian cancer. Am. J. Obstet. Gynecol. 119:991, 1974.

Hester, L.L., White, L.: Radioactive colloidal chromic phosphate in the treatment of ovarian malignancies. Am. J. Obstet. Gynecol. 103:911, 1969.

Keetel, W.C., Fox, M.R., Longnecker, D.S., Latourette, H.B.: Prophylactic use of radioactive gold in the treatment of primary ovarian cancer. Am. J. Obstet. Gynecol. 94:766, 1966.

Meyers, M.A.: The spread and localization of acute intraperitoneal effusions. Radiology 95:547, 1970.

Moore, D.W., Langley, J., II.: Routine use of radiogold following operation for ovarian cancer. Am. J. Obstet. Gynecol. 98:624, 1967.

Müller, J.H.: Curative aim and results of routine intraperitoneal radiocolloid administration in the treatment of ovarian cancer. Am. J. Roentgenol. Radium Ther. Nucl. Med. 89:533, 1963.

Priver, M.S.: Radioactive colloids in the treatment of stage Ia ovarian cancer. Obstet. Gynecol. 40:42, 1972.

Reid, G.W., Watson, E.R., Chester, M.S.: A note on the distribution of radioactive colloidal gold following intraperitoneal injection. Br. J. Radiol. 34:323, 1961.

20

The Role of Chemotherapy in Ovarian Cancer

In contrast to surgery plus radiation (which is considered to be the definitive therapy for cancer), chemotherapy—the treatment of cancer with drugs and hormones—can be used effectively for disseminated as well as localized cancer. Chemothereapy has become a reality only in the past 32 years. In 1945 nitrogen mustard was found to be effective against lymphomas. Each of the three decades since then has seen important advances in the number of compounds available and in the spectrum of their usefulness. Since that time many drugs have been added to the therapeutic armamentarium. Within the last decade it has become clear that, although chemotherapy had long been considered largely a palliative procedure capable of extending but not saving lives, certain kinds of cancer can now be cured by anticancer drug therapy (chemical treatment). A major goal of current cancer chemotherapy is to achieve cures by prompt and vigorous treatment of such cancers. Combinations of antineoplastic drugs have been used with success, particularly when each drug used acts on the cancer cell in a different way. Progress has been made by using multiple drugs simultaneously as well as in sequence.

In patients whose cancers are limited to a bodily region that has an accessible separate blood supply, the introduction of chemotherapeutic agents into an artery which supplies the cancer tissue has provided substantial benefits.

Certain cancers can be cured by chemotherapy. Chemotherapy now constitutes a major and indispensable therapeutic approach capable of producing cures in particular kinds of widespread cancers. Among those cancers responding to chemotherapy are choriocarcinoma, metastatic hydatidiform mole, Burkitt's tumor, acute lymphatic leukemia of children, Hodgkin's disease, embryonal carcinoma of the testis, embryonal carcinoma of the ovary, extraembryonal carcinoma of the ovary, adenocarcinomas of the uterine corpus, and carcinomas in the superficial layers of the skin. Chemotherapy has provided therapeutic benefits but not cures in a number of other types of cancer. Chronic myelocytic leukemia and chronic lymphocytic leukemia, lymphosarcoma, reticulum cell sarcoma, multiple myeloma, polycythemia vera, mycosis fungoides, malignant melanoma, Wilm's tumor, and neuroblastoma are other forms of cancer in which palliation and clinical improvement can be achieved by chemotherapy, and for which in the disseminated state, chemotherapy is the preferred means of treatment.

In addition, several types of carcinoma are also significantly benefited by anticancer drug therapy. Clinical improvement and significant palliation occur but long-term freedom from the disease has not been observed in any appreciable fraction of the patients. Carcinomas of the breast, large intestine, stomach, pancreas, prostate, epithelium of the head and neck, thyroid, ovary and adrenal gland are all subject to palliation in a proportion of the patients when the appropriate anticancer chemotherapeutic drugs are used. The drug regimens differ widely for the several different types of cancer mentioned.

With some cancers the effects of the anticancer drugs that have been used so far have been notably unpredictable. Although the tumors may show some response and decrease in size, major clinical benefit has not ordinarily accompanied this regression in patients with carcinomas of the lung, cervix, kidney, or bladder.

STRUCTURE OF THE CELL

Cancer is a disease of the cell. Structures within the cell are visible with the electron microscope. The important structures that have been identified and whose functions have been studied are briefly outlined.

The *nucleus* contains the master chemical deoxyribonucleic acid (DNA) in the chromosomes; the *nucleolus* found in the nucleus is considered the storehouse of DNA as well as the transport mechanism for messenger RNA (mRNA). The *cytoplasm* contains the protein-making sites or ribosomes. The *endoplasmic reticulum* is the network to which the ribosomes adhere. *Mitochondria* are the site of energy metabolism and probably have a limited production of protein. The *Golgi complex* is thought to play a key role in intracellular synthesis and mobilization of certain proteins and carbohydrate components. The *plasma membrane* is a complex structure through which materials pass in and out of the cell. Plasma membrane is the area of contact between a cell with its neighbors; it permits the passage of ions and molecules, influences the movement of the cell, and probably plays an important role in controlling growth.

Of all cell parts that theoretically may become transformed in malignancy, the cell surface is currently the most suspect. Changes in the cell surface control the uptake and release of material from the cell as well as controlling adhesiveness and cohesiveness. These properties may influence invasion and metastasis. It is not surprising that cell surface transplantation antigens are altered in malignancy. Although such tumor-specific antigens are not confined to the surface, it is on the surface of the intact cell that they are most readily detected. The tumor-specific transplantation antigens (TSTA) present on the cell surface are responsible for and sensitive to the immune response in the host which may result in tumor destruction.

CELL KINETICS OR CELL DIVISION

Cellular reproduction (cell division cycle or cell kinetics) is divided into five phases: (1) *growth 1* (G1), which is postmitotic and takes up at least one-half the life cycle of the cell; (2) *synthesis* (S), in which the DNA content is doubled and takes up about 29 to 30% of the life cycle of the cell; (3) *growth 2* (G2), which occurs just before mitosis and takes up about 19 to 20% of the life cycle of the cell; (4) *mitosis* (M), which takes up about 1% of the cell cycle; and (5) *growth 0* (G0), the resting or nondividing phase of the cell. This phase is variable and depends upon the type of cancer.

Studies on cell kinetics reveal that certain anticancer drugs have a more predictable effect on different phases of the cell. The alkylating agents attack cells in all phases of the division cycle; antimetabolites attack the cell in the S phase, as does actinomycin D. Vincristine is a mitotic inhibitor and works best in the late G2 phase. Bleomycin has its most significant effect in the G2 phase. The cell is relatively resistant to attack by the anticancer drugs during the resting phase (G0). Many cells in a tumor population are at one time or another in G0, are at rest, and do not divide until some stimulus triggers the mitotic mechanisms of cell division. Therefore, according to the nature of the cytotoxic agent, cells in the G0 stage are not susceptible to the drug's action. The reserve compartment of the hematopoietic system consists of cells in G0. Most of the drugs now used to treat cancer have little effect in the G0 phase. Approximately 40 to 80% of the marrow stem cells are in G0 at any given time. When chemotherapeutic agents cause lowering of the white blood cell count, the resting marrow cells temporarily enter the cell cycle and proliferate rapidly (Figure 61).

One of the principles of modern anticancer chemotherapy is the use of drugs in relation to the cell cycle or cell kinetics, in order to insure maximum therapeutic response and minimum toxicity. Currently, no single treatment, whether with one or several drugs, eliminates all the tumor cells of a neoplasm. Nevertheless, the anticancer drugs reduce a constant percentage of tumor cells. This reduction, which is constant regardless of the first order of kinetics, is in accordance with the first order of kinetics representing its peculiar rate of reduction. Applying this principle, it is just as easy to reduce 1,000,000 cancer cells to 10,000 as it is to reduce 100 cancer cells to 1. Both represent a 99% reduction. The ultimate goal of cancer chemotherapy is to eradicate the last cancer cell. This is theoretically possible with constant chemotherapy. General toxicity, however, is a limiting factor. Cancer cells may eventually become resistant to the drugs, as a result of selection from a mixed cell population. This resistance has been shown to result from the loss of activating enzymes, from the induction of synthetic enzymes, or from an increase in repair processes. Resistance can be minimized by the use of suitable drug combinations.

Cancer cell population studies have concluded that each tumor cell divides into two cells once each generation time, that is, the time for one entire division cycle. The time required for this cycle is about the same for all cells in a given population of cells. Since each tumor cell divides into two cells at each generation time, it is evident that by 10 generations a single cell

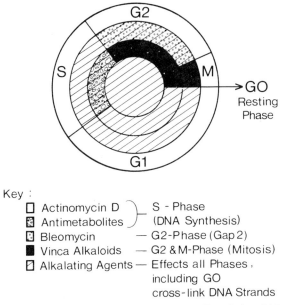

Key :

☐ Actinomycin D ⟩ S - Phase
▨ Antimetabolites ⟩ (DNA Synthesis)
▨ Bleomycin — G2-Phase (Gap 2)
■ Vinca Alkaloids — G2 & M-Phase (Mitosis)
▨ Alkalating Agents — Effects all Phases ,
including GO
cross-link DNA Strands

Figure 61. The cell division phases and the phase of the cell cycle in which anticancer drugs function.

proliferates into 1,000 (10^3) cells. Therefore the growth of many cells following this pattern will result in a thousandfold increase every 10 generations.

This growth pattern is referred to as exponential or logarithmic. When the log cells are charted against time, the pattern is a smooth curve. It is possible to gain insight into the effects of drugs on cancerous and normal cells by comparing the growth characteristics of each type. In order to be detected, a tumor must have a volume of at least 1 cc ($1 \times 1 \times 1$ cm) consisting of about 10^9 cells (one billion). The volume of cells necessary to kill a patient (critical volume) is 1000 cc ($10 \times 10 \times 10$ cm), or about 10^{12} cells (one trillion). Since these values are a thousandfold (10^3) apart, their separation in time represents ten generations of growth.

Currently, well-prescribed anticancer chemotherapy can reduce the population of lymphocytic leukemia cells from 10^{12} to 10^6 in acute lymphocytic leukemia of childhood. Although the patient is not cured at this point, the disease is in remission. The goal of anticancer chemotherapy is to reduce the last million cells (10^6) to zero. It is accepted that 100% cell kill of leukemic cells is necessary to achieve cure. The assumption is based on work with the mouse leukemic cell. A single leukemia cell implanted into a mouse can multiply and eventually cause the death of the animal. The mouse leukemic cell reproduces in about 12 hours. After an interval of 20 days, one cell can multiply to approximately one billion cells, which is enough to kill the mouse. Since one cell can rapidly become a lethal number of cells, it is probably necessary to kill every leukemia cell to achieve a cure.

Studies have shown that a given dose of drug kills the same percentage of cells, no matter how many are present. For example, the same dose will kill 99% of 100,000 leukemia cells or 99% of 100 cells, whichever number of leukemic cells is present in the animal. Therefore 1,000,000 cells can be reduced to 10,000, and 10,000 reduced to 100, and 100 to 10 or less, then 10 cells to 0. In leukemic mice cures can be produced if the drug is administered on an intermittent schedule to allow for recovery of normal cells, and if the dose is large enough so that the percentage of the cell population killed outpaces the multiplication of surviving leukemic cells. If the anticancer chemotherapy does not reduce the cell population by at least 75%, each day's multiplication of surviving cancer cells will outpace the inhibiting effect of the drug and will soon kill the animal.

Similar observations in leukemia studies in the human subject have been recorded. Estimates of the doubling time of human leukemic cells have ranged from 2 to 8 days, but a 4-day doubling time has been more often assumed. Further calculations indicate that it takes about 160 to 170 days for one cell doubling every 4 days to reach one trillion cells, the number considered lethal for man.

A brief outline is given of the principal groups of anticancer drugs used in practice (Figure 62).

ANTIMETABOLITES:

FOLIC ACID ANTAGONISTS

Chemistry
1. Derivatives of folic acid
2. The component parts of the folic acid molecule are
   A.   Plexidine nucleus
   B.   *p*-Aminobenzoic acid
   C.   Glutamic acid
3. Folinic acid is the formyl-containing analogue of reduced folic acid. It is called synthetic citrovorum factor of Leucovorin.

Mechanism of Action
1. Blocks folic and reductase to prevent availability of single carbon fragment. This blocks purine ring biosynthesis.
2. By a lesser action it inhibits methylation of deoxyuridylic acid to thymidylic acid, blocking pyrimidine synthesis.

Toxicity
1. Mouth lesions
2. Ulceration of the gastrointestinal tract
3. Bone marrow depression
4. Susceptibility to infection
5. Alopecia
6. Hyperpigmentation
7. Teratogenic properties

Formation

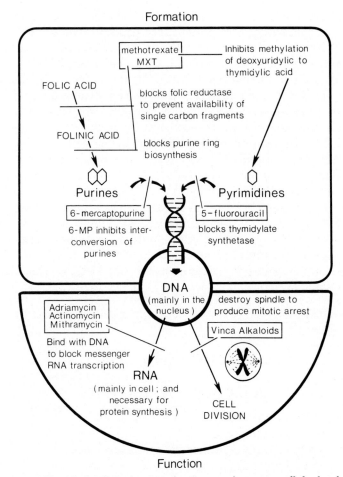

Figure 62. Mechanism of action of anticancer drugs at a cellular level.

Method of Administration and Dosage

1. 4 Amino-N^{10}-methyl-   Oral   2.5–5.0 mg/day
    pteroylglutamic acid
    Amethopterin, methotrexate   IV or IM   5–25 mg/day for 5 days

Uses

1. Choriocarcinoma
2. Cancer of the ovary
3. Cancer of the breast
4. In combination with other anticancer drugs for treating cancer of the cervix

PURINE ANTIMETABOLITES

Chemisty

6-Mercaptopurine

Mechanism of Action
1. Blocks purine ring biosynthesis
2. Inhibits interconversion of purines

Toxicity
1. Leukopenia
2. Thrombocytopenia
3. Stomatitis
4. Nausea and vomiting

Method of Administration
Usual dose: 2.0–2.5 mg/kg/day orally or 500 mg/m^2/day intravenously for 5 days every 10 to 14 days.

Uses
1. Acute lymphatic leukemia
2. Occasionally in choriocarcinoma

PYRIMIDINE ANTIMETABOLITE:

Fluorouracil (5-FU)

Mechanism of Action
1. Blocks thymidylate synthetase
2. Inhibits methylation of deoxyuridylic to thymidylic acid blocking pyrimidine synthesis

Toxicity
1. Myelosuppression
2. Stomatitis
3. Gastrointestinal ulceration
4. Nausea and vomiting
5. Alopecia
6. Cerebellar ataxia

Method of Administration
12 mg/kg/day × 3
Smaller dose, 1–2 times weekly for maintenance.

GLUTAMINE ANTAGONISTS

Azaserine (0-diazoacetyl-1-serine)
DON (6-diazo-5-oxo-1-norleucine)

Chemistry
1. Diazo compounds, closely related in structure to glutamine
2. Derived from both filtrates of a streptomyces

Mechanism of Action
1. Interference of the donation of an amino group by glutamine to various biochemical needs in the body, thereby blocking the conversion of formyl glycineamide ribonucleotide (FGAR) to formyl glycineamidine ribonucleotide (FGAM)

2. A step in purine biosynthesis in which glutamine acts as an amine donor under the influence of an amidotransferase

Toxicity
1. Mouth lesions
2. Gastrointestional tract disturbances
3. Leukopenia
4. Thrombocytopenia
5. Liver damage

Methods of Administration and Dosage

1.	Azaserine	IV	5–10 mg/kg/day
		Oral	× 10 or more
2.	DON	IV	0.2 mg/kg/day

Uses
1. Choriocarcinoma (rarely now)
2. Childhood acute leukemia

POLYFUNCTIONAL ALKYLATING AGENTS

Chemistry

$$H_3CN \begin{array}{c} CH_2CH_2Cl \\ \diagup \\ \diagdown \\ CH_2CH_2Cl \end{array} \longrightarrow CH_3N \begin{array}{c} CH_2 \\ \diagup \\ \diagdown \\ R^l \end{array} \longrightarrow \begin{array}{c} CH_2 \\ \diagup \\ CH_2 \\ \diagdown \\ CH_2 \end{array}$$

Mechanism of Action
1. Important sites of action appear to be on the nucleic acids, probably within the nucleus; this is suggested by the following observations:
   A. They are mutagenic
   B. They are carcinogenic
   C. Preferentially deactivate DNA-containing viruses
   D. Inactivate the pneumococcal and *H. influenzae* transforming principles
2. Alkylation (insertion of an alkyl group) may interfere with synthesis of cross-linking in a number of places. Prevents H bonding between chains of DNA
3. A monofunctional compound produces nuclear energy by a sheet mass effect
   A. Has only one active alkyl group
4. Polyfunctional agents are 50 to 100 times more active than the monofunctional group
   A. They are cross-linking agents
   B. Reactive atoms bridge across two chromosomal strands or react at two points on a chromosome

Toxicity
1. Delayed deaths may occur 3 to 7 days after exposure to LD50
2. Decrease in antibody production

3. Increased susceptibility to infection
4. Diarrhea
5. Ulceration of the gastrointestinal tract
6. Hemorrhagic cystitis
7. Involution in size of lymph nodes, thymus, and spleen
8. Progressive fall in the leukocytes and platelets in the peripheral blood
9. Decrease in spermatogenesis
10. Teratogenic effect

Methods of Administration and Dosage

1.	Mechlorethamine HCl (HN$_2$CHl, Mustargen)	IV	0.4 mg/kg, single or divided doses
2.	Chlorambucil (Leukeran)	Oral	0.1–0.2 mg/kg/day (6–12 mg/day)
3.	Melphalan (Alkeran) (L-phenylalanine mustard, L-PAM) (L-Sarcolysin)	Oral	0.2 mg/kg/day x 5 2–4 mg/day maintenance
4.	Cyclophosphamide (Endoxan, Cytoxan)	IV or Oral	200 mg/day IV for 5 days 50 mg/BID orally
5.	Triethylenethiophosphoramide (TSPA, Thio-Tepa)	IV	0.2 mg/kg × 5 days
6.	1,4 Dimethanesulfonyloxybutane (Busulfan, Myleran)	Oral	2–6 mg/day 150–250 mg/course
7.	Nitroso-urea alkylating agents		
A.	1,3-bis (2 chloroethyl)-1-nitroso-urea (BCNU)	IV	100 mg/m² every 6 weeks Next course in 4 to 6 weeks
B.	Chloroethyl-cyclohexyl-nitroso-urea (CCNU)	Oral	120–150 mg/m² every 6 weeks

Uses

1. Carcinoma of the ovary
2. Hodgkin's disease
3. Lymphomas
4. Burkitt's tumor
5. Multiple myeloma
6. Cancer of the breast
7. Neuroblastoma
8. Carcinoid
9. Leukemias

ANTIBIOTICS

Mechanism of Action

1. Form a complex with DNA involving selective binding at the guaninecystosine segments, with a specific block in the DNA-

dependent RNA synthesis (inhibits formation of messenger RNA [mRNA]).

Toxicity
1. Damage to bone marrow and intestinal epithelium
2. Nausea and vomiting
3. Diarrhea
4. Skin eruption

Methods of Administration and Dosage

1.	Actinomycin D or Dactinomycin (Cosmegen)	IV	0.01 mg/kg/day × 5 days or 0.04 mg/kg weekly
2.	Daunomycin	IV	0.8–1.0 mg/kg/day × 3 to 6 days; total dose never to exceed 25 mg/kg
3.	Mitomycin C (Mutamycin)	IV	0.06 mg/kg × 2 weekly if blood counts permit
4.	Adriamycin	IV	50–75 mg/m² in single or divided doses every 2 weeks
5.	Mithramycin	IV	25 μg/kg every other day × 3–4 days

Uses
1. Lymphomas
2. Leukemias
3. Solid tumors
4. Embryonal tumors
5. Trophoblastic disease
6. Carcinoid
7. Lower calcium level (Mithramycin)

MITOTIC INHIBITORS

Vinka Alkaloids

Chemistry
1. Dimeric indole-dihydroindole alkaloids
2. Periwinkle plant

Mechanism of Action
1. Arrest of mitosis in metaphase by destruction of spindles

Toxicity
1. Nausea and vomiting
2. Diarrhea
3. Leukopenia
4. Neurotoxic paresthesias
5. Palsies
6. Peripheral neuritis
7. Alopecia
8. Ileus

Methods of Administration and Dosage

1.	Vinblastine	IV	0.1–0.15 mg/kg/weekly

	(Velban)		
2.	Vincristine (Oncovin)	IV	0.03–0.075 mg/kg/weekly

Uses
1. Choriocarcinoma
2. Lymphoma
3. Leukemia
4. Hodgkin's disease

ENZYMES

L-asparaginase
1. Normal cells can synthesize their own supply of asparagine. It appears that asparagine-dependent cells lack an enzyme, asparagine synthetase, which in normal cells converts aspartic acid to asparagine. Certain types of leukemia (such as acute lymphoblastic) have an asparagine dependence. This provides an explanation for the effect of L-asparaginase. The tumor activity of L-asparaginase is also found with transplanted rat tumors and with primary dog lymphosarcoma. The final indications for the use of the enzyme in the treatment of malignancy remain to be determined.

Method of Administration and Dosage

1.	L-asparaginase	IV	50–200 IU/kg/day or 200–1000 IU/kg 3–7 days each week for 28 days

Uses
1. Acute lymphoblastic leukemia

NONALKYLATING AGENT THERAPY

Methods of Administration

1.	Hexamethylmelamine	8 mg/kg/day PO
2.	Cis-Platinum II (Diamine dichloride)	30 mg/m^2 IV × 3 every 28 days with mannitol diuresis

New Agents and Other Agents That Have Not been Evaluated in Ovarian Cancer

Cytembena
Porfiromycin
Porcarbazine
F Torafur
Bleomycin
Streptozotocin
DTIC

Traditionally, the treatment for ovarian cancer has been surgery followed by x-ray therapy. Chemotherapy was reserved for the far-advanced and recurrent ovarian cancers. The results from this treatment have been poor, despite the facts that a more aggressive surgical program has been carried out and that supervoltage has been introduced with innocative plans for administering the radiation. Ovarian cancer is a surface spreader and is found over the kidneys and liver in stage III. Because it is necessary to shield the liver and kidneys with lead to prevent radiation hepatitis and nephritis, these patients are selected for therapeutic failure when radiation therapy is given to the whole abdomen. Metastatic cancer has been found between the liver and diaphragm in about 10 to 12% of stage I ovarian cancer. It is obvious that x-ray therapy would not help these patients. As a consequence of the inability to control ovarian cancer in most instances with surgery and radiotherapy alone, chemotherapy is being increasingly employed in the management of this cancer.

Whether chemotherapy has increased the overall survival is difficult to estimate, but it has made life more comfortable for a great number of these unfortunate patients. Each center has its own criteria but, in general, patients with metastases and ascites have been chosen for chemotherapy. Chemotherapy given in a well-controlled manner does not produce as much morbidity as radiation therapy delivered to the upper abdomen. Following response, and in the absence of palpable disease, a second look may be undertaken to determine whether the patient is a candidate for (1) excision of any remaining cancer, or (2) continued chemotherapy.

Laparoscopic examination has been employed to evaluate and monitor the response of the tumor to therapy. The presence of tumor that is confirmed by biopsy appears to have more significance than negative findings following laparoscopic examination.

Single agent chemotherapy of the alkylating group has proved most valuable for the treatment of common epithelial ovarian cancers. Combination chemotherapy at this time does not produce better results than a single alkylating agent, except in the treatment of germ cell and gonadal stromal tumors.

Two methods are selected more often than any others for the administration of the chemotherapeutic drugs—the continuous or maintenance method and the intermittent plan. When the continuous method is followed, the alkylating agent, such as cyclophosphamide (Cytoxan), is given in 200 mg doses intravenously for 5 days, followed by 50 mg orally twice a day. The white blood count and differential, as well as the hemoglobin, should be checked after 2 to 3 weeks, and the drug should be discontinued if the WBC drops below 3,000 per mm^3 or polys below 1500 per mm^3. Although the platelets are not often affected by Cytoxan, it is wise to make a platelet count every 6 weeks. The number of platelets can be estimated from the blood smear. Although the intermittent treatment with L-phenylalamine mustard (Melphalan, Alkeran) is considered superior, it may be given continuously by using 2 to 4 mg a day as long as the white count remains over 3,000 and the platelet count over 100,000.

The second method is the intermittent approach and the drug can be given orally or intravenously by bolus. When the intermittent oral method is followed, L-phenylalamine mustard (Melphalan) in a dosage of 0.2 mg/kg of body weight is given each day for 5 days. In the intermittent intravenous method, cyclophosphamide in a dosage of 6 mg/kg of body weight is given for 5 days. It is anticipated that this plan can be followed at 4- to 6-week intervals. However this plan often depresses the bone marrow adversely and a longer interval is required between treatments. Blood chemistries and a complete blood count, including a platelet count, should be made before the drug is administered.

Because Bruce has shown that when chemotherapeutic agents lower the white blood count, the resting marrow stem cells temporarily enter the cell cycle and proliferate rapidly, it follows that spacing of chemotherapeutic agents as in the intermittent regimen should give the best results. However a study of several investigations using either the continuous or intermittent regimen produced essentially the same results.

The combination of chemotherapy and radiation therapy has not proved any more successful than when each is given alone, and in fact there is increased morbidity.

The alkylating agents cyclophosphamide and Alkeran are probably employed more than any other drugs in that group. Although not used as often, chlorambucil and thio-tepa have given similar results in carefully controlled series.

Hexamethylmelamine is a derivative of the alkylating agent triethylene-melamine but probably does not act primarily as an alkylating agent. The drug is given in a dosage of 6 to 8 mg/kg/day in divided doses orally. The drug causes occasional nausea and vomiting but appears to have less bone marrow depression complications than other alkylating agents. The principal toxicity is peripheral neuropathy, which usually prevents the drug from being given for more than 8 or 9 months. Smith and coworkers have reported that it is effective in an occasional patient who does not respond to Melphalan or Act Fu Cy regimens.

Recently a platinum compound, cis-dichlorodiamineplatinum (II) (cis-platinum II diamine dichloride) has been under investigation. Cis-platinum was first introduced as a possible anticancer drug by Rosenberg and colleagues in 1965. It has been shown to have antineoplastic activity in many in vitro and in vivo animal systems. As a single agent its response rate in previously treated patients is not impressive, but when combined with adriamycin it holds promise as an additional modality of therapy in recurrent and advanced ovarian cancer. The toxicity noted has been typical of that found with heavy metals and includes elevated blood urea nitrogen, tinnitus, anemia, nausea, vomiting, and myelosuppression.

Two dosage schedules have been explored. A high-dose schedule, 30 mg/m² daily on 3 successive days (these courses were repeated every 4 weeks), and a low-dose schedule, 30 mg/m² once every 2 to 3 weeks. The high-dose schedule proved to be more toxic without any therapeutic advantage. However reevaluation of the high-dose schedule after adequate hydration and attention to the nutritional status of the patient has demonstrated additional control of the cancer. Mannitol should be given to produce a diuresis.

Cis-platinum has many biologic properties similar to alkylating agents in its effect on DNA synthesis and its cross-linking of DNA.

Adriamycin is an antitumor antibiotic. It has been the subject of a great deal of research and clinical evaluation in the past few years. Studies have shown that it is active as a single agent in previously untreated patients and in those in whom alkylating agent therapy fails. Adriamycin has produced a great deal of alopecia, gastrointestinal toxicity, and stomatitis. Several ongoing trials comparing adriamycin alone and in combination with an alkylating agent or cis-platinum should provide important information on the relative activity of this important agent in advanced ovarian cancer. In combination with cyclophosphamide and cis-platinum, it has displayed increased anticancer activity in comparison to its use as a single agent or in combination with one other anticancer drug.

COMBINATION CHEMOTHERAPY IN OVARIAN CANCER

One of the most widely accepted hypotheses in cancer research is that the initial event leading to malignancy is a change in a single cell. Following this, there may be a series of events within succeeding generations of cells, finally culminating in many malignant cells which may develop into a mass as a solid tumor or may be at once widespread throughout the body, as in leukemias.

A major problem in cancer chemotherapy has been the development of resistance to the action of a specific drug to which a cancer was initially susceptible. Resistance is apparently caused by the development of mutant or genetically altered cells that are no longer subject to damage by the drug. However, such cells may be responsive to a different drug.

Many of the recent advances in the treatment of the leukemias and lymphomas have been associated with schedules consisting of two or more drugs given concomitantly or sequentially. Agents that produce toxicity in different organs are said to have independent toxicity. They can be combined frequently at full doses to produce increased damage to the tumor but little or no increased toxicity to the patient. Methotrexate and 6-mercaptopurine, both antimetabolites and both producers of damage to the bone marrow and gastrointestinal tract, would be expected to have additive toxic effects. Data show, however, that when 60 to 70% of the normal doses of the two drugs are combined, the combined toxicity is not greater than the toxicity of either drug alone.

Only a few published studies of combination chemotherapy have included more than a small number of patients with ovarian carcinoma. Smith compared the response to melphalan alone with the response of a three-drug combination, including cyclophosphamide, actinomycin D, and 5-fluorouracil (Act Fu Cy) for the treatment of common epithelial ovarian tumors, and he found no significant difference in the response rate. The toxicity of the combination was greater than that of melphalan alone. New knowledge of the action of the drug as well as new drugs and better control of the nutritional and metabolic status of the patient may demonstrate the value of multiple drug therapy given either in combination or in sequence.

Currently no combination regimen has been clearly demonstrated to be superior to alkylating agents used alone in the treatment of common epithelial ovarian cancer. DeVita and Schein have reported that there are important reasons to consider combination anticancer therapy in ovarian carcinoma. Ideally the combination should include drugs with proven antitumor activity against epithelial ovarian tumors and should have an acceptable toxicity. The drugs should have different mechanisms of action. Several studies are underway to test the designated combinations and to compare them directly with a parallel group treated by a single alkylating agent. This approach should answer the question of whether combination therapy is superior to alkylating agents used alone.

INTRAAORTIC INFUSION

The credit for introducing intraarterial infusion into clinical medicine belongs to Klopp and coworkers, who reported the use of nitrogen mustard injected directly into the artery supplying a tumor site. The technique used at Lenox Hill Hospital employs a catheter passed by way of the femoral and threaded into the aorta to any desired level, or by way of the brachial artery into the aorta. The latter method is preferred because the patient has more mobility. Multiple anticancer drugs are pumped into the aorta with an infusion pump. The drugs are given sequentially in antcipation of blocking tumor cells at different phases of the cell cycle. The drug schedule is:

1. Cytoxan, 200 to 400 mg, to run for 24 hours and is then repeated for a second 24 hours.
2. Actinomycin D, 1 mg to run for 8 hours.
3. Vincristine, 1 mg, to run for 6 hours.
4. Adriamycin, 50 mg, to run for 24 hours.
5. The patient does not receive any anticancer drug for 48 hours.
6. The entire cycle of drug therapy is repeated. Multiple cycles are given in anticipation of controlling the cancer.

There has been only one cure with this method. However pain has been relieved in most instances, and most had an improved feeling of well being. The tumor disappeared in 3 of 10 patients for more than 2 years, and the bone marrow depression has been less than with intravenous or oral therapy. To date, there is no direct evidence that intraaortic chemotherapy has any advantage over the intravenous route as far as survival is concerned.

Progestational agents have been employed in the management of endometrioid ovarian cancer. The results are controversial. If this type of medicine is given it should be used in pharmacologic doses, i.e., depo-provera, 400 mg, intramuscularly each day for 10 days and then once a week, or delalutin, 1250 mg (5 ml) intramuscularly each day for 10 days and then once a week for long periods of time. Megace, 40 mg three times a day by mouth, is given daily. In the presence of an elevated FSH and/or LH titer, the same regimen has been used. Depo-provera has a more predictable action on the suppression of gonadotropins. The progestogens may be used concurrently with any of the anticancer drugs.

SUMMARY

Unfortunately, progress in the management of ovarian cancer has been painfully slow. It is a tragedy that 100,000 women have succumbed to this disease in the past decade. Ovarian cancer is now the leading cause of death from gynecologic cancer. These women literally vomit themselves to death. They are often ravishingly hungry and one bit of food or a drink causes them to vomit. Unlike the terminal stage of many other cancers, during which the patient gradually becomes comatose, the ovarian cancer patient is usually alert right up to the time of death. In spite of this, the best therapy for each stage of the disease is not known.

The impressive responses of some patients to a single alkylating agent has suggested an expanded role for chemotherapy. There is an urgent need to explore the potential of multiple drug therapy as new anticancer drugs prove to have activity against ovarian cancer. It will be important to compare standard alkylating agents with new active agents as well as combination chemotherapy regimens. The newer chemotherapeutic agents must be systematically investigated in patients who have failed existing standard methods of treatment in order to identify new agents of promise in the management of this disease. Subsequent clinical trials should compare newer therapies to optimal existing treatment within each stage. Such studies will define the role of chemotherapy in the managment of ovarian cancer and will enable patients to enjoy the benefits of continually improving forms of therapy.

Chemotherapy now constitutes a major and indispensable therapeutic approach, capable of producing cures, in particular kinds of widespread cancer. It has produced some spectacular results in ovarian cancer. In contrast to surgery and radiation therapy, chemotherapy—the treatment of cancer with drugs and hormones—can be used effectively for disseminated as well as localized cancer. Chemotherapy has become an accepted modality of treatment only in the past 30 years. Each of these three decades has seen the addition of new drugs with a wide spectrum of usefulness. Originally it was used only for palliation, but now is the primary treatment for several malignancies. A major goal of current cancer chemotherapy is to achieve cures by prompt and vigous treatment of those cancers that have responded to anticancer drugs.

It remains for the gynecologist and the chemotherapist to explore the best method and regimen to control ovarian cancer as well as its role in prophylaxis as well as therapy. Combinations of chemotherapeutic agents have been used with substantial success in certain cancers, particularly if each of the drugs used acts on the cancer cell in a different way. Major improvements in the treatment of certain cancers have been achieved by using several of the active drugs simultaneously, as well as by using different drugs in sequence. This approach must be thoroughly explored by systemically investigating these regimens in the various families of ovarian cancer.

Chemotherapy can occasionally produce a cure in a broad spectrum of cancers, including ovarian cancers. The cancers that can be cured by chemotherapy are not always those that grow most rapidly. Not all are from the same primitive embryonic tissue; many organ classes are represented. Furthermore, curative chemotherapy is not usually a product of a single drug or a single technique of drug use. Rather, many different drugs are involved, sometimes in combination with each other, sometimes with surgery or radiation. Ovarian cancer was previously treated with a single alkylating drug, and if that failed the second and then third-line drugs were added. Currently, programs have been established to study systematically and in detail the value of multiple drug therapy for the initial chemotherapeutic regimen. The high degree of specificity between a particular tumor and a particular drug or drug combination implies that no universal chemotherapeutic cure can be anticipated. The complexity of special drugs and regimens for special tumors can also be construed to mean that a drug that fails in treatment of one kind of cancer may exhibit major activity against another. Until a laboratory test is established to idenfity the best anticancer drug or combination of drugs for a given tumor, treatment will continue to depend on empirical factors as well as on past and present clinical experience.

The sensitivity of cancer cells to drug action depends on a variety of possible factors. Many of these are not known and there are few tests to guide the clinician in selecting and administering anticancer drugs. The anticancer drug must reach the cancer cell surface in the right concentration, enter the cell, remain active or become active through enzymes present in the cell, reach a critical target site, and combine with it. It is ideal if the anticancer drug combines with the critical target site at a time when chemical processes on which the cell depends for its viability or reproduction are in progress. It is important to eliminate the bypass pathways in the cell that would negate the effect of the anticancer drug. The chain is no longer than its individual links, and failure of the whole chain can result from the failure of any one step. Thus any anticancer drug given by the wrong regimen to a mass of cancer cells that is biologically insusceptible to its action at that time is a failure of chemotherapy. Such an error introduces a degree of toxicity without any therapeutic help. Better drug design and better understanding of the biologic characteristics of each cancer type, and indeed of each cancer, will advance the effectiveness of chemotherapy. But studies on the treatment of ovarian cancer only recently have been directed toward these goals.

It is obvious that much work remains to be done before the use of chemotherapy in ovarian cancer reaches the stage that it has in choriocarcinoma, leukemias, and many embryonal tumors. However many studies now underway should provide guidelines for the chemotherapeutic treatment of ovarian cancer that will give a predictable chance for cure in an increased number of patients.

BIBLIOGRAPHY

Bagley, C. M., Young, R. C., Canellos, G. P., et al.: Treatment of ovarian carcinoma: Possibilities for progress. New Engl. J. Med. 287:856, 1972.

Barber, H. R. K.: Editorial Comment, in Surgical Disease in Pregnancy. Edited by H. R. K. Barber, E. A. Graber, Saunders, Philadelphia, 1974, p. 718.

Bruce, W. R.: A model system for examining the action of anticancer agents at the cellular level in vivo. Natl. Cancer Inst. Monogr. 24:249, 1967.

Bruce, W.R., Meeker, B.E., Valenote, F.A.: Comparison of the sensitivity of normal hematopoietic and transplanted lymphoma colony-forming cells to chemotherapeutic agents administered in vivo. J. Nat. Cancer Inst. 37:233, 1966.

Brulé, G., Eckhardt, S. J., Hall, T. C., Winkler, A.: Drug Therapy of Cancer, World Health Organization, Geneva, 1973

Connors, T. A., Roberts, J. J. (Eds.): Platinum coordination complexes in cancer chemotherapy, in Recent Results in Cancer Research, Vol. 48. Springer-Verlag, Berlin, 1974.

DeVita, V. T., Schein, P. S.: The use of drugs in combination for the treatment of cancer. New Engl. J. Med. 288:998, 1973.

Hryniuk, W. M., Bertino, J. R.: Rationale for selection of chemotherapeutic agents. Adv. Intern. Med. 15:267, 1969.

Klopp, C. T.: Fractionated intraarterial cancer chemotherapy with methylbisamine hydrochloride, Preliminary report. Ann. Surg. 132:811, 1950.

Parker, R. T., Parker, C. H., Wilbanks, G. D.: Cancer of the ovary: Survival studies based upon operative therapy, chemotherapy, and radiotherapy. Am. J. Obstet., Gynecol. 108:878, 1970.

Rosenberg, B., Van Camp, L. Kregas, T.: Inhibition of cell division in Escherichia coli by electrolysis products from a platinum electrode. Nature 205:698, 1965.

Smith, J.P.: Chemotherapy in advanced ovarian cancer. Nat. Cancer Inst. Monograph 42:141, 1975.

Smith, J.P., Rutledge, F., Wharton, J. T.: Chemotherapy of ovarian cancer: New approaches to treatment. Cancer 30:1565, 1972.

Van Eden, E. B., Falkson, G., Van Dyk, J. J., et al.: 5-fluorouracil, imidazole-4-carboxamide, vincristine and BCNu given concomitantly in the treatment of solid tumors in man. Cancer Chemother. Rep. 56(I):691, 1972.

Wallace, H. J., Higby, D. J.: Phase I evaluation of cis-platinum II diammine chloride (PDD) and a combination of PDD plus adriamycin, in Recent Results in Cancer Research. Vol. 48. Springer-Verlag, Berlin, 1974, p. 167.

Watkins, E., Jr., Sullivan, R.D.: Cancer chemotherapy by prolonged arterial infusion. Surg. Gynecol. Obstet. 118:3, 1964.

Webb, M. J., Malkasian, G. D., Jorgensen, E.O.: Factors influencing ovarian cancer survival after chemotherapy. Obstet. Gynecol. 44:564, 1974.

Wiltshaw, E., Kroner, T.: Phase II study of cis-dichlorodiamineplatinum (II) in advanced adenocarcinoma of the ovary. Cancer Treat. Rep. 60:55 1976.

Young, R. C.: Chemotherapy of ovarian cancer: Past and present. Semin. Oncol. 2:267, 1975.

Young, R. C., Hubbard, S. P., DeVita, V. T.: The chemotherapy of ovarian cancer. Cancer Treat. Rev. 1:99, 1974.

21

The Role of Radiation Therapy in the Management of Ovarian Cancer

T he protocol for the management of ovarian cancer at Lenox Hill Hospital has phased out external radiation therapy as a therapeutic modality for the common epithelial ovarian cancer. Radiation therapy has been reserved for selected stage IV patients in whom the disease involves supraclavicular and/or inguinal nodes. It is not given in stages I, II, or III for reasons stated in other chapters of this book.

Because external radiation therapy is frequently employed by a great number of doctors in the management of ovarian carcinoma, a discussion of the use of radiation therapy and of the two most frequently employed methods of giving the therapy will be presented.

Ovarian cancer is not a single entity but encompasses a group of diseases with different biologic behaviors, all spreading diffusely over the surface of organs throughout the abdominal cavity. It may also spread to the retroperitoneal lymph nodes, particularly along the paraaortic chain. Even in early disease, when the tumor has been limited to one ovary and has been completely removed, there is the possibility of potential contamination of the peritoneal cavity. It is therefore accepted by many physicians that irradiation of the entire abdomen is the logical therapy for ovarian carcinomas.

Kottmeier's technique is to administer the therapy through two large anterior and two corresponding posterior fields, while protecting the kidneys and liver. His protocol has progressed from the conventional x-ray therapy (200 to 400 Kv) aimed at the large fields as described above (with the occasional addition of later fields), to the use of supervoltage. Kottmeier's results do not indicate that supervoltage radiation gives improved results, but from a physical point of view, it has several advantages. The wide field technique attempts to deliver a total dose of 2,000 rads over 6 weeks and no more than 3,000 rads can be delivered in 5 to 6 weeks to such a large volume of the abdomen. A daily dose of 200 rads to the lower abdomen is well tolerated, but it is inadvisable to exceed 100 rads per day to the upper abdomen.

Delclos reports on another technique using three or four fields. It is a modification of the static field method. The treatment, which is given with megavoltage, is not better tolerated than the static field method because the tissue volume irradiated at any one time is the same. Although a higher dose is given to the central volume, which may be desirable in selected situations in which a higher dose is warranted around the paraaortic area, this can be better accomplished by the use of a megavoltage unit at an 18 to 25 MEV level, with a field within a field, or with an additional boost after completion of whole abdominal irradiation. There is an increased incidence of gastrointestinal complication with this method of treatment.

Often treatment has to be interrupted because of nausea, diarrhea, malaise, temperature elevation, fatigue, loss of appetite, and a considerable drop in the blood count. It is unlikely that this dose will be lethal in any significant number of tumors, except the pure dysgerminoma.

The other technique, popularized by Delclos, is the moving strip technique for treating the whole abdomen from the pelvic floor to the diaphragm over the course of 30 to 40 days. The technique was introduced in Manchester, England, in 1957. It can be used with any supervoltage unit by proper correction of depth dose and penumbra effect, provided that the beam is wide enough to cover the abdomen from side to side.

This technique treats a volume of tissue eight times by the beam and four times by the penumbra (12 days total). The whole treatment time, to cover the area from the pelvic floor to the diaphragm, extends from 30 to 40 days. A tumor dose of 2,500 to 2,700 rads, measured at the midline of the patient along a sagittal plane, can be delivered safely. The dose delivered to the tumor has a much greater biologic efficiency because it is given in a much shorter time than with the static field technique. Because only a fragment of the abdominal cavity and surrounding tissues is irradiated at any one time, tolerance is also better. The dose given by this technique is equivalent to about 3,200 to 3,400 rads given in 3.5 weeks by the static field technique. After irradiation of the whole abdomen, Delclos adds 2,000 rads in 2 weeks to the pelvis (15 × 15 cm fields) by means of a 25 MEV photon beam (from a Betatron or Linear Accelerator).

The volume of tissue to be irradiated by the strip technique described by Delclos is divided into a series of contiguous segments, and the field is moved from one end of the volume to the other. Lines 2.5 cm apart are marked on the front and back of the patient. On the first day a single strip is treated from the front, and on the second day an identical opposite field is irradiated from the back. Thereafter, one 2.5 cm wide strip is added daily until four strips have been irradiated front and back. Next the 10 cm strip is moved 2.5 cm up every day by alternating front and back until the last strip is reached. The field is then reduced by one strip of 2.5 cm daily. In the last two days a single 2.5 cm strip is irradiated. The kidneys are shielded from the posterior beam by two half value layers (HVL) of lead placed on a satellite platform (which will reduce the dose to the kidneys to about 50% of the tumor dose). The right side of the liver (three strips) is shielded both front and back with one HVL of lead. To compensate for the lower dose at both ends of the irradiated volume, the treatment is started one strip below the lower margin of the pelvic field (placed at midpubis), and completed one strip above the diaphragm which should be localized by fluoroscopy. As reported above, the pelvis then receives an additional 2,000 rads.

The patients tolerated the moving strip technique better than they did the static field method. There was very little weight loss during treatment despite the high incidence of nausea and diarrhea. The hemoglobin and hematocrit remained fairly constant, but the lymphocytes and platelets dropped by 60% of the original value during the first two weeks and then started to return toward normal after therapy was completed. The diarrhea tended to appear by the second week of treatment and then decreased, whereas the nausea was more marked in the fifth week during the most intense treatment to the upper abdomen.

The common epithelial ovarian carcinomas arise from the germinal epithelium. This histogenetic origin might imply a high degree of radiosensitivity. However experience has showed that in general these tumors have limited radiosensitivity. Among the germ cell tumors the dysgerminoma has a high radiosensitivity response, and among the gonadal stromal tumors (granulosa cell) the response in general is excellent but does not equal that of the dysgerminoma. The other germ cell tumors (embryonal teratomas) and the extraembryonal tumors (endodermal-sinus tumors and the choriocarcinoma ovarian tumors) are relatively radioresistant. Thus, for the common epithelial ovarian tumors, radiation therapy is severely handicapped by frequent widespread anatomic distribution of tumors of limited radiovulnerability.

Consequently, for those physicians who use radiation therapy on patients whose ovarian cancer is grossly limited to the pelvis, it seems preferable to irradiate this restricted tumor and tissue volume to a potentially cancericidal dose. This approach is chosen in preference to treating the entire peritoneal cavity to a lower and likely ineffective dose limited by patient tolerance.

The patient does not tolerate radiation therapy of the entire peritoneal cavity to cancericidal dosage. Therapy is initially limited by the nausea, vomiting, diarrhea, weight loss, fatigue, lack of appetite, and drop in the blood count. These complications are reversible, but the most serious problem is nonreversible damage to the kidneys and liver by doses required to control cancer (Figure 63).

Currently, a moving strip technique has been employed to irradiate the entire peritoneal cavity. This technique has been proposed in an attempt to improve the dose-time relationship, but such improvement is achieved at the expense of delivering a homogenous dose of irradiation to anatomic structures and the tumor. This results from the daily variation in position. Hot spot damage to the intestines may result.

Experience indicates that radiation should have its optimal application for patients with stage II ovarian cancer. The results in stage I do not show any advantage to the addition of external x-ray therapy. The radioactive isotopes play a significant role in increasing the 5-year survival rate in stage

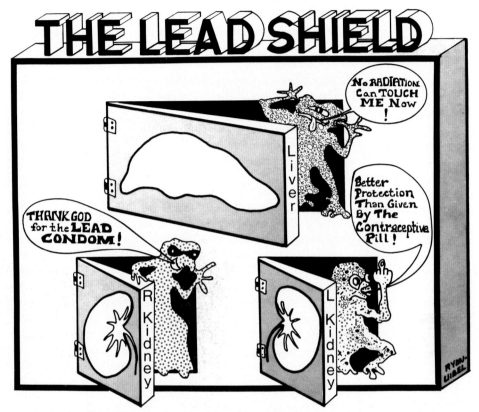

Figure 63. Schematic representation of the cancer cell being protected by a lead shield and thereby avoiding a cancericidal dose during abdominal radiation therapy.

I common epithelial ovarian cancers. Use of external radiation therapy in patients with stage III disease is compromised by the necessity of reducing the dosage to large tissue volumes. Local irradiation for palliative purposes occasionally is useful in patients with stage III and IV disease.

Since laparotomy is necessary for the diagnosis of tumors in situations in which radiation therapy is likely to be useful, irradiation has followed definitive surgery. Therefore preoperative irradiation, frequently preferred in other clinical problems, has not been adequately evaluated. The work reported on the poor response rate to radiation therapy when tumor masses are larger than 2 cm would preclude the use of preoperative x-ray therapy except in very highly selected cases.

In the past, in some institutions the uterus has not been removed so that it might be used as a container for radium. But now, available external radiation therapy allows adequate close distribution throughout the entire pelvis. Therefore the uterus, which is frequently involved by ovarian cancer, should be removed at the time of initial definitive therapy.

External radiation therapy is supplied by machines producing x-rays, gamma rays, or electrons. In addition, machines producing protons, neutrons, and mesons are under intense investigation. X-ray machines range from very low to very high voltages (10,000 volts=10 KEV, to 70,000,000 volts=70 MEV). In general, the higher the voltage, the greater the penetration of the x-rays. X-ray therapy with voltage over 1 MEV is called supervoltage therapy and is used for deep-seated cancers. The principal advantage of supervoltage machines compared with ordinary 250 KEV machines is the greater penetration and less severe skin reaction.

The most common teletherapy machine is the cobalt 60 unit. Practically every department of radiation therapy now has a cobalt machine. These units produce a fairly homogenous (clean) beam of 1 MEV and 1.3 MEV gamma rays.

Radiation therapy makes use of the ionizing radiations—x-rays and electrons produced by man-made machines, and gamma rays which emanate from naturally or artificially radioactive elements—to destroy cells by injuring their capacity to divide. The "law" for Bergonie and Tribondeau, formulated in 1906, stated that x-rays are more effective on cells that have a greater reproductive activity; the effectiveness is greater on those cells that have a larger dividing future, and on those cells whose morphology and function are least fixed. The radiosensitivity of cells and tissues is proportional to their reproductive capacity and inversely proportional to their degree of differentiation. Since the central attribute of cancer cells is their sustained, uncontrolled, lawless proliferation, injury to this property is precisely what is desired. Although some rapidly dividing normal cells are also killed during the radiotherapeutic eradication of a cancer, the large reservoir of similar normal cells outside the irradiated field is readily able, in most instances, to replenish the supply and to repair the irradiated tissues. Thus, in favorable cases, the cancer gradually disappears completely during treatment, the acute radiation reaction in the normal tissues then slowly subsides, and 1 or more years later the patient may present no external evidence whatever of having been treated.

OXYGEN AND RADIOSENSITIVITY

It has long been known that cells are nearly threefold more radiosensitive in the presence of oxygen than in its absence. Many cancers outgrow their blood supply, and the presence within them of necrotic foci strongly suggests that those cancer cells that have come to be more than 150 to 200 microns from the nearest capillary are severely hypoxic or anoxic. Oxygen concentration diminishes as the distance from the capillary increases. Cells near the necrotic center may actually be anoxic. Oxygen concentration will fall to zero 150 microns from capillaries, and cells more distant than this will be anoxic. This anoxia may underlie the observation that the zone of living cells is rather constant in width. Diffusion of oxygen across the zone, and its eventual exhaustion of cells in it, may determine how many cells can live as the tumor mass increases. The source of oxygen and nutrients may be pushed too far away from cells at the center and many of the cells may die. Such hypoxic or anoxic cells would be quite radioresistant when compared to normally oxygenated ones adjacent to the stroma. It may well be that, in the usual course of events, they die and become part of the necrotic center of the tumor, but because they are extremely hypoxic they may survive a normal course of radiotherapy.

The radiation therapists have reported that a tumor mass of 2 cm or larger has a large residue of hypoxic cells after x-ray therapy. These hypoxic cells may not die, and in fact may begin to divide and give rise to a recurrence of the tumor. This possibility has caused therapists to reevaluate their positions and has resulted in their reluctance, if not refusal, to treat such patients. Thus it is suggested that the recurrent growth of many cancers after an initially good radiotherapeutic response may be due to the survival of microscopic foci of such hypoxic, radioresistant tumor cells which, after shrinkage of the tumor, are once again brought into proximity with blood vessels, can obtain oxygen and nutrients, and thereupon resume active proliferation (Figure 64).

RADIOBIOLOGY

It is now established that the killing of cells by ionizing radiation, both in vivo and in clonal cell culture, is an exponential function of dose, beyond an initial low-dose range in which the survival curve exhibits a "shoulder."

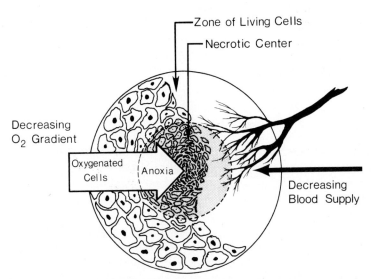

Figure 64. Tumors have ectopic regions. The mass of cells grows outward from its interior. Oxygen concentration diminishes as the distance from the capillaries increases. Cells near the necrotic center may actually be anoxic. Such hypoxic or necrotic cells would be quite radioresistant when compared to normally oxygenated ones near the periphery.

When the same total dose is split into two fractions separated in time by an increasing interval, survival increases for the first 2 to 4 hours, then decreases during the next 3 to 4 hours, and finally increases again with concomitant restoration of the shoulder to the survival curve. It is thus apparent that the shoulder represents a recovery process, which is operative at low doses but becomes overwhelmed as the dose increases. Split dose recovery is diminished by low temperature, and by certain chemical agents such as actinomycin D, and at least in some cells by hypoxia. This suggests that it is an energy-consuming enzymatic process, but neither the identity of the molecular lesion nor the mechanism of its repair is known at this time.

DNA BREAKS

The linear energy transfer (LET) is a measure of the average rate of energy loss along the track of an ionizing particle. It is the energy released (usually in KEV) per micron of medium (tissue) along the track of any ionizing particle. LET is not a static or constant value; it will be different even for the same particle over different portions of the track because, although charge on a particle is a constant factor, the velocity will be continually changing (decreasing) all along the particle track. Each interaction (excitation or ionization) involves a loss of energy from the particle and a concomitant deceleration. As a result, LET gradually increases along a particle track, and increases dramatically just before the particle comes to rest. This peak in the rate of energy dissipation is called the "Bragg peak." Particles with different degrees of charge will produce different tracks. Highly charged particles interact frequently; consequently they have a high LET and the ionization along their tracks is very dense. Particles with lesser degrees of charge are sparsely ionizing, and they have a lower LET.

The radiobiologic effects on cells may be due to molecular, enzyme, or nuclear damage. The principal macromolecular target in the cell is its nucleus, and particularly the DNA. The nuclear damage includes inhibition of cell division, chromosome mutation, and nuclear damage. In bacteria it has been shown that ionizing radiation produces both single and double-strand breaks in DNA, and several lines of evidence suggest that the double-strand breaks account for most of the lethal events. X-rays can go through a chromosome like a Gigli saw, and if conditions are right the two portions of the chromosome join as they were before and no damage results. However potentiators such as the halogenated thymidine analogs (5-bromodeoxyuridine), if given during x-ray therapy, may be incorporated into DNA in place of thymidine and inhibit cell growth. Other potentiators such as hydroxyurea bind to DNA and may thus interfere or compete with the binding of a repair enzyme to a site of injury. Certain nuclear particles, notably protons, neutrons, and negative pi mesons, have attracted attention as substitutes for x-rays and electrons because they are much less dependent on oxygen and, in the case of pi mesons, have unique properties which would make possible a much more precise and selective localization of the beam energy to the volume occupied by the cancer. Unlike x-rays, which cut through a chromosome like a Gigli saw, the particles such as protons, neutrons, and pi mesons are large particles, and when they pass through a chromosome a large piece of the chromosome is torn loose, making it more difficult for that chromosome to reestablish itself.

SUMMARY

In our protocol for common epithelial ovarian cancer, external x-ray therapy has been reserved for selected patients with stage IV cancer of the ovary in whom the disease involves supraclavicular and/or inguinal nodes. Radiation therapy is not given in stages I, II, or III. Some centers routinely give irradiation therapy to all stage II ovarian cancer patients.

The natural history of germ cell and gonadal stromal ovarian cancers permits a more rational external x-ray therapy program. Indeed, both groups (except for the embryonal and extraembryonal germ cell cancers) respond well to x-ray therapy. The dysgerminoma spreads to paraaortic nodes, and a limited part of the abdomen can then be radiated to cancericidal doses. The gonadal stroma are characterized by local spread, late recurrence, and recurrence within the pelvic cavity. This provides the opportunity to successfully treat the patient with external therapy.

An attempt has been made in this chapter to review briefly the types of radiation therapy and radiobiology that may help the clinician in managing patients with ovarian cancer.

BIBLIOGRAPHY

Bleehen, N.M.: Prospects from radiobiology, *in* Recent Advances in Cancer and Radiotherapeutics: Clinical Oncology. Edited by K.E. Halman. Williams & Wilkins, Baltimore, 1972.

Buschke, F., Parker, R.G.: Radiation Therapy in Cancer Management. Grune & Stratton, New York, 1972, p. 276.

Delclos, L., Braun, E.J., Herrera, J.R., Sampiere, V., Van Roosenback, E.: Whole abdominal irradiation by cobalt 60 moving strip technique. Radiology 81:632, 1969.

Delclos, L., Fletcher, G.H.: Postoperative irradiation for ovarian carcinoma with the cobalt-60 moving strip technique. Clin. Obstet. Gynecol. 12:993, 1969.

Delclos, L., Murphy, M.: Evaluation of tolerance during treatment, late tolerance, and better evaluation of clinical effectiveness of the cobalt 60 moving strip technique. Am. J. Roentgenol. Radium Ther. Nucl. Med. 96:75–80, 1966.

Delclos, L., Smith, J.P.: Tumors of the ovary, *in* Textbook of Radiotherapy, Second edition. Edited by G. Fletcher. Lea & Febiger, Philadelphia, 1973, pp. 690–702.

Delclos, L., Smith, J.P.: Ovarian cancer, with special regard to types of radiotherapy. Natl. Cancer Inst. Monogr. 42, 1975.

Fazehas, J.T., Maier, J.G.: Irradiation of ovarian carcinoma. A prospective comparison of the open field and moving strip techniques. Am. J. Roentgenol. Radium Ther. Nucl. Med. 120:118–123, 1974.

Fletcher, G.H.: Clinical dose-response curve of subclinical aggregates of epithelial cells and its practical application in the management of human cancers, *in*

Biological and Clinical Basis of Radiosensitivity. edited by Friedman. Thomas, Springfield, 1974, pp. 485–501.

Fuks, Z.: External radiotherapy of ovarian cancer: Standard approaches and new frontiers. Semin. Oncol. 2:253, 1975.

Kjellgren, O., Jonsson, L.: Bone marrow depression in the pelvis after megavoltage irradiation for ovarian carcinoma. Obstet. Gynecol. 105:849–855, 1969.

Kottmeier, H.L.: Radiotherapy in the treatment of ovarian carcinoma. Clin. Obstet. Gynecol. 4:865, 1961.

Kottmeier, H.L.: Ovarian cancer with special regard to radiotherapy, in Gynecological Cancer. Edited by D.J. Deely. Butterworths, Appleton-Century-Crofts, New York, Boston, 1971, p. 186.

Perez, C.A., Bradfield, J.S.: Radiation therapy in the treatment of carcinoma of the ovary. Cancer 29:1027, 1972.

Pizzarello, D.J., Witcofski, R.L.: Basic Radiation Biology. Lea & Febiger, Philadelphia, 1970.

Pizzarello, D.J., Witcofski, R.L.: Medical Radiation Biology. Lea & Febiger, Philadelphia, 1972.

Rosenhoff, R., Young, R., Bagley, C., et al.: Peritoneoscopy: A valuable tool for initial staging and "second look" in ovarian cancer. Proc. Am. Assoc. Cancer Res. 15:171, 1974.

Wharton, J.T., Delclos, L., Gallagher, S., et al.: Radiation hepatitis induced by abdominal irradiation with cobalt 60 moving strip technique. Am. J. Roentgenol. Radium Ther. Nucl. Med. 117:73–80, 1973.

22

Autoimmune Disease

A dvanced and recurrent cancer of the ovary may display clinical features similar to those found in an autoimmune response. For this reason a brief discussion on autoimmune disorders is included here, and a correlation of the findings in advanced and recurrent ovarian cancer discussed.

Clinical and experimental observations show that individuals can sometimes respond immunologically to certain of their own antigens (self-antigens). These important exceptions to the principle of self-tolerance help analyze its fundamental mechanisms, and they are frequently associated with disease. It is often not clear, however, whether these anomalous responses cause, or are the result of, disease. Hence it is necessary to emphasize the distinction between an *autoimmune response*, in which an individual makes antibodies or becomes allergic to a self-antigen, and an *autoimmune disease*, which is a pathologic condition arising from an autoimmune response. Autoimmune reactions can be both antibody-mediated and cell-mediated. Autoimmunity reflects a loss of immunologic tolerance to tissue and cellular antigens. Immunologic tolerance is the result of an active physiologic process and is not simply the lack of an immune response. Before the pathogenetic processes that lead to autoimmunity are discussed, it is important to review the role of B cells, T cells (suppressor and helper), as well as the mechanisms involved.

BACKGROUND

Experiments, clinical observations, and studies of experiments of nature (Bruton's agammaglobulinemia, Di George syndrome, Swiss agamma-globulinemia) have led to the concept of two cell systems of immunity, namely, T (thymus-derived) lymphocytes concerned with cell-mediated immunity, and B (probably bone-marrow-derived) lymphocytes represent independent lines of differentiation but have a common precursor stem cell.

Pluripotent stem cells originate in the yolk sac and migrate to the fetal liver and then to the bone marrow. These stem cells differentiate into the cells of all the major hematopoietic elements. Lymphocytes, the primary cells involved in all immunologic reactions, are classified in two subpopulations according to their origin and functions. T lymphocytes derive their immunologic maturity from the thymus and are responsible for cell-mediated

237

immunity, and B lymphocytes mature in an unknown site, probably in the bone marrow, and are responsible for antibody-mediated immunity. In recent years a number of receptors and antigens have been identified on the surface of human lymphocytes. These surface markers serve to evaluate lymphoid cell populations in a variety of human diseases.

Lymphoid stem cells can function as prethymic cells and are processed in the thymus under the influence of thymosin or thymopoietin to differentiate into T cells. T lymphocytes represent 80% of the circulating peripheral blood lymphocytes and are responsible for protection against certain infective agents such as fungi, intracellular facultative bacteria and most of the viruses, rejection of tissue transplants, and delayed-type hypersensitivity. The effector functions are performed by the pharmacologically and biochemically active chemical mediators, the lymphokines, which are produced by the T cells when they are exposed to specific antigens or nonspecific mitogens. These lymphokines (transfer factor [TF], lymphocyte transforming activity [LTA], migration inhibition factor [MIF], and lymphotoxin [LT]) probably have both specific and nonspecific functions. The immunocompetent T lymphocyte produces sensitized T lymphocyte subpopulations. These sensitized T lymphocytes release a helper factor which enables immunocompetent B cells to respond to antigens which they are otherwise unable to recognize.

The sensitized subpopulation of lymphocytes may produce suppressor T cells which regulate the B-cell response to some antigens. Accumulated data indicates that the interaction of certain antigens with the thymocytes during tolerance induction results in a turning off of B cells so that they no longer cooperate with T cells to produce antibodies. Suppression by T cells can be mediated by both specific and nonspecific means. It has not been determined whether there are two distinct subpopulations of lymphocytes for helper and suppressor functions. The same T-cell population under different circumstances may function as either helper or suppressor T cells. It may be that specialized populations of T lymphocytes send "on and off" signals to effector cells.

Lymphoid stem cells are processed by an alternate pathway which is poorly understood in man, but which has been extensively studied in birds and in the bursa of Fabricius. The precursor cells under the influence of a hormone-like substance (bursin) are processed in the liver and later in the body marrow to differentiate into B lymphocytes. In response to antigenic stimulation, the immunocompetent B cells differentiate into plasma cells that produce antibody. These immunocompetent B cells may be stimulated by a helper factor from a sensitized T-lymphocyte population to produce a K cell. The K cell can act in the presence of an antibody to destroy a cell. It does not need complement to accomplish this. B lymphocytes are responsible for protection against bacteria.

In addition to the T cells (helper T cells and suppressor T cells) and B cells (variant K cells), there is also a D cell. This cell has the characteristics of both

T and B lymphocytes, but its role in the immune mechanism has not been clarified.

An autoimmune disease can generally be defined as one in which an autoantibody or a sensitized lymphocyte reacts with host tissue. This does not mean that the autoantibody or lymphocyte plays a causative role in the disease. In light of recent work, autoimmunity may arise whenever there exists a state of immunologic imbalance in which B-cell activity is excessive and suppressor T-cell activity is diminished. This imbalance occurs as a consequence of viruses, drugs, genetic factors, environmental factors, carcinogens, or cancer itself. A central mechanism in this concept involves a disturbance of the delicate balance between suppressor and helper activity of the regulatory T cells. Either an excess of helper T-cell activity or a deficiency of suppressor T-cell activity could lead to the development of autoimmunity. The mechanisms by which such a balance may be upset are complex but may involve many factors, including viral factors and the abnormal production of thymic hormones. It is the imbalance between B-cell production and suppressor T cells that is important in autoimmune diseases. The impaired immunoregulation is then expressed by the production of an increased number of B cells.

In autoimmune disease in man, similarities to the disease in the New Zealand black mouse can be seen, particularly in reference to genetic susceptibility, immune deficiency, and thymic injury.

Genetic susceptibility to autoimmunity is reflected by the high incidence of autoimmune phenomena in families of patients with immunologic deficiencies and in families of patients with systemic lupus erythematosus. Inherited immunodeficient syndromes are associated with a high incidence of autoimmunity as well as increased risks of infection and malignancy.

It has repeatedly been reported that there is a connection between immune disorders and malignant transformation of lymphoid tissue. This connection is illustrated by the higher incidence of reticulum cell sarcoma in certain autoimmune disorders, such as Sjögren's syndrome, and the association of Coombs-positive hemolytic anemia with reticulum cell sarcoma, chronic lymphocytic leukemia, and malignant lymphomas.

Finally, viruses are associated with autoimmune syndromes in man. Although viruses have not been reported as a causative agent of malignancy in man, there is indirect and suggestive evidence that a virus or viruses may play an etiologic role in Burkitt's lymphoma and possibily in myelogenous leukemia. Work in progress with the enzyme reverse transcriptase may answer this question. Not only has it been established that a virus can cause a malignancy such as Marek's disease in chickens (a lymphomatosis), but a vaccine has been produced that immunizes chickens against the disease.

Cancer of the ovary is usually advanced when first diagnosed. Between 60 and 80% of the cases are in stages III and IV when the diagnosis is made. It has been well established that cancer is markedly immunosuppressive. In animal models and in humans it has been shown that cancer that is growing is accompanied by a high titer of suppressor serum. The serum blocks the cancer so that the T lymphocytes are unable to attack the cancer cells. This is an in vivo response and does not occur in vitro unless suppressor serum is added to the culture. This action involves the humoral mechanism and is the result of a cell-free antibody being secreted by the B cell or plasma cell. The hypothetical question raised is whether advanced cancer of the ovary is ever an autoimmune disease. To my knowledge there is no documentation that there is an excess of helper T-cell activity or a deficiency of suppressor T-cell activity in patients with cancer of the ovary.

In an ovarian cancer project at Lenox Hill Hospital, it has been possible to isolate an autologous antibody by eluting it from the surface of the tumor cell. An antigen has been identified but has not yet been purified. While working on the project we observed that these patients were difficult to cross-match and that they possessed an antibody that interfered with the typing and cross-matching of these patients. The research associate (B.D.) has identified an antibody that reacts with normal tissue but does not recognize the ovarian cancer antigen. On the other hand, the ovarian cancer antibody identifies the ovarian carcinoma but does not recognize normal tissue. After treatmentwith cortisone for 2 or 3 days, it has been possible to suppress the antibody that was interfering with the cross-match, and successful cross-match was then possible. This observation suggests but surely does not prove that an autoimmune disease is present in those patients with advanced and recurrent ovarian cancer. The use of anticancer drugs often gives these patients a sense of well-being long before there is any anticipated effect. The combination of all of these factors raises the question of the production of an autoimmune disorder or disease in these patients.

SUMMARY

Autoimmunity is both a major immunologic phenomenon in clinical medicine and an important immunobiologic clue to the workings of the immune system. It may arise whenever there exists a state of immunologic imbalance in which B-cell activity is diminished. This imbalance occurs as a consequence of genetic, viral, and environmental mechanisms acting singularly or in combination. A central mechanism has also been postulated and involves an imbalance between suppressor and helper T cells. Either an excess of helper T activity or a deficiency of suppressor T activity could lead to the development of autoimmunity. If the B cell is overstimulated or under-regulated, autoimmunity may result. If the imbalance of regulatory signals results in excessive B cell proliferation, malignant lymphomas may develop as they do in some New Zealand mice.

Aging, the response to bacterial and viral infections, and specific immunologic diseases may give rise to a condition similar to autoimmunity. The individual may respond immunologically to certain of his or her own antigens (self-antigens). These important exceptions to the principle of self-tolerance help to analyze its fundamental mechanisms and are frequently associated with disease. It is important to emphasize the distinction between an autoimmune *response,* in which an individual makes antibodies or becomes allergic to a self-antigen, and an autoimmune *disease,* which is a pathologic condition arising from an autoimmune response. Autoimmune reactions can be both antibody-mediated and cell-mediated. Autoimmunity reflects a loss of immunologic tolerance to tissue and cellular antigens. Immunologic tolerance is the result of an active physiologic process and is not simply the lack of an immune response.

In treating patients with ovarian cancer, we observed that it was often difficult to cross-match their blood before transfusions. At first it was felt that previous transfusions had stimulated antibodies to the platelets and leukocytes of the original donors. However it was noted that some had antibodies present but had not been transfused before. The research associate (B.D.) identified the presence of an antibody which did not recognize the cancer antigen but which reacted to the normal tissue of the host. Treatment with a corticosteroid suppressed the antibody and permitted a compatible cross-match of blood. At this time the antibody has not been studied in more detail. This observation suggests but does not prove that an autoimmune disorder or disease may accompany an advanced or recurrent ovarian cancer.

BIBLIOGRAPHY

Allison, A.C.: Unresponsiveness to self-antigens. Lancet 2:1401, 1971.

Allison, A.C., Denman, A.M., Barnes, R.D.: Cooperating and controlling function of thymus-derived lymphocytes in relation to autoimmunity. Lancet 2:135, 1971.

Altman, A., Cohen, I.R., Feldman, M.: Normal T cell receptors for alloantigens. Cell Immunol. 7:134, 1973.

Barnes, E.W., Irvine, W.J.: Clinical syndromes associated with thymic disorders. Proc. R. Soc. Med. 66:151, 1973.

Belohradsky, B.H.: Meeting report of the second international workshop on primary immunodeficiency diseases in man. Clin. Immunol. Immunopathol. 2:281, 1974.

Bretscher, P.: A model for generalized autoimmunity. Cell. Immunol. 6:1, 1973.

Christian, C.L., Phillips, P.E.: Viruses and autoimmunity. Am. J. Med. 54:611, 1973.

Cooper, M.D.: Meeting report of the second international workshop on primary immunodeficiency diseases in man. Clin. Immunol. Immunopathol. 2:416, 1974.

Fudenberg, H.H., Stites, D.P., Caldwell, J.R., Wells, J.V.: Basic and Clinical Immunology. Lange Medical Publications, Los Altos, 1976.

Gershon, R.K.: T cell control of antibody production, *in* Contemporary Topics in Immunology. Vol. 3. Edited by M.D. Cooper, N.L. Warner Plenum, New York, 1974.

Glasser, D.L., Silvers, W.K.: Genetic determinants of immunological responsiveness. Adv. Immunol. 18:1, 1972.

Harris, J.E., Sirkovics, J.G.: The Immunology of Malignant Disease. Mosby, St. Louis, 1970.

Levy, J.A.: Autoimmunity and neoplasia: The possible role of C-type viruses. Am. J. Clin. Pathol. 62:258, 1974.

Marx, J.L.: Slow viruses: Role in persistent disease. Science 181:1351, 1973.

McDevitt, H.O., Bodner, W.F.: Histocompatibility antigens, immune responsiveness and susceptibility to disease. Am. J. Med. 52:1, 1972.

Paterson, P.Y.: Multiple sclerosis: An immunologic reassessment. J. Chronic Dis. 26:119, 1973.

Rowley, D.A. Specific suppression of immune responses. Science 181:1133, 1973.

Siegel, M.M., Good, R.A. (Eds.): Tolerance, Autoimmunity and Aging. Thomas, Springfield, 1972.

Steinberg, A.D., Baron, S., Talal, N.: The pathogenesis of autoimmunity in New Zealand mice: Induction of antinucleic acid antibodies by polymosinic polycytidylic acid. Proc. Natl. Acad. Sci. U.S.A. 63:1102, 1969.

Stutman, O.: Lymphocyte subpopulations in NZB mice: Deficit of thymus dependent lymphocytes. J. Immunol. 109:602, 1972.

Thomas, L.: Experimental mycoplasma infections as models of rheumatoid arthritis. Fed. Proc. 32:143, 1973.

Wybran, J.L., Levin, A.S., Spitler, L.E., Tudenberg, H.H.: Rosette-forming cells, immunological deficiency diseases and transfer factor. N. Engl. J. Med. 288:710, 1973.

23

Tumor Markers in Ovarian Cancer

A ll vertebrates have a defense system which protects them from disease-causing microorganisms. Its deliberate exploitation has conquered many infectious diseases and has long been a major achievement of medical science in terms of preventing suffering and saving lives.

The progressive and inexorable nature of cancer has led many physicians and laymen alike to believe that humans are incapable of defending themselves against it. There was a time, however, when many infectious diseases that are now easily eradicated or cured, seemed almost as inevitable in their course as cancer does today. Attempts to fight cancer immunologically go back to the early days of immunology.

A primary goal of cancer research is to define differences between normal and neoplastic cells that can be used as a point of attack in tumor diagnosis, prophylaxis, and therapy. Even if no qualitative differences exist, quantitative differences may be large enough to serve the same purpose.

Early in this century the hope was held that dissimilarities between normal and neoplastic cells could be demonstrated by immunologic methods, and that vaccination against cancer could be demonstrated. However work with outbred animals showed that the rejection of tumor by previously immunized animals was, in a great number of instances, attributable to sensitization to the normal alloantigens (HL-A) that were present in the animal in which the tumor originated (and therefore in the tumor), but not in the recipients.

Recognition of this response to the normal alloantigens rather than to a specific tumor antigen set back the field of tumor antigens. An accepted view followed that tumor-specific antigens could not possibly exist, because they would confer a selective disadvantage on the cells that carried them and lead to their immediate elimination by immunologic mechanisms. The fact that neoplasms often metastasize to the lymph nodes was viewed as an additional indication that an immunologic defense against cancer could hardly play a role.

When inbred strains of mice were developed in quantity, the pieces of the puzzle began to fall into place. It was now possible to analyze the conditions that either allowed transplants of normal and neoplastic tissues to grow in their hosts or led to their rejection.

The modern scientific study of the relationship of immunity to cancer was undertaken by Gross in the 1940s and later by Prehn and Main in the 1950s with extensive work on experimental transplantable tumors and the phenomena causing a rejection of grafted normal and cancerous tissue in inbred animals. A major conceptual advance in cancer research was achieved when it was established that cancers do arouse a specific immune response in the organism within which they appear. The background for the identification of tumor markers will be reviewed.

Immunology is a relatively new medical discipline. However the concept of immunity is an ancient one and is properly termed the study of resistance to infection. The term *immunity* has taken on an expanded role; it is now defined as the property whereby the lymphoreticular system makes a memorized response to an antigenic stimulus. This may result in a state of positive reaction known as sensitization, or in one of negative reaction known variously as immunologic tolerance, immunologic paralysis (acquired tolerance), or immunosuppression. It is a complex state arising from the properties of the individual, the community, the race, and the species; but the most striking thing about it is the specific nature of its protection in individuals after recovery from infection.

The future of modern immunology was born when Jenner discovered that inoculation with cowpox crusts protected man against smallpox. The next advancement in immunology was made through the contributions of Louis Pasteur. Roux and Yersin then demonstrated the existence of an exotoxin elaborated by diphtheria bacillus. The existence of tumor-specific antigens was suspected by the medical scientists of that era. In 1895 Héricourt and Richer attempted passive immunization with antisera produced in animals injected with human tumors. The results were highly unpredictable. In 1906 Bashford claimed that prior inoculations of tumor and whole blood in mice prevented the growth of transplants of a mammary adenocarcinoma. He noted that established transplants of spontaneous cancers were not affected. Seventy years later and millions of dollars spent on research have not resolved the problem. However the advances made in the last three decades arouse hopes of cure with certain cancers and promise the opportunity for early diagnosis in others, all within the foreseeable future.

Cancer-specific antigens were first identified in a little-quoted study by Gross in 1943. He described the failure of mice to accept transplants of a specific cancer after they had been immunized with material from the same cancer growing upon syngeneic mice. The rebirth of tumor immunology as an active field of research may be said to have occurred in 1957 when Prehn discovered that mice who were immunized against syngeneic methylcholanthrene-induced fibrosarcomas by inoculation of living sarcoma tissue followed by surgical removal of the growing tumor, were resistant to subsequent grafts of the same tumor. In addition, immunization with normal tissue did not confer resistance to the tumor grafts. The mice that had become resistant to the tumors still accepted skin grafts from the primary hosts of these tumors. Different methylcholanthrene-induced sarcomas were found to have individually distinct antigens; mice that were immune against one tumor still accepted the grafts of other tumors.

Tumor-specific transplantation antigens (TSTA) have been demonstrated not only in chemically induced tumors but also in tumors induced by viruses. A great number of tumor-associated antigens have now been identified. Although the syngeneic donor-host relationship seldom pertains in man, other experimental methods have clearly shown that many different types of human tumors have tumor-associated antigens. These tumor types are colonic (Gold and Freedman, 1965); ovarian (Levi, Keller, and Mandl, 1969; Ioachim, Dorsett, and Barber, 1972); bronchial (Yashi et al., 1968); mammary (Edynak et al., 1971); urothelial carcinomata (Bubenik et al., 1970); neuroblastoma (Hellström et al., 1968); melanoma (Morton et al., 1968; Jehn et al., 1970); lymphomata (Smith, Klein, and Klein, 1967; Klein et al., 1969; Buffe et al., 1970; Order, Porter, and Hellman, 1971); leukemia (Harris et al., 1971); and sarcomata (Morton et al., 1969; Wood and Morton, 1971).

The progressive nature of cancer has led many physicians and laymen alike to believe that human beings are incapable of defending themselves against cancer. Until closely inbred mice were available for studies, the results of tumor transplants were unpredictable and difficult to explain. However, when genetically pure strains of animals became available for study, experiments on tumor immunity using the techniques employed in the earlier studies showed clearly that previous success was related to the presence in the tumor of genetically imcompatible transplantation antigens of the original host, and that tumor regression, when it occurred, was consequent to homograft rejection rather than to immunity to tumor-specific antigens.

With this tool available extensive work on experimental transplantable tumors and the phenomenon causing the rejection of grafted normal and cancerous tissue in animals was carried out. A major conceptual advance was established when it was demonstrated that cancers do arouse a specific immune response in the organism within which they appear. Antigenic differences represent the first known qualitative distinctions between cancer cells and their normal counterparts. These qualitative differences between normal and cancer cells had escaped other methods of investigation but were revealed by immunologic techniques. These techniques took advantage of the extraordinary power of discrimination of the immune defense mechanism itself. Cancer immunology appears to be on the threshold of an era in which it will be possible to establish an early diagnosis. It was these advances that prompted us to undertake a multidisciplined approach to the problem of ovarian cancer, and to make early diagnosis through an immunologic method the keystone of the project.

Cancer of the ovary is the leading cause of death from gynecologic cancer. The constant challenge presented by ovarian cancer is that almost 11,000 women die from ovarian cancer each year and the results were no better in 1976 than they had been in the previous two decades. Since early diagnosis is a matter of chance rather than a scientific method, it follows that it is not possible to treat ovarian cancer with any predictable degree of certainty for cure. In the present state of our knowledge, early diagnosis is the key to successful treatment.

The definition of an ovarian tumor is difficult because of the diversity of histogenetic types of neoplasms originating in the ovary. It is considered a family of diseases rather than a single, distinct entity. The ovary is complex in its embryology, histology, steroidogenesis, and potential for malignancy. It is made up of germ cells, gonadal stromal cells, and mesenchymal tissue, each with its own potential to form tumors. The ovary is unique not only because it gives rise to a variety of cancers, but also because it is itself a favorite site for metastases from other organs.

This chapter summarizes work on tumor markers concerning the immunology of cancer. The application of immunologic methods to the study of human tumors has made significant progress. It has been demonstrated that there is immunity to autologous tumors manifested by both tumor and cellular reactions. Tumor-specific antigens have been discovered, two of which, carcinoembryonic antigen (CEA) and alpha fetoprotein (AFP), have already been introduced in practice as a method of monitoring the treatment of tumors of endodermal origin or of tumors arising from the primitive vitelline duct.

IMMUNOLOGIC MEANS OF CANCER DETECTION

In the cancer cells of animals or, more specifically, on the cell membrane of these cancer cells, there are antigens (associated with DNA and RNA viruses) which are shared by all cancer cells produced by a particular virus. These antigens are referred to as *common antigens.* Cancer cells produced by chemical carcinogens also have antigens on their cell membranes, but these are different in each tumor produced by the carcinogen and have been referred to as *unique antigens.* Recently this rigid separation of antigens has been challenged, and now it is felt that both can be present with one or the other playing the major role.

Antigens have also been found in human cancers. Burkitt's tumor has antigens that have been identified, and this same antigen is associated with infectious mononucleosis. A common as well as a unique antigen has been found in melanomas. The finding of a common antigen in melanomas suggests a possible viral origin for this type of cancer. An antigen which appears to be a common antigen has also been identified in epithelial ovarian cancers.

FETAL ANTIGENS

A new type of antigen, called *fetal antigen,* has been identified in association with human cancers. These antigens are released from the cancer cells and can be detected in the blood stream. They are found in the fetus, most often during the first two trimesters, and disappear before birth. But they reappear later in cancerous cells. Apparently during the first two trimesters a gene is functioning which is repressed in the third trimester or at birth. Later it is derepressed during carcinogenesis.

The two most commonly studied fetal antigens are the carcinoembryonic (CEA) and the alpha fetal protein antigens (AFP). Other fetal antigens are leukemia-associated antigen (LAA), fetal sulphoglycoprotein antigen (FSA), and placental-alkaline phosphatase. All of these antigens offer promise as useful agents in the development of diagnostic tests.

Of great interest has been the discovery of one particular group of materials—the embryonic-specific fetal antigens. It has been shown that they are associated with human and animal tumors and that they can be released into the body fluids. These antigens have been found in diverse tumors of the mouse, rat, and hamster, where they occurred spontaneously or were induced by physical, viral, and chemical agents. It has been proposed that this is a universal oncologic phenomenon termed *retrogenetic expression.*

Tumor-associated macromolecules fall into two groups. The first group comprises those macromolecules which reside within or on tumor cells, which have not yet been shown to be released, and which may be detected because of their influence upon the host's cellular and humoral systems. That is, they are present in tumors and body fluids without known metabolic effects— carcinoembryonic antigen (CEA), leukemia-associated antigens (LAA), fetal sulphoglycoprotein antigen (FSA), and polypeptides—and they are present in tumors and body fluids with metabolic effects—placental alkaline phosphatase, placental-type hormones, and related products. The other group is constituted by those macromolecules which are not present in or on tumor cells but are also released from the tumor cells into the body fluids. The ectopic production of hormones, their subunits, and related materials and fetal- associated macromolecules are the principal examples.

CARCINOEMBRYONIC ANTIGEN

The carcinoembryonic antigen (CEA) was first described by Gold and Freedman in 1965. The heterologous (produced in another species) antibodies to the carcinoembryonic antigen were produced by injecting saline extracts of colon cancer into rabbits. Adenocarcinoma of the human colon does not extend for more than 6 or 7 cm beyond the tumor. Because the resection always includes some of the surrounding normal tissue, it was possible to obtain both normal and tumor tissue from the same person. Therefore it was possible subsequently to absorb the rabbit antiserum with the corresponding normal bowel obtained during resection of the primary tumor mass. This permitted the researchers to circumvent the problem of distinguishing tumor-specific from individual specific antibodies in the final antiserum preparations.

Initially, an antigen common to all adenocarcinomas of the bowel was demonstrated by a variety of immunologic techniques. Subsequently, a similar antigen was found in the embryonic gut and was called *carcinoembryonic antigen.* The antigen was identified in the first two trimesters but was absent at birth. It was suggested that the gene producing the antigen in early embryonic life had been repressed. Later in adult life when it was found in association with adenocarcinoma of the gut, it was felt that the repressed gene had been derepressed. The stimulus for the derepression may have been a virus, a carcinogen, failure of the immunologic survillance mechanism, age, or some unknown factor.

Recently it has been reported that CEA has been found in association with a variety of tumors, both entodermal and nonentodermal. Because the serum from patients with both entodermally and nonentodermally derived carcinomas had elevated levels of CEA, an antigenic site common to several tumors was hypothesized to exist on CEA.

The carcinoembryonic antigen has been characterized as a glycoprotein with a molecular weight of 200,000. Recent studies raise doubts that CEA is a homogeneous material. It appears to have similarities in its activity to blood group A substance. Chemical analysis reveals a repeating unit of N-acetyl glucosamine which appears to be partly responsible for the antigenicity of CEA. The correlation between blood groups and malignancies is now receiving a great deal of attention.

RADIOIMMUNOASSAY TESTS

There are several modifications of this test being used. Todd uses a so-called triple-isotope–double-antibody assay. The Hansen method uses a Zirconyl phosphate gel (Z-gel), whereas the Gold test uses ammonium sulfate to precipitate the antibody-bound CEA. In general, antigens combine with their appropriate antibody to form an antigen-antibody complex. In the Roche method of using the radioimmunoassay procedure, the unknown sample is first added to the antibody and incubated. Then the radioactive-labeled antigen is added and incubated. The reaction of antigen with antibody is essentially irreversible. The test can be summarized in this manner: A radioimmunoassay is basically a standard antigen that has been tagged with an isotope and an antibody that is going to react with it. Anything that interferes with that reaction is measured in terms of the amount of isotope that does not come down. This is translated and called CEA or whatever is being tested.

CONCLUSION ON CEA

The normal value for CEA is 2.5 ng/ml. It is now accepted that CEA is not a method for screening for cancer of the colon. However it does provide a means of monitoring the results of therapy. If the CEA level is elevated before surgery and within 2 to 18 days after complete resection of a colonic tumor falls to a baseline level, any rise can be interpreted as suggestive of reactivation of the cancer. CEA is not specific for the diagnosis of cancer, and the amount present has significance in making a diagnosis. It is possible to divide CEA into three groups: below 2.5 ng/ml is normal; 12.5–40 ng/ml is intermediate; and above 40 ng/ml is high. Patients with benign disease, malignant tumors, or inflammatory and regenerative disorders may fall into the normal or intermediate groups, while levels in excess of 40 ng/ml are practically diagnostic of malignancy.

ALPHA FETOPROTEIN (AFP)

Serum AFP assays have currently gained an important place in the diagnosis and differential diagnosis of hepatocellular and testicular tumors. The observation that elevated AFP may occur before the detection of tumors by other means has important implications. In addition, successful therapy is associated with a decline in AFP to normal, and it rises again when the tumor recurs.

AFP is known to be a product of the human fetal liver, gastrointestinal tract, and yolk sac. It has been shown that the endodermal sinus tumor which is of vitelline origin invariably gives a positive test for AFP. Since the outcome of disease does not appear to depend on the level of AFP, there is a suggestion that a homeostatic control exists for AFP production in the tumor cells. This does not seem to be true for teratocarcinoma. It has its greatest value in the study of hepatomas of the liver, endodermal sinus tumors of the ovaries, as well as teratocarcinomas of the ovary. Besides the alpha fetoprotein, there are α_2H-fetoprotein (α_2HF), βS fetoprotein, and γ (gamma) fetoprotein (γFP).

AFP is a specific protein of embryonal and fetal serum in mammals. It is an alpha globulin and is the dominant serum protein during embryonic development and in early life. The level of AFP in fetal blood is 4 to 5 mg/liter, but during development the concentration gradually falls. In adult life the titer ranges from 2 to 15 ng/ml. It is a well-characterized protein with a molecular weight of about 70,000, and it comprises a single polypeptide chain. Its physio-chemical properties are very close to those of serum albumin.

AFP acts as an albumin substitute early. It also binds estrogen and may suppress lymphocyte activity. The synthesis of AFP starts at the same time as embryonic hemopoiesis. In the yolk sac where the first blood islets are formed, AFP is synthesized, and is the principal source of AFP in the embryo. During this time fetal hepatocytes are responsible for AFP synthesis. As the process of liver hemopoiesis begins to fade and hepatocytes progressively differentiate, AFP synthesis ceases, or to be more precise, falls to between one hundred-thousandth and one millionth of its maximal value. It can be concluded that AFP is one of the most distinct and well-defined biologic makers of certain tumors. Its presence in adult serum is evidence of hepatocellular carcinoma (HC) or teratocarcinoma of the ovary and testes (TC). AFP can be used as a specific diagnostic indication of these tumors, and because there is usually a specific correlation between AFP dynamics in the patient's blood and/or tumor progression or regression, it can be used to monitor the effectiveness of treatment.

FETAL SULPHOGLYCOPROTEIN ANTIGEN (FSA)

FSA occurs in the gastric juice in the fetus and in 96% of patients with gastric carcinoma. Certain immunologic studies indicate that FSA and CEA share common antigenic determinants. FSA production has also been reported to precede the development of overt carcinoma. The difficulty in interpreting this is that the incidence of FSA-positive patients with peptic ulceration far exceeds their known incidence of malignant change of approximately 2%. The successful removal of gastric cancer need not be followed by a decline of FSA levels in gastric juice.

Alpha α_2H-fetoprotein (α_2HF) is detected in the fetal liver and serum up to the end of the second postnatal month. It is elevated in adults with various tumors, including hepatoma, cholangiocarcinoma, and lymphoma. After the third postnatal month, raised levels are uncommon in children with noncancerous conditions.

The βS fetoprotein is elevated in the serum of patients with hepatocarcinoma, cholangiocarcinoma, gastric carcinoma, leukemia, and lymphoma. It is present in the serum until the seventh postnatal month.

Leukemia-associated antigen (LAA) is derived from the tumor cell membrane and is not found in the sera of normal persons or of patients with hepatomas. Unfortunately, serum LAA need not decline during remission.

There are two types of αfetoprotein (αFP): αFP-1 and αFP-2. The αFP-1 type does not occur in the serum of healthy persons, pregnant women, or patients with nonneoplastic disease, but it may be found in the fetus as well as in the sera of a minority of patients with tumors. The αFP-2 type has been found not only in breast carcinomas themselves, but also in normal breast tissue.

TISSUE POLYPEPTIDE ANTIGEN (TPA)

TPA has been shown to be a component of the endoplasmic reticulum and plasma membrane. It is a polypeptide with specific antigenic properties which now have been identified in a variety of species. It is a tumor-associated antigen occurring in human placenta, in human cancer tumors, and in body fluids of cancer patients. TPA is present in the membrane structures of human cancer cells. It can be detected there by the effects of cytotoxic antibodies or by the localization of fluorescent, monospecific anti-TPA antibodies.

TPA is released from growing and multiplying human cancer cells in vitro and can be specifically demonstrated in the culture medium hemagglutination inhibition technique. Because TPA is produced by propagating tumor cells, it could be expected to appear also in placenta and fetuses, and indeed it does, particularly in the placenta. High levels of TPA were found in all of the individual placentas.

Further studies of TPA have disclosed that the antigenic specificity of the TPA molecule is not limited to the human species; it is present in a wide variety of different animal species, ranging from apes through hoof-bearing animals and rodents, down to different fishes.

TPA has the ability to inhibit stimulation of lymphocytes by PHA in cell culture and to stimulate the uptake of radioactive thymidine in cultures of peripheral blood lymphocytes from immunized horses. It has also been found in patients with inflammatory changes of other origin. In studies carried out there is close agreement between TPA level and the clinical course of patients with metastases from mammary carcinoma. It has proved to be a good method to monitor the progress of the patient during therapy. In most cases the TPA was reduced to normal levels before remissions were evident from the clinical parameters studied. Therefore the test is considered to be worthwhile in governing the treatment of critically ill patients. Useless drugs can be discarded and replaced by more potent or more specific drug therapy before evidence of further progress of cancer is detected by x-ray or scintigram studies.

HORMONES (ECTOPIC HORMONE PRODUCTION AND MALIGNANCIES SUSCEPTIBLE TO HORMONE INFLUENCES)

The ectopic hormone syndromes represent an important aspect of oncology. Inappropriate hormone production can also serve as an index of tumor activity as their levels decline with successful therapy.

There are certain similarities between hormones and neoplasia. The immunologic defenses are decreased among the very young and the very old. It is the same age group in which we find a decreased production of hormones. In addition, tumor antigens are most often found on the cell membranes, and antigens in this position are considered to be the most important in producing antibodies specific for mounting a defense against that particular cancer. The similarity to hormone synthesis has a similar cell pattern of action. The specificity of hormonal response depends on the existence of unique receptors in the cell membrane. The peak incidence of tumors occurs at a time when there is maximum hormone imbalance, i.e., during puberty and the prepubertal months as well as during the perimenopausal and early menopausal years.

Attempts to explain why nonendocrine tumors should produce ectopic hormones has given rise to a great deal of discussion. It is generally, if not totally, accepted that if humans start from one cell, that cell must carry all the potential genetic and phenotypes of the body. The next question raised is why some genes function and others are repressed. Only time and additional studies will give us these answers. One theory that has aroused a great deal of interest is the so-called depressor-deletion hypothesis, proposed by Gellhorn. This theory proposes that as a tumor becomes progressively less well differentiated it loses the depressor which modifies the biosynthetic mechanisms present in the multipotential or embryonic cell. Another theory suggests that embryonic cells at a very early stage of development migrate into the mucosa of the alimentary tract and may give rise to endocrine glands. These scattered neuroendocrine cells have the potential to develop into a variety of hormone-producing tumors.

There are also other hypotheses concerning the origin of the nonendocrine neoplasms producing hormones, i.e., the derepression of existing genes and the random production of "new" material. In the genetic hypothesis it should be restated that all cells of an organism may contain the same DNA information and therefore are capable of synthesizing an unlimited number of proteins. As cellular differentiation progresses, the cell is limited to the production of a limited number of proteins and enzymes. As neoplasia develops the gene is derepressed and its capability to synthesize a particular protein or hormone may be restored. The hormone should be similar to the original hormone. This has been reported in erythemia, hypercalcemia, and Cushing's syndrome. The aberrant protein synthesis hypothesis suggests that with the development of neoplasia, abnormal cells develop which would synthesize new or altered DNA. In most instances it would be anticipated that the hormones produced by the neoplasms would be different from the natural hormones. This is confirmed in patients with neoplasms causing hypoglycemia or hyperthyroidism. In these cases the hormone produced by the neoplasm is immunologically different from the natural hormone.

PARAENDOCRINE TUMOR ACTIVITY

There are several humoral syndromes associated with neoplasia: hyperadrenocorticism, hypercalcemia, hypoglycemia, erythremia, hyperthyroidism, precocious puberty, inappropriate secretion of antidiuretic hormones, atypical carcinoid syndrome, and ectopic human chorionic gonadotropin secretion. The last syndrome will be discussed in detail.

Ectopic Human Chorionic Gonadotropin Secretion

Human chorionic gonadotropin (HCG) and human luteinizing hormone (HLH) are two glycoproteins with similar biologic activity. Both hormones are composed of an α and β subunit. The β subunit confers immunologic and bioloic specificity. The placenta normally secretes human chorionic gonadotropin and is found normally during pregnancy. Human luteinizing hormone is secreted by the pituitary and is found in the peripheral blood of both males and females after puberty. Since human chorionic gonadotropin is found normally only during pregnancy, its detection under any other circumstance implies that a human chorionic gonadotropin secreting tumor is present. Until recently most antisera to human chorionic gonadotropins could not discriminate between human chorionic gonadotropin and human luteinizing hormone. The development of an antisera specific for the beta subunit has been described and documented. It is specific for human chorionic gonadotropin.

It has been shown that approximately 40% of all tumors, including those in men, secrete human chorionic gonadotropin, and the percentage climbs to 90% among embryonal ovarian tumors and testicular tumors. This finding confirms reports that differentiated somatic cells do carry information for all the potential cell phenotypes of the body, and this has been demonstrated by the technique of nuclear transplantation into an enucleated egg and this egg with a transplanted nucleus can support the development of a fertile adult.

Precocious sexual maturity has followed the production of a gonadotropin-like material elaborated by a tumor. In these tumors there were no teratoid or trophoblastic elements that could have produced the gonadotropin. One is left with the conclusion that it represents cellular dedifferentiation and derepression of a gene.

A radioimmunoassay has been developed which selectively measures HCG in serum or plasma samples containing both HCG and HLH. Using that assay system, a large number of serum or plasma samples from patients with documented tumors have been assayed for the presence of immunoreactive HCG. Adenocarcinoma of the stomach, ovary, pancreas, and hepatoma are the tumors most commonly associated with ectopic HCG secretion. The incidence of ectopic HCG secretion ranged between 17 and 40% in those selected tumor types. Significantly, 30% of epithelial ovarian cancers and up to 90% of the embryonal ovarian carcinomas are associated with measurable amounts of this hormone.

Heterogeneity has been observed among the hormonal peptides secreted by tumors. Human chorionic gonadotropin (HCG) is composed of two dissimilar, noncovalently linked subunits. In a variety of tumor tissue extracts, samples of serum or urine contained not only HCG, but either or both subunits of HCG. A few rare tumors have had only free α or free β subunits present.

Lymphocyte function in vitro is altered by human chorionic gonadotropin. High concentrations of HCG inhibit the response of lymphocytes to phytohemagglutinin. The trophoblasts have antigens on their surfaces which have a negative charge, as does the lymphocytes. The fact that like charges repel each other may explain why the pregnancy (allograft) is not rejected. In addition, the antigens of the trophoblast stimulate an antibody response. These antibodies have been shown to function as blocking or enhancing antibodies in a great number of instances. Since it has been shown that a great number of tumors produce chorionic gonadotropin, the blocking antibodies formed may protect the tumor from the killer lymphocytes. Whether or not HCG, encountered during normal pregnancy or in patients with tumors ectopically secreting HCG, exerts any physiologic effect on the immune system in the human is unknown. If HCG were to exert a significant immunosuppressive effect, one might expect to see a significant difference in the clinical course of patients with tumors that ectopically secrete HCG when compared to patients with comparable tumors not ectopically secreting HCG. These findings have not yet been implemented.

Ferritin

A purified antigen identified as ferritin by electrophoretic, chemical, and immunologic criteria has been studied by Marcus. It has been found in breast cancer. Studies in the laboratory at Lenox Hill Hospital found that both normal ovary and the common epithelial tumors contained ferritin. There was no reaction between the purified ferritin and the antisera raised in the rabbit or the antibody extracted from ascitic fluid. It was concluded after additional studies that the common epithelial ovarian cancer antigen was not ferritin.

Regan Alkaline Phosphatase Isoenzyme

The Regan isoenzyme is heat stable, and at least one component of the enzyme has a molecular weight in the 200,000 range. The alkaline phosphatase enzymes are known to occur in serum and are derived from the liver, bones, lung, intestinal tract, and placenta. The placental alkaline phosphatase enzyme does not occur in fetal tissues, blood, or serum but does occur in maternal serum during the third trimester of pregnancy. It is never found in the serum of normal male subjects. The enzyme was first detected in a patient named Regan who had lung cancer. It has been found in association with a variety of cancers. When alkaline phosphatase is present it is a useful method to monitor tumor progression or regression. It can be detected in malignant serosal exudates. In any patient with an elevated serum alkaline phosphatase level found by routine methods, reexamination should be carried out to see if the placental alkaline phosphatase is responsible for the elevation. If it is, a careful evaluation should be carried out to detect or eliminate a latent neoplasm.

Stolbach found the isoenzyme in the serum of 30 to 40% of patients with cancer of the ovary and in 50 to 70% of malignant fluids from patients with carcinoma of the ovary.

Ovarian Cancer Antigen

This subject is covered in chapter 24. However, a short description is included here with the tumor markers.

Heterologous antisera produced against pools of ovarian carcinoma tissue have reacted consistently and specifically with the tissues of origin in immunodiffusion and immunofluorescence tests. The highly absorbed sera showed no reaction with normal ovarian tissues, normal human serum components, and various other neoplasms. These investigations have suggested the presence of a specific antigenic component in carcinomas of the ovary. This antigen did not cross-react with the carcinoembryonic antigen (CEA) and was not revealed in fetal tissues. Present attempts to purity and fully characterize this antigen are aimed toward its possible use in a much needed diagnostic test for the early detection of carcinoma of the ovary.

Recently it was demonstrated that effusions of patients with ovarian cancer contain sizable amounts of free and complexed immunoglobulins. Salt precipitation procedures recovered antibodies which, after purification and concentration, displayed a high degree of specificity against ovarian cancer cells. It is hoped that autologous antibodies recovered from peritoneal effusions will be utilized in sensitive radioimmunoassay tests, which are greatly needed for the early detection of ovarian cancer, the leading cause of death from gynecologic neoplasia.

SUMMARY

The presence of tumor-associated markers (macromolecules) in association with human tumor is now well established and accepted. They occur either on the surface of the cell membrane or within the cell. The tumor markers (antigens) may be released into the body fluid. Many are also known to be present in fetal tissues, and some possess biologic activity.

To be clinically useful, tumor antigens must meet the following criteria:

1. The antigen must pass from the tumor into the body fluids at a very early point in the life of the tumor.
2. The antigen must aid in the differential diagnosis.
    A. The tumor markers must be found only with tumors.
    B. Ideally, it should be site-specific or tumor-site-specific.
3. The titer or amount of tumor marker or antigen should decline with successful therapy.
4. The titer should rise early when recurrence develops.
5. It must be readily measurable by routine laboratory methods

Tumor markers are being identified at an increasingly rapid rate. Confusion will result if the same marker receives different names. Obviously, the ideal plan to coordinate the work of various investigators would include a registry with liberal exchange of material, and a committee to identify the marker with an acceptable name.

None of the currently recognized tumor-associated markers that occur in body fluids are specific for malignant tumors; quantitative rather than qualitative differences exist among inflammatory disease and benign and malignant tumors. In spite of this, CEA and AFP have an accepted clinical role at this time. They aid in tumor diagnosis (especially AFP) and in monitoring the effects of therapy.

A number of tumor markers are frequently recognized in elevated amounts with particular types of tumors. Measurement of each marker, hormones, and their products will make available a group of tests which, studied collectively, may supply help in detection, differential diagnosis, and prognostic assessment. Immunological Parameters Laboratories have developed the capacity to quantify each of the known means by which man immunologically resists infections and intoxications as well as cancer.

By outlining the immunologic parameters or spectra, it may be possible to observe functional heterogeneity between tumors of identical morphology or between cells of the same tumor. Such a finding could have behavioristic, histogenetic, and etiologic significance.

Ectopic production and secretion of hormones by a wide variety of tumors were initially recognized by signs and symptoms of excess circulating biologically active hormones. The development of more sensitive techniques has made it evident that not all tumors secrete biologically active hormones. Some of the forms of polypeptide hormones may not be active biologically even though present in high concentrations, whereas others secrete very low titers which are not detected clinically. Modern technology has made it possible to test for the ectopic production and secretion of hormones produced by a wide variety of tumors. Several new syndromes have been identified, and it is easier to identify ones previously described. Every hormone known to be normally secreted by endocrine organs or the placenta has been documented to be secreted ectopically by a great number of tumors. Several of these hormones may be used as biochemical markers of malignancy for both screening and monitoring patients with documented or suspected tumors.

There are certain striking similarities between hormones and neoplasia:

1. Immunologic defenses are decreased among the very young and the very old.
2. Hormone production is low among the very young and the very old.
3. Tumor antigens are most often on the cell membrane.
4. Hormone action starts on the cell membrane.
5. Human chorionic gonadotropin (HCG) may represent a surface antigen.
6. The peak incidence of many tumors, especially of the urogenital tract, occurs at the prepubertal or pubertal years.
7. The peak incidence of many tumors (breast, uterus, and ovary) occurs at the peri- and postmenopausal years, during the time when there are marked hormone changes.

Endocrine-active substances that are of interest to the gynecologist and are produced by aberrant hormone activity by tumors include gonadotropins, lactogens, thyrotropins, and adrenocortropins, as well as calcium mobilizing and erythropoietic substances.

BIBLIOGRAPHY

Abelev, G.I.: Alpha fetoprotein in oncogenesis and its association with malignant tumors. Adv. Cancer Res. 14:295–358, 1971.

Alexander, P.: Fetal "antigens" in cancer. Nature 235:137, 1972.

Alpert, M.E., Uriel, J., DeNechaud, B.: Alpha feto globulin in the diagnosis of human hepatoma. N. Engl. J. Med. 278:964, 1966.

Baldwin, R.W.: Tumor specific antigens associated with chemically induced tumors. Rev. Eur. Etudes Clin. Biol. 25:593, 1970.

Baldwin, R.W., Erubleton, M.J.: Demonstration by colony inhibition methods of cellular and humoral immune reactions to tumor-specific antigens associated with aminoazo-dye-induced rat hepatomas. Int. J. Cancer 7:17, 1971.

Barber, H.R.K., Kwon, T.: Hormones and cancer (ectopic hormone production and malignancies susceptible to hormone influences). J. St. Barnabas Med. Center, Symposium on The Current Status of Hormonal Therapy, 1975, p. 22.

Barlow, J.J., Bhattacharya, M.: Tumor markers in ovarian cancer: Tumor-associated antigens. Semin. Oncol. 2:203, 1975.

Braunstein, G.D., Vaitukaitis, J.L., Carbone, P.P., et al.: Ectopic production of human gonadotropin by neoplasms. Ann. Intern. Med. 78:39, 1973.

Bubenik, J., Perlmann, P., Helmstein, K., Moberger, G.: Immune response to urinary bladder tumors in man. Int. J. Cancer 5:39, 1970.

Buffé, D., Rimbault, C., Lemerle, J., Schweisguth, O., Burton, P.: Presence d'une ferroproteine d'origin. Tissulaire, Lα_2H dans le serum des enfants porteurs de tumeurs. Int. J. Cancer 5:85, 1970.

Coligan, J.E., Eagan, M.L., Todd, C.W.: Detection of carcinoembryonic antigen by radioimmune assay. Natl. Cancer Inst. Monogr. 35:427–432, 1972.

Dorsett, B.H., Ioachim, H.L., Stolbach, L., Walker, J., Barber, H.R.K.: Isolation of tumor-specific antibodies from effusions of ovarian carcinomas. Int. J. Cancer 16:779, 1975.

Edynak, E.M., Hirshant, Y., Old, L.J., Trempe, G.L.: Antigens of human breast cancer. Proc. Am. Assoc. Cancer Res. 12:75, 1971.

Fishman, W., Raam, S., Stolbach, L.L.: Markers for ovarian cancer: Regan isoenzyme and other glycoproteins. Semin. Oncol. 2:211, 1975.

Freedman, S.O.: Carcinoembryonic antigen: Current clinical applications. J. Allergy Clinl Immunol. 50:348, 1972.

Gall, S.A., Walling, J., Pearl, J.: Demonstration of tumor-associated antigens in human gynecologic malignancies. Am. J. Obstet. Gynecol. 115:387, 1973.

Gold, P.: Antigenic reversion in human cancer. Ann. Rev. Med. 22:85, 1971.

Gold, P., Freedman, S.O.: Demonstration of tumor-specific antigens in human colonic carcinomata by immunologic tolerance and absorption techniques. J. Exp. Med. 121:439, 1965.

Gross, L.: Intradermal immunization of C3H mice against a sarcoma that originated in animals of the same line. Cancer Res. 3:326, 1943.

Haber, E.: Radioimmunoassay: Principles and Practical Applications. Little, Brown, Boston, 1974.

Harris, R., Viza, D., Todd, R., Phillips, J., Sugar, R., Jennison, R.F., Marriott, G., Gleeson, M.H.: Detection of human leukaemia associated antigens in leukaemic serum and normal embryos. Nature, London 233:556, 1971.

Helström, I., Hellstrom, K.E., Pierce, G.E., Bill, A.H.: Demonstration of cell-bound and tumoral immunity against neuroblastoma cells. Proc. Nat. Acad. Sci. U.S.A. 60:1231, 1968.

Ioachim, H.L., Dorsett, B.H., Sabbath, M., Andersson, B., Barber, H.R.K.: Antigenic and morphologic properties of ovarian carcinoma. Gynecol. Oncol. 1:130–142, 1973.

Jehn, U.W., Nathanson, L., Schwartz, R.S., Skumen, M.: In vitro lymphocyte stimulation by a soluble antigen from malignant melanoma. N. Engl. J. Med. 283:329, 1970.

Laurence, D.J.R., Munro, N.: Fetal antigens and their role in diagnosis and clinical management of human neoplasms: A review. Br. J. Cancer 26:335, 1972.

Levi, M.M., Keller S., Mandl, J.: Antigenicity of a papillary serous cystadenocarcinoma tissue homogenate and its fractions. Am. J. Obstet. Gynecol. 105:856, 1969.

LoGerfo, P., Krupey, J., Hansen, H.J.: Demonstration of an antigen common to several varieties of neoplasia. N. Engl. J. Med. 283:138, 1971.

Mitchison, N.A.: Immunologic approaches to cancer. Transplant Proc. 2:92, 1970.

Morton, D.L., Malmgren, R.A., Holmes, E.C., Ketcham, A.S.: Demonstration of antibodies against human malignant melanoma by immunofluorescence. Surgery, St. Louis 64:233, 1968.

Neville, M.A.: Human tumor antigens and their potential usefulness in modern medicine, in Immunological Techniques for Detection of Cancer. Edited by S. Björklund. Stockholm, 1973, p. 15.

Order, S.E., Porter, M., Hellman, S.: Hodgkin's disease: Evidence of a tumor associated antigen. N. Engl. J. Med. 285:471, 1971.

Shuster, J.: Immunologic diagnosis of human cancers. Am. J. Clin. Pathol. 62:243–257, 1974.

Smith, J.B.: Alpha fetoprotein: Occurrence in certain malignant diseases and review of clinical applications. Med. Clin. North Am. 54:797–803, 1970.

Smith, R.T., Klein, G., Klein, E.: Studies of the membrane phenomenon in cultured and biopsy cell lines from the Burkitt lymphoma, *in* Advances in Transplantation. Edited by J. Dausset, J. Hamberger, G. Mathé. Williams & Wilkins, Baltimore, 1967, p. 483.

Stolbach, L.L., Krant, M.J., Fishman, W.H.: Ectopic production of an alkaline phosphatase isoenzyme in patients with cancer. N. Engl. J. Med. 281:757, 1969.

Tee, D.E.H., Wang, M., Watkins, J.: Antigenic properties of human tumors: Tumor-specific antigens. Eur. J. Cancer 1:315, 1965.

Vaitukaitis, J.L.: Peptide hormones as tumor markers. Cancer 37:567, 1976.

Van Nagell, J.R., Meeker, W.R., Parker, J.C., Jr., Harralson, J.D.: Carcinoembryonic antigen in patients with gynecologic malignancy. Cancer 35:1372, 1975.

Wood, W.C., Morton, D.L.: Host immune response in common cell-surface antigen in human sarcomas. N. Engl. J. Med. 284:569, 1971.

Yashi, A., Matsumura, Y., Carpenter, C.M., Hyde, L.: Immunochemical studies on human lung cancer antigens soluble in 50% saturated ammonium sulfate. J. Nat. Cancer Inst. 40:663, 1968.

24

Ovarian Cancer Project

C ancer of the ovary is the leading cause of death from gynecologic cancer. An ovarian cancer project was undertaken at Lenox Hill Hospital to explore areas that needed study and possibly could provide information to control ovarian cancer. The project was divided into three main parts to launch an attack toward understanding the ovary that had developed a malignant potential and to apply this knowledge towards the development of a test for early diagnosis. The study included (1) ultrastructural examination of the common epithelial ovarian tumors by the electron microscope; (2) tissue culture of the epithelial ovarian cancers; (3) immunologic study proper in an attempt to raise a heterologous antibody against a common epithelial ovarian cancer antigen.

Ultrastructure of Common
Epithelial Ovarian Cancers

The ultrastructural study of the various types of ovarian carcinoma showed heterogeneity within the same tumor with coexistence of more than one cell type and with variations from differentiation to anaplasia. The coexistence of serous and mucinous cells in ovarian carcinoma, also noted by Gondos, can be satisfactorily explained by the histogenetic theory of Hertig, which attributes the origin of all epithelial tumors of the ovary to the multipotential ovarian surface germinal epithelium. This was a significant observation in that it suggested that the epithelial ovarian cancers might share a common antigen. When the results of our study indicated that there is a shared antigen, the possibility of an immunologic test using pooled antigens for the main epithelial tumors moved closer to a reality than it had been before this observation.

Tissue Culture of Ovarian Cancer

The culture of common epithelial ovarian cancer cells in vitro has proved to most useful in comparing their morphology and behavior. In addition, tissue cultures are indispensable for any work on tumor virology and immunology. With few exceptions, all tumors showed signs of initial growth in vitro, manifested by cellular attachment to the glass, spreading, and aggregation. Within the next 2 or 3 days more cells attached and spread on the glass, forming small colonies of epithelioid or polyhedral cells. At about 10 to 14 days a clear growth pattern was most often noticeable, becoming better expressed as the cellular density increased. Some of the cultures never grew enough to permit subculturing and died off after 2 to 3 weeks, while others grew quite abundantly for a period of several months.

It was noted that cultures that exhibited a certain pattern of growth maintained that pattern consistently after many months in vitro, numerous subcultures, and even after freezing and resuscitation. A comparative study of tissue cultures in light and electron microscopy led to the conclusion that the ovarian cancer cells have preserved in vitro most of their salient features. In addition, the cells grow in an immune-free environment. These conclusions were essential in permitting us to use confidently the cultures of ovarian carcinomas in immunologic studies.

Raising an Antibody to a Tumor-Associated Antigen in Common Epithelial Ovarian Cancers

The application of immunologic methods to the study of human tumors has made significant progress. It has been demonstrated that there is immunity to autologous tumors manifested by both tumor and cellular reactions. Tumor-specific antigens have been discovered, two of which, carcinoembryonic antigen (CEA) and alpha fetoprotein (AFP), have already been introduced in practice as a method of monitoring treatment for these tumors.

The accumulated knowledge of tumor immunology indicates a degree of antigenic specificity in regard to each type of tumor and suggests the existence of etiologic agents and pathogenic mechanisms. It follows that each type of tumor should be studied individually. Some tumors have not received the attention that their clinical importance demands. Ovarian cancer is such an example. Although it is a constant challenge to the clinician because of its lack of early symptoms and rapid growth, little basic research has been carried out. Therefore, within the framework of a multilateral study on carcinoma of the ovary, common epithelial ovarian cancers were studied. This chapter deals with immunologic investigation of these epithelial ovarian carcinomas in comparison with normal ovaries and various other tumors. Using immunofluorescence and immunodiffusion, we found that epithelial ovarian carcinomas share a common antigenic component not present in the other tissues assayed. The immunologic studies included cytotoxicity assays using the patient's own serum, and they indicated the presence of specific humoral antibodies.

A search for specific antigens in various malignant tumors, undertaken earlier by Witebsky, Rose, and Shulman, included the production of antisera raised in rabbits against two ovarian carcinomas. Both antisera gave positive complement-fixation tests with extracts of ovarian tumors, whereas neither reacted with extracts of normal ovaries. More recently, Levi raised antisera in rabbits against papillary serous cystadenocarcinoma of the ovary and isolated an antigenic component in the tumor homogenates. With this background and the expanded work reported on the carcinoembryonic antigen (CEA), the present study on the common epithelial ovarian cancer antigen was established.

MATERIALS AND METHODS

The tumors were brought to the laboratory under sterile conditions within 10 minutes of their removal, fixed for light and electron microscopy, processed for tissue cultures, and either prepared immediately for tumor extracts or frozen for later use.

Preparation of Antisera

Tumor extract for immunization was prepared by using homogenized, pooled, common epithelial ovarian cancer tissues in equal volumes of saline 4°C. The homogenates from the pooled epithelial ovarian cancers were mixed with an equal volume of complete Freund's adjuvant and emulsified by brief sonication at 4°C. Heterologous antisera was raised by injecting the tumor–Freund's adjuvant emulsion subcutaneously in multiple sites once a week for 4 weeks, followed by a boosting dose at the sixth week and collection of the sera 5 days later. The resultant antiserum was screened against pooled soluble antigen from normal and neoplastic cells in double diffusion studies. Although in studies with CEA normal colon removed from 7 cm or more from the cancer can serve as a control possessing the same HLA antigens as the cancer, this is not possible in studies on ovarian cancer. Therefore the sera had to be serially absorbed by using a variety of tissues, a process which will be described later.

Preparation of Soluble Antigen

The soluble antigen extracts of tissue to be used in the immunoprecipitation tests and absorption of antisera were prepared from the previously homogenized tissue, which was sonicated with an equal volume of phosphate-buffered saline at pH 7.2 for 60 seconds at 4°C. The resultant sonicates were centrifuged at 48,000 g for 2 hours at 4°C. The supernatant was stored at −80°C and used as 50% tissue extracts, or dialyzed against distilled water and concentrated by lyophilization. Blood substances and other tissue extracts either were prepared for absorption of antisera or were purchased.

Absorption of Antisera

The heterologous antisera was absorbed by suspending from 10 to 100 mg of lyophilized tissue extract per 1.0 ml of antisera and storing for 15 hours at 4°C. The sera were then centrifuged at 70,000 g for 1 hour at 4°C. The absorption process was carried out against a variety of tissues. The supernatant was used as the absorbed antisera in the immunodiffusion studies.

Immunodiffusion Test

The immunodiffusion test was performed by the method of Ouchterlony in either Hyland pattern C plates (Hyland Laboratories, Costa Mesa, California), or Cordis IDF I and II cells (Cordis Laboratories, Miami, Florida). Precipitation patterns were read after 1, 2, and 5 days.

Results of the Immunodiffusion Test

Sera from rabbits immunized with tumor material were screened in gel diffusion against soluble antigen extracts of ovarian tumors and normal tissues. Multiple precipitin lines against both types of tissue were obtained with sera of two rabbits. Those sera showing additional activity against tumor extracts were exhaustively absorbed with lyophilized soluble antigens from a pool of normal ovaries, as well as with normal human sera and AB blood group substance. Absorbed serum from one rabbit retaining activity against ovarian carcinoma pools was then screened against a variety of normal and neoplastic tissue extracts in double gel diffusion and indirect immunofluorescence. This serum reacted specifically with ovarian carcinomas in immunodiffusion and showed no activity with normal tissues, neoplasms of other origin, benign tumors of the ovary, or fetal ovary extracts.

Immunofluorescence Test

Cells for examination by immunofluorescence were either grown directly on slides in short-term tissue cultures or prepared by mincing fresh tissue in Hank's balanced salt solution and adjusting the cell concentration in 1 to 2 million cells per ml before application of cell suspension to clear spots on microscopic slides sprayed with Fluoroglide (Chemplast, Inc., Wayne, New Jersey). Cryostat thin sections of tumor tissue were also successfully examined but not routinely used because of occasional nonspecific attachment of fluorescent conjugates. Dried slides were fixed for 10 minutes in acetone and were examined immediately or stored at $-80\,^{\circ}$C. Immunofluorescence tests were performed by incubating prepared slides with the appropriate dilution of antisera for 1 hour at $37\,^{\circ}$C in a moist chamber, followed by two 5-minute washings in normal saline and two 5-minute washings in distilled water. The slides were then air-dried.

The individual fluorescent antibody test was carried out to produce a sharp end point for reading with the ultraviolet microscope. The tumor antigen that had been prepared with the untagged heterologous absorbed antibody now received an application of fluorescein-conjugated goat antirabbit immunoglobulin antisera (Hyland Laboratories) at a dilution of 1:10. The slide was again incubated for 1 hour at $37\,^{\circ}$C and washed as before. They were then stained for 5 minutes in a 0.6% Evans blue solution to remove autofluorescence, then washed for 5 minutes with 20% phosphate-buffered saline at pH 7.4 in glycerol. The slides were examined under a Leitz fluorescence microscope using an HBO 200 mercury light source with a BG 12 exciter filter and a K 540 barrier filter. The heterologous absorbed antisera consistently gave reactions of 1:16 and of 1:32 with tissues of all other types, but with carcinoma of the ovary the cancers maintained in tissue culture for periods up to 1 year retained their ability to fix antibody when stained by this procedure.

Material, Methods, and Results of Study with Ascitic Fluid

Cells from ascitic fluid found in patients with common epithelial ovarian cancers have been found to grow well in tissue culture. Stolbach has been able to extract a tumor antigen from the surface of ovarian cancer cells obtained from ascitic fluid by utilizing hypertonic KC1. He was also able to obtain an IgG fraction from the ascitic fluid by using the Rivanol extraction method. In addition, each of the IgG fractions from patients with the common epithelial ovarian cancers reacted with the KC1 extract. The extracts from patients with other malignancies did not react.

The project on ascitic fluid by one of the researchers (B.D.) was carried out be extracting the antibody by a salt precipitation method rather than the conventional Rivanol technique. The studies on ascitic fluid revealed that the tumor cells, as opposed to other cells, showed a large amount of bound antibody as well as complement. There are two unanswered questions at this time, namely, how much specific antibody is present and why doesn't the complement contribute to tumor cell destruction?

The tumor antibody is a natural antibody against an epithelial ovarian tumor and is extremely helpful in identifying the antigen. When ascitic fluid was tested for antitumor antibody activity by indirect immunofluorescence and counterelectrophoresis, none was found. This result might be anticipated if tumor antigen were present in excess, because then all the tumor-specific antibody would logically be bound as an immune complex. This possibility was explored by dissociation of the antigen-antibody and recovery of the antibody alone. Under these conditions it was found that ascitic fluid from malignant common epithelial tumors of the ovary contained antibody specifically reacting with ovarian tumor cells, both in cytoplasm and membrane, by indirect immunofluorescence. A common epithelial ovarian cancer cell extracted from ascitic fluid and reacted against heterologous antirabbit sera is included for comparison. Thoracentesis fluid from lung effusions failed to demonstrate the presence of such antibody.

In pursuing the work with the antibody isolated from the ascitic fluid an attempt was made to block its reaction with the common epithelial ovarian antigen by first reacting the antigen with fluorescein-tagged heterologous antisera raised in the New Zealand white rabbit. The result revealed a more intense fluorescent reaction at the cell membrane. It may be explained by accepting the premise that the heterologous antibody and the homologous antibody attach to different antigenic determinants on the same molecule. Additional work will be carried out to prove or disprove this hypothesis.

Less work is being done on the heterologous antibody in this project at present, and more attention has been directed to the homologous antibody extracted from the ascitic fluid. It had been demonstrated that antibodies can be eluted at low pH from the surface of neoplastic cells derived from either solid tumors or cells in ascitic fluid. These antibodies are capable of blocking specific cell-mediated cytotoxicity against autologous tumor cells.

In this project tumor cells collected from peritoneal effusions of patients with ovarian carcinomas, when stained with fluorescein-labeled antihuman immunoglobulins, showed strong, diffuse fluorescence of tumor cells, suggesting the presence of sizable amounts of antibodies on their surface. Consequently, we have assumed that peritoneal effusions in carcinomas of the ovary, which usually include numerous tumor cells, might also contain specific antibodies either free or bound in antigen-antibody complexes. The recovery of antibodies from specific complexes appears to be a most desirable aim because they represent pure, autologous immunoglobulins that do not require exhaustive absorption preparations and because they can be used as highly specific reagents to detect the presence of tumor antigens. In addition, the amount of antibodies that can be recovered from ascitic fluid is much greater than that obtainable from serum. The use of the Amicon TCT-10 tangential flow ultrafiltration cell has proved to be a more efficient procedure for the processing of large quantities of antibody. The concept of obtaining antibodies by breaking antigen-antibody complexes seems to hold more promise because antibodies thus obtained will most likely exhibit the highest specificity and will therefore represent the most sensitive reagents for the detection of tumor antigens. The amount of antigen and antibody extracted has provided the opportunity to explore new approaches to the application of a sensitive radioimmunoassay for the detection of ovarian carcinoma antigens.

The present phase of the project differs from attempts in the past to isolate tumor-associated antigens and to develop antibodies against these antigens for use as diagnostic reagents. In these studies the antisera were developed in laboratory animals and their specificity was enhanced by absorption with normal human tissue extracts.

In the case of ovarian cancer antigens, crude tumor extracts injected into animals have been used by previous investigators to produce poly-specific antisera. These antisera were subsequently absorbed with nontumor tissue extracts as well as nonovarian tumor extracts to make them specific for ovarian tumor antigens.

In contrast to the approach usually followed by investigators who have utilized heterologous antisera to identify ovarian cancer antigens, the basic principle of the ovarian cancer project is to use autologous antitumor antibodies as probes to identify ovarian cancer antigens. The recovered tumor-specific antibodies will be used to prepare an immunoadsorbant for the purification of the antigen or antigens. The antigen isolated and purified will be used to raise high affinity antibodies (monospecific) in an appropriate animal system; this is essential for developing diagnostic assays such as radioimmunoassays. The antigen will further be utilized to detect circulating tumor-specific antibodies, or antibodies in the effusion fluids of patients. In addition, the separation of antigen-antibody complexes by low pH treatment and ultrafiltration might also be applied to serum and may possibly result in a test system for the direct measurement of this immune complex (possibly blocking factors) in the serum. The proposed radioimmunoassay would involve use of polymerized antibody of high affinity and potency. Although much work needs to be done, the concept of utilizing autologous antibodies as probes for isolating specific ovarian tumor antigens has great potential.

SUMMARY

The results of these experiments, using both heterologous and human antibody, are that the common epithelial ovarian tumor produces at least one surface-specific tumor antigen. An additional cytoplasmic tumor-specific antigen is suggested but not proved at this point. Work on the melanoma indicates that each melanoma may have a unique surface antigen, in addition to the common intracellular antigen. There is a precedent in experimental work for the coexistence of shared and unshared tumor antigens in the same cell. Two types of antigens are also found in tumors induced by viruses. In all these cases the presence of the individual antigen may be masked by the common antigen. The current project on common epithelial ovarian tumors has not advanced to the point at which a comparison can be made.

A purified antigen identified as ferritin by electrophoretic, chemical, and immunologic criteria was supplied by Marcus. Although both normal ovarian as well as the common epithelial tumors contained ferritin, there was no reaction between the purified ferritin supplied to us and the antisera raised in the rabbit or the antibody extracted from ascitic fluid. It was concluded after additional studies that the common epithelial ovarian cancer antigen was not ferritin.

The results of the experiments employing immunodiffusion and immunofluorescence with heterologous sera raised in rabbits against the common epithelial ovarian tumors suggest the existence of a cross-reacting antigen specific to epithelial ovarian tumors. This possibility is supported by findings from the ultrastructural study of various types of epithelial ovarian carcinoma, which show heterogeneity within the same tumor and the coexistence of more than one cell type with variations from differentiation to anaplasia. The coexistence of serous and mucinous cells in ovarian carcinoma noted by Gondos can be satisfactorily explained by the histogenetic theory of Hertig, which attributes the origin of all epithelial tumors of the ovary to the multipotential ovarian surface germinal epithelium, referred to as the mesothelial lining.

The consistently positive reaction of ovarian carcinoma and the negative reaction of normal tissues, including normal human serum components, with highly absorbed antisera make it improbable that the observed phenomenon is caused by normal tissue alloantigens. A possible explanation may be that the antigenic difference between ovarian carcinoma and normal tissue is quantitative in nature. However the negative results in immunofluorescence and the inability of relatively large amounts of normal tissue to absorb out the specific activity of the antiserum do not support this possibility.

A comparison by immunodiffusion and immunoelectrophoresis between the common epithelial ovarian antigen and the carcinoembryonic antigen (CEA) as well as the alpha fetoprotein antigen (AFP) showed a lack of cross-reactivity. Unlike CEA, the common epithelial ovarian antigen counld not be detected in fetal tissue. Although CEA is associated with different titers related to a variety of inflammatory and metabolic disorders as well as to malignancy (suggesting a quantitative and almost nonspecific response), the common epithelial ovarian antigens give a specific and qualitative response.

The results of the current investigation suggest the presence of a specific antigenic component in the common epithelial ovarian cancers. The purification and characterization of this antigen, presently underway at Lenox Hill Hospital, are necessary steps toward establishing baselines that will serve as important background material toward the possible demonstration of a specific ovarian tumor antigen, antibody, and/or antigen-antibody complex in the blood of patients with ovarian cancer. The additional studies carried out in ascitic fluid have reinforced our accumulated data. The next logical step is to purify the antigen so that it can be used in radioimmunologic studies. This may give us a sensitive and practical assay that can be used for early diagnosis of ovarian cancer.

The current project at Lenox Hill Hospital is to process malignant effusion fluids from patients with carcinoma of the ovary with the following specific aims: (1) to isolate and purify tumor-specific antibodies and/or antibody-antigen complexes from effusion fluids; (2) to dissociate the antibody-antigen complexes and separate the tumor-associated antigens and antibodies making up these complexes; (3) to determine the immune specificity of antibodies isolated from effusion fluids by indirect immunofluorescence techniques using malignant and nonmalignant cells of different origins; (4) to detect tumor-associated antigen and/or tumor-specific antigen in the effusion fluid and tumor extracts; (5) to utilize the recovered tumor-specific antibodies to prepare an immunoadsorbent for the purification of the antigen(s); and (6) to develop a diagnostic assay for detecting circulating antibody, antigen, and antigen-antibody complexes in patients with various stages of ovarian malignancy. The ultimate aim is to develop a screening test for the early diagnosis of ovarian cancer in asymptomatic women. The present approach of utilizing autologous antibodies as probes for isolating specific tumor antigens overcomes some of the major problems encountered when working with crude tumor extracts to develop heterologous antibodies in animals.

Radioimmune assay techniques based on tumor-associated antigens are finding application in the diagnosis of human cancer. There are two basic forms of radioimmune assay. One is based on complete saturation of the antibodies with antigen, and the other is based on progressive filling of the antibody-binding sites. The specificity and sensitivity of any assay depend primarily on the antiserum used. For a high sensitivity, a high binding constant for the antibody is important. The preparation of a suitable antiserum, particularly a monospecific antiserum, is very important. Specificity in a radioimmune assay is never absolute, but it may be improved through knowledge of the structure of the antigen. The model for these principles is the carcinoembryonic antigen.

BIBLIOGRAPHY

Abelev, G.I.: Alpha fetoprotein in oncogenesis and its association with malignant tumors. Adv. Cancer Res. 14:295, 1971.

Alexander, P.: Fetal "antigens" in cancer. Nature 235:137, 1972.

Alpert, M.E., Uriel, J., DeNechaud, B.: Alpha feto globulin in the diagnosis of human hepatoma. N. Engl. J. Med. 278:964, 1966.

Baldwin, R.W.: Tumor specific antigens associated with chemically induced tumors. Rev. Eur. Etudes Clin. Biol. 25:593, 1970.

Baldwin, R.W., Erubleton, M.J.: Demonstration by colony inhibition methods of cellular and humoral immune reactions to tumor-specific antigens associated with aminoazo-dye-induced rat hepatomas. Int. J. Cancer 7:17, 1971.

Bhattacharya, M., Barlow, J.J.: An immunologic comparison between serous cystadenocarcinoma of the ovary and other human gynecologic tumors. Am. J. Obstet. Gynecol. 117:849, 1973.

Bhattacharya, M., Barlow, J.J.: Immunologic studies of human serous cystadenocarcinoma of ovary. Demonstration of tumor-associated antigens. Cancer 31:588-595, 1973.

Battacharya, M., Barlow, J.J.: Tumor-associated antigen(s) from human cystadenocarcinoma of the ovary. Proceedings of the 11th International Cancer Congress, 1974, p.105.

Coligan, J.E., Eagan, M.L., Todd, C.W.: Detection of carcinoembryonic antigen by radioimmune assay. Natl. Cancer Inst. Monogr. 35:427-432, 1972.

Dorsett, B.H., Ioachim, H.L., Stolbach, L., Walker, J., Barber, H.R.K.: Isolation of tumor-specific antibodies from effusions of ovarian carcinomas. Int. J. Cancer 16:779-786, 1975.

Edynak, E.M., Hirshant, Y., Old, L.J., Trempe, G.L.: Antigens of human breast cancer. Proc., Am. Assoc. Cancer Res. 12:75, 1971.

Gall, S., Walling, J., Pearl, J.: Demonstration of tumor-associated antigens in human gynecological malignancies. Am. J. Obstet. Gynecol. 115:367, 1973.

Haber, E.: Radioimmunoassay: Principles and Practical Applications. Little, Brown, Boston, 1974.

Ioachim, H.L., Dorsett, B.H., Sabbath, M., Andersson, B., Barber, H.R.K.: Antigenic and morphologic properties of ovarian carcinoma. Gynecol. Oncol. 1:130-142, 1973.

Knauf, S., Urbach, G.H.: Ovarian tumor-specific antigens. Am. J. Obstet. Gynecol. 119:966-970, 1974.

Laurence, D.J.R., Munro, N.: Fetal antigens and their role in diagnosis and clinical management of human neoplasms: A review. Br. J. Cancer 26:335, 1972.

LoGerfo, P., Krupey, J., Hansen, H.J.: Demonstration of an antigen common to several varieties of neoplasia. N. Engl. J. Med. 283:138, 1971.

Mitchison, N.A.: Immunologic approaches to cancer. Transplant Proc. 2:92, 1970.

Shuster, J.: Immunologic diagnosis of human cancers. Am. J. Clin. Pathol. 62:243-257, 1974.

Stolbach, L.L., Krant, M.J., Fishman, W.H.: Ectopic production of an alkaline phosphatase isoenzyme in patients with cancer. N. Engl. J. Med. 281:757, 1969.

Van Nagell, J.R., Meeker, W.R., Parker, J.C., Jr., Harralson, J.D.: Carcinoembryonic antigen in patients with gynecologic malignancy. Cancer 35:1372, 1975.

25

Immunotherapy and Immunopotentiation

Immunotherapy of human tumors is a highly promising modality that is still a subject of investigation and may pose unforeseen risks. It should be performed in patients brought into remission by conventional anticancer therapy and against the background of a complex, reliable monitoring system capable of quantitatively measuring the patient's antitumor immune reactions. It is important to differentiate between *immunoprophylaxis,* which is the administration of an immunostimulator or immunopotentiator when all gross disease has been removed, and *immunotherapy,* which is given to control or eradicate macroscopic disease. A more detailed discussion of this subject is presented in the book, *Immunobiology for the Clinician.*

Immunotherapy is the treatment of disease by active or passive immunization. Immunity is the property whereby the lymphoreticular system makes a memorized response to an antigenic stimulus. This may result in a state of positive reaction known as sensitization, or in one of negative reaction (diminished or absent), known variously as immunologic tolerance, immunologic paralysis (acquired tolerance), or immunosuppression. Therefore it is not strictly correct to follow the common usage of the word *immunization* as a synonym for *sensitization* or *stimulation.*

The most efficient cures of diseases that our philosophy can conceive involve the potentiation of normal, biophysical, or biochemical processes, or the countering of abnormal processes which lead to or accompany disease. Cancer presents few examples of this ideal at present, but studies of what has become known as host resistance are clearly an early step in this apparently logical direction. These are multitudinous factors—such as intercellular communication, metabolic peculiarity, biochemical selection, and hormonal requirement—which may be involved in host resistance. The immune activities of the lymphoreticular system have received the greatest attention and will be the main topic of this discussion.

THE IMMUNE DEFENSE SYSTEM

The antigens on the surface of cancer cells are generally weak antigens, and although they do arouse a specific response in the host, the response is also weak. If the tumor cell has the ability to stimulate a specific immune response, why does the cancer continue to grow in the presence of a mechanism designed to control its growth? The explanation may be that the rate of growth exceeds the capacity of the immune response. However studies in animals have disclosed more specific reasons for the failure of the immune response to prevent the start and growth of cancer. These reasons are discussed in the next section.

FAILURE OF THE IMMUNE RESPONSE

Immunosuppression

Many factors contribute to immunosuppression, including aging, the neoplastic process itself, anticancer drug therapy, radiation therapy, genetic defects, neonatal thymectomy, and, to a lesser extent, antibiotics, anesthetics, analgesics, and hypnotics. In reality, it is difficult to separate the contributions of drugs and disease in bringing about immunosuppression. One of the most potent of these factors to bring about a state of immunosuppression is the cancer itself, and as it progresses the degree of immunosuppression increases. In any attempt at the use of immunotherapy, the disease must first be debulked.

Immunologic Tolerance

In a broad sense, immunologic tolerance may represent a specific form of immunosuppression. It is usually associated with exposure to an antigen during embryonic or early neonatal life, before the immune system has matured. It may, however, occur later in life. The tolerance theory for the progress of cancer is offered as an explanation for the theory cancer arises from a single cell clone. Work on choriocarcinoma has suggested this mechanism. When it occurs, the host is not immunologically tolerant in general, but only tolerant for that specific tumor antigen.

Immune Paralysis (Acquired Tolerance)

The currently preferred term is *acquired tolerance.* It is induced by injecting very small or very large doses of antigen. The tolerance persists as long as that antigen remains in the body. In clinical practice it has been suggested that immune paralysis occurs in the host with large tumors. Following the removal of such a large tumor mass, the host exhibits resistance to the reimplantation of her own tumor cells. This fact suggests that the intrinsic failure of the immune response was not the cause of the original lack of immune reaction. Rather, the temporary paralysis resulted from the system's inability to cope with too big a challenge.

Immunologic Enhancement (Blocking Antibodies)

This phenomenon was discovered in the course of transplantation experiments. It was anticipated that animals transplanted with grafts of foreign cancer cells, then given injections of antiserum against cancerous cells, would rapidly reject the grafts. However it was found that the cancer cells were not only tolerated, but that the rejection was delayed. The antibody produced and then injected was an enhancing or blocking antibody, as opposed to a cytotoxic antibody. These antibodies may have coated the tumor by forming an antigen-antibody complex at the surface membrane. This complex covering the surface would prevent the killer lymphocytes from attacking the tumor.

Immunoselection

Cancer develops from a clone of cells. Some mutate and form more antigen than other cells. These cells attract more antibodies and are eliminated from the cell population, leaving the cells with weaker antigens as survivors. The colony of cells with weak antigens grows slowly and may sneak through the immunologic defenses of its host. When the host is finally sensitized, it may be too late to mount an effective attack against an already established and fast-growing tumor.

Antigen Modulation

As soon as antibody is formed, cancer cells of certain animal leukemias cease synthesizing antigens. As a result, the immunologic defense becomes ineffective. In humans this response has not been documented.

It is a tribute to the prepared minds of scientists that they observed that cancer regression occasionally followed when the host had an infection. Bacille Calmette-Guérin (BCG), an antituberculosis vaccine introduced in 1921, is presently under controlled observation in the field of immunotherapy. For more than 100 years the disappearance of cancer after severe infection has been reported. In the early 1900s Coley noted the disappearance of cancer after a severe streptococcus infection. He therefore began to treat cancer patients with a variety of bacterial toxins, but despite a few promising results found no consistent therapeutic benefit. Interest in the use of toxins as an immunopotentiator waxed and waned until the present time. Clinically, the observation was made and repeatedly observed that those patients with empyema following pneumonectomy for lung cancer did better than those who had an uncomplicated postoperative course. In addition, it has been reported that the simultaneous injection of certain bacteria with an antigen increased the immune response to the antigen. Tubercle bacilli were found to be among the most effective bacterial adjuvants for immune stimulation. Complete Freund's adjuvant is a water-in-oil emulsion adjuvant in which killed, dried tubercle bacilli are suspended in the oil phase. This adjuvant is especially effective in stimulating cell-mediated immunity, and in some animals, e.g., the guinea pig, it potentiates production of certain immunoglobulin classes.

For orientation purposes the immunotherapy of cancer can be outlined as follows:

1. Active immunization against cancer
   A. Active immunization *against oncogenic virus*
   B. Active immunization *against cancer cells*

Autochthonous or autologous cells
Allogeneic cells
Attenuated cells
Soluble tumor antigens
C. Modification of antigenicity
2. Passive immunization against cancer
A. Passive immunization
B. Adoptive immunization
Allogeneic lymphocyte transfer
Transfer factor
Immune RNA
Autologous lymphocyte stimulated in vitro with a mitogen
is phytohemagglutinin (PHA)
Bone marrow transplant
Thymosin
3. Nonspecific and miscellaneous
Coley's toxin
BCG (bacille Calmette-Guérin)
Vaccinia, pertussis vaccine, poly-IC
MER (methanol extraction residue of BCG)
Maruyama vaccine
Cornybacterium parvum
Levamisole
DNCB (dinitrochlorobenzene)
Chalones
Interferon and interferon inducers
Deblocking factor
Neuraminidase, vibrocholerae (VCN)
Concanavalin A (Con A)
Viruses

MECHANISMS OF ACTION

The approaches being undertaken in immunotherapy are directed toward increasing the resistance of the patient to her tumor, augmenting those components of the immune response that effectively combat the malignancy, and suppressing or eliminating those that interfere with immune resistance. The tumor has the ability to defend itself against host immunity by producing and shedding large amounts of antigen into the circulation. There are several methods for immunotherapy, as outlined above. At present a great deal of attention is directed to the nonspecific methods for stimulating the immune mechanism. Among these methods, BCG has received the greatest amount of attention, and its mechanism of action will be briefly reviewed.

BCG induces a local, sustained, chronic, granulomatous, inflammatory response. Lymphocytes, macrophages, and a variety of polymorphonuclear cells are attracted into the site of injection, and an immune response against the BCG organism is initiated. The lymphoid response releases a variety of lymphokines (transfer factor, lymphocyte transforming activity, migration inhibition factor, and lymphotoxin). Macrophages activated into a state of increased phagocytic and metabolic function seem able to kill tumor cells by as yet unknown mechanisms. The tumor cells may be killed as a result of the activated macrophages or through the local release of cytotoxic materials.

OPTIMUM REQUIREMENTS FOR IMMUNOTHERAPY

1. The tumor must possess proven antigenicity. It must be sufficiently different from the corresponding normal cells of the host to be antigenic and capable of producing an immune response. These include melanoma, sarcoma, neuroblastoma, carcinoma of the breast, Burkitt's lymphoma, leukemia, colonic cancer, ovarian cancer, and others.

2. Identical antigens must be present when allogeneic tumors are used. It has been reported that melanomas, sarcomas, and common epithelial ovarian cancers share common tumor-specific antigens within their own group of tumors. If the tumors are processed it is important to protect the tumor antigens so that they will not be altered.

3. Tumor cells must be free of blocking antibodies or antigen-antibody complexes that might inhibit the production of an immune response.

4. Viable tumor cells should not be injected. Even though allogeneic cells with a different HL-A antigen may be rejected, the risk of dissemination is always present in the immunodepressed patient.

5. The patient must be immunologically capable of responding to the stimulus provided by immunotherapy. Tests employed include skin tests to common antigens, DNCB, or the responsiveness of lymphoid cells to mitogens. Surgery, radiation, and chemotherapy may cause an immunosuppression. Therefore if immunotherapy is to be employed it should be started before the definitive therapy as outlined above and discontinued when the immunologic competence falls. It can be resumed when the competence rises. Reports indicate that the secondary immune response is more resistant to immunosuppression than is the primary response.

6. Immunotherapy is relatively ineffective in the presence of extensive tumor. It is therefore important to reduce the tumor mass to a minimum by conventional methods before instituting immunotherapy. A test that will indicate what the critical volume of tumor is before therapy is instituted is essential for the selection of patients for this treatment.

7. The tumor itself acts as an immunosuppressant. It is obviously more likely to be effective when a large tumor is present. Therefore removal of tumor bulk by surgery, radiation, or chemotherapy indirectly represents a method of immunotherapy.

8. A growing tumor puts the immune response at a marked disadvantage. Therefore, if immunotherapy is to be successful, it must be carried out early on a grand scale.

9. It is important to augment the cellular immunity while suppressing the

production of antibodies. One of the theories advanced to explain the effect of chemotherapeutic agents is that they inhibit the action of the blocking antibodies and allow the killer lymphocytes to work. Work with K cells (killer cells) has caused this statement to be modified. The K cell is a variant of the B cell and is able to attack tumor target cells after they have been exposed to a specific antibody, and does not require the presence of complement.

METHODS OF IMMUNOTHERAPY

The well-documented occurrences of spontaneous regressions of human neoplasms has led to widespread interest in host defenses against tumors, particularly the immune defense. The demonstration that cancers do arouse a specific immune response in the organism within which they appear has strengthened the evidence for an immune response to tumors. It has been demonstrated in a variety of tumors that they possess tumor-associated antigens that stimulate an antibody response. Attempts have been made to apply this knowledge to the control of tumors by employing immunotherapy. Immunotherapy is still in the embryonic and experimental stage. It is obvious from accumulated data that there are several ways in which immunotherapy may be administered. Before discussing each type of immunotherapy it is important to point out the importance of the in vitro evaluation of immune responses. Immunotherapy should be monitored in the laboratory. In gynecologic cancer only BCG and *C. parvum* have been subjected to extensive and intensive investigation. Therefore only these two will be discussed as representatives of the nonspecific and miscellaneous group.

NONSPECIFIC AND MISCELLANEOUS

Coley, working in the early part of this century at Memorial Hospital, noted the regression of a malignancy in a patient whose course was complicated by erysipelas. He began to treat patients with various bacterial toxins (*Streptococcus* and *Serratia marcescens*). Although there were a few promising results, there was no predictable cure rate among the patients treated with bacterial toxin.

BCG (Bacille Calmette-Guérin)

Among the nonspecific methods of immunotherapy, bacille Calmette-Guérin (BCG) and *Cornybacterium parvum* have received the most extensive clinical trials. Nonspecific immunotherapy has been reported to promote both cell-mediated immunity and antibody production and may be effective in partially reversing the immunosuppressive effects of both the tumor and the immediate stress suppression of conventional therapy. BCG may be given orally or by scarification, or directly into the tumor (intralesionally). Its mechanism of action is not entirely clear. BCG does induce a sustained chronic granulomatous inflammatory response. Lymphocytes, macrophages, and polymorphonuclear leukocytes are attracted to the site of injection and an immune response is initiated. Cytotoxic factors are also produced which damage not only cancer cells but also the normal cells. The suggestion has been made that the sensitized lymphocytes also release a nonspecific macrophage activating factor (MAF) that creates a cytotoxic population of macrophages which appears to distinguish malignant from normal cells, killing only malignant ones. Sensitized T lymphocytes also release a helper factor that enables immunocompetent B cells to respond to antigens which they otherwise would be unable to recognize. The hard data relative to the survival rate following the use of BCG must await the results of the protocols established by the National Cancer Institute. BCG administration is associated with complications. Among these are draining abscesses, fever, malaise, hypotension, bacteremia, granulomatous lesions of the liver, and even two fatalities thought to be due to hypersensitivity to the organism. The growth of the neoplasm is rarely accelerated after giving BCG. The complications of BCG immunotherapy can be classified as local or systemic.

Local	*Systemic*
Ulceration	Fever, chills, malaise
Induration	Nausea, myalgia
Pruritus	Arthralgia
Serous drainage	Hepatitis
Regional lymphadenopathy	Progressive mycobacterial infection
	Erythema nodosum
	Vitiligo
	Uveitis
	Thrombocytopenia
	Anaphylaxis
	Tuberculin shock
	Death

MER is a methanol extraction residue of BCG. It is being tried as an immunopotentiator. This is part of an effort to develop nonliving derivatives of BCG that can be chemically defined and purified. The Maruyama vaccine is a water-soluble extract of human tuberculosis organism. Chemical trials are under way to evaluate its usefulness.

Cornybacterium parvum

Immunologic interest in the gram-positive anaerobe, *Cornybacterium parvum*, was stimulated after the demonstration of its remarkable stimulatory effect on the reticuloendothelial system when administered as a killed vaccine.

There are several strains of *Cornybacterium* reported in the literature, but only two strains have been explored in current tumor work—*C. parvum* and *C. granulosum*. These strains are similar in their reticuloendothelial system. The result is the emergence of a great number of highly activated macrophages. Macrophages activated by *C. parvum* show an augmented phagocytic capability and an increased lysosomal enzyme activity.

C. parvum boosts the antibody response to a variety of antigens. Both IgM and IgG antibody levels are augmented and relative binding affinities are enhanced. *C. parvum* can boost antibody levels to T-cell-independent antigens as well as to T-cell-dependent antigens. Evidence indicates that it is the activated macrophage that provides the added proliferative stimulus to the antigen-sensitive and ultimately antibody-producing B lymphocyte. In addition, the macrophages activated by *C. parvum* encourage chronic retention of lymphocytes within lymphoid organs. Because *C. parvum*-stimulated splenic macrophages may result in T-cell depression, the strategic local injection of *C. parvum* is important so that the macrophages from the lymph nodes can carry out their antitumor effect. The macrophages from the stimulated spleen and lymph node cells have different responses. A pertinent finding relative to the delayed type hypersensitivity following *C. parvum* therapy is that it must precede antigen sensitization to produce this effect. Because treatment of established tumors means that sensitization with tumor antigens must in large part precede *C. parvum*, the usual depression of cell-mediated immunity is circumvented.

While it is not the intent of this section to be comprehensive, some other factors reported for *C. parvum* are listed: protection against viral infection and graft versus host diesease, induction of autoimmunity evidenced by hemolytic anemia, fetal resorption, and an increased sensitivity to endotoxin and histamine.

C. parvum has been reported to have its greatest effect when there is a reduced amount of tumor volume. It is more effective if the patient has immunocompetence and can respond to therapy. Intravenous *C. parvum* probably localizes in the lungs and liver and may prove to be highly effective against tumors or metastases in these organs and result in systemic immunity. It has been observed that there is at least a temporary drop in cell-mediated immunity following systemic (IV) injection of *C. parvum*.

Subcutaneous or intradermal injection of *C. parvum* is not toxic and may be highly effective if used strategically. It should be noted that too high a dose of *C. parvum* may overstimulate draining lymph nodes and impair their efficiency.

BCG has been the most widely studied nonspecific stimulant in cancer therapy. It is now apparent that BCG and *C. parvum* may be similar with respect to their modes of antitumor activity. Macrophages activated by either vaccine demonstrate nonspecific antitumor activity in vitro; in addition, in vivo antitumor effects of both apparently result in part from the fallout from an immune response to the organisms themselves. It should be emphasized that augmentation of specific antitumor responses is common to the ways in which their antitumor activities are effected. *C. parvum* is fully effective when administered in the form of killed vaccine, whereas killed BCG is apparently ineffective. Therefore BCG is difficult to control as far as the loss of viability during storage or transportation is concerned, whereas this is not a problem with *C. parvum*.

Considerable data is accumulating on the antitumor activities of various fractions of BCG (MER) which may be as effective as viable organisms. It is anticipated that material fractionated from *C. parvum* will become available, and time will determine whether there is a relationship between the nature and activity of both *C. parvum* and BCG antitumor fractions. It has been shown that degrees of stimulation induced by both *C. parvum* and BCG are different in inbred strains of mice. It is also suggested that genetic constitution may be another intrinsic source of variability in using these agents.

Although immunotherapy offers an exciting approach to the control and treatment of cancer, it has not provided additional help to the conventional methods of treating cancer of the ovary. Currently, there is no method for monitoring the volume of cancer or the effect of treatment, and this makes it difficult to know how much treatment should be given. In addition, the treatment is nonspecific and the results are not predictable.

SUMMARY

The well-documented occurrence of spontaneous regressions of human neoplasms has led to widespread interest in host defenses against tumors, particularly the immune defenses. The demonstration that cancers do arouse a specific immune response in the organism within which they appear has strengthened the evidence for an immune response to tumors. It has been demonstrated in a variety of tumors that they possess tumor-associated antigens that stimulate an antibody response. Attempts have been made to apply this knowledge to the control of tumors employing immunotherapy. Immunotherapy is still in an embryonic and experimental stage. It is obvious from accumulated data that there are different ways in which immunotherapy may be developed or given.

In general, immunization implies a method of protection, rather than an active form of treatment. Traditionally, an antigen has been given to stimulate an immune response to that antigen and is called active immunity. The administration of an antibody provides passive immunity. In work carried out in animals, immunization with an oncogenic virus gives complete protection against the later development of a tumor.

The long hoped for and ultimate goal of tumor immunology is effective immunization of the cancer patient against his or her own tumor. The approaches being taken in immunotherapy are directed toward increasing the resistance of the patient to his or her tumor, augmenting those components of the immune response that effectively combat the malignancy, and suppressing or eliminating those that interfere with immune resistance. Attention is also being given to the possibility that the tumor may defend itself against host immunity by producing and shedding large amounts of antigen into the circulation.

It is important to evaluate the immune competence of the host when considering immunotherapy. In addition, one must select a form of immunotherapy based on clinical factors, including other modalities of therapy to be employed. Furthermore, immunotherapy has a practical role only when the amount of residual or remaining tumor cells is extremely small. In animal model systems, immunotherapy is most beneficial when less than 10^5 residual cells remain after surgery.

The following guidelines have been established for the clinical and practical application of immunotherapy based on human and animal studies.

1. A tumor should be entirely removed or debulked so that the residual volume of cancer is small.

2. A method to judge the return of immunocompetence following surgery or irradiation will provide a timetable to help in administering the immunotherapy at the optimum time. The immunotherapy will then provide even more resistance to disease.

3. The immunotherapy should be administerd in areas where the lymphatic drainage is felt to be free of tumor. This will minimize the danger of acquired tolerance and immunologic enhancement.

4. An attempt should be made to stimulate cell-mediated immunity without producing antibodies. The T lymphocytes have the potential to act as killer lymphocytes, while the antibodies may be blocking or enhancing antibodies.

5. A method for monitoring the volume of cancer is necessary.

6. Methodology for monitoring both cell-mediated and humoral immunity, as well as blocking activity, should be available and utilized to insure that the benefit outweighs any harm that may follow immunotherapy.

The application of immunotherapy is presently under constant change. New advances are made almost daily, but immunotherapy is still considered experimental. Methods applied in the past, as well as those now under trial, may be classified as active, passive, adoptive, and nonspecific immunotherapy.

BIBLIOGRAPHY

Alexander, P.: Immunotherapy of cancer: Experiments with primary tumors and syngeneic tumor grafts. Prog. Exp. Tumor Res. 10:23, 1968.

Anderson, J.M.: Immunotherapy of Cancer. Clinical Oncology, Williams & Wilkins, Baltimore, 1972, p.193.

Barber, H.R.K.: Immunobiology for the Clinician. John Wiley & Sons, New York, 1977, p. 231.

Bast, R.C., Jr., Zbar, B., Borson, T., Rapp, H.L.: BCG and cancer. New Engl. J. Med. 290:1413–1420, 1974.

Biggs, P.M., Churchill, A.E., Rootes, D.G., Chubb, R.C.: The etiology of Marek's disease in oncogenic herpes-type virus, in Perspectives of Virology, Academic Press, New York, 1968, p. 211.

Cunningham, T.J., Olson, K.B., Laffin, R., et al.: Treatment of advanced cancer with active immunization. Cancer 24:932–937, 1969.

Currie, G.A.: Eight years of immunotherapy: A review of immunological methods used for the treatment of human cancer. Br. J. Cancer 26:141–153, 1972.

Currie, G.A., Bagshave, K.D.: Active immunotherapy with cornybacterium parvum and chemotherapy in murine fibrosarcoma. Br. Med. J. 1:541, 1970.

Haddsen, J.W.: Levamisole: A synthetic immunopotentiator under evaluation. Memorial Sloan-Kettering Cancer Center Clinical Bulletin 5:32, 1975.

Hellström, K.E., Hellström, I.: Immunological defenses against cancer. Hosp. Pract. 3:45, 1970.

Humphrey, L.J., Jewell, W.R., Murray, D.R., et al.: Immunotherapy for patients with cancer. Ann. Surg. 173:47–54, 1971.

Hunter-Craig, I., Newton, K.A., Westburg, G., at al: Use of vaccine virus in the treatment of metastatic malignant melanoma. Br. Med. J. 2:512–513, 1970.

Isaacs, A., Lindenmann, J.: Virus interference. The interferon. Proc. R. Soc. Lond. (Biol.) 147:258, 1957.

Israel, L., Halpern, B.: Le cornybacterium parvum dans les cancers avancés: Première évaluation de pactirité therapeutique de cette immuno-stimuline. Nouv. Presse Med. 1:19–23, 1972.

Kersey, J.H., Spector, B.D., Good, R.A.: Immunodeficiency and cancer Adv. Cancer. Res. 18:211–230, 1973.

Klein, E.: Hypersensitivity reactions at tumor sites. Cancer Res. 29:2351–2362, 1969.

Lawrence, H.S.: Transfer factor. Adv. Immunol. 11:195, 1969.

Levis, W.R., Kraemer, K.H., Klinger, W.G., et al.: Topical immunotherapy of basal cell carcinoma with dinitrochlorobenzene. Cancer Res. 33:3036–3042, 1973.

Marligit, G., Gutterman, J.N., Burgess, M.A., et al.: Immunotherapy. Its possible application in the management of large bowel cancer. Digest. Dis. 19:1047–1053, 1974.

Mathé, G.: Active immunotherapy for acute lymphoblastic leukemia. Lancet 1:697–699, 1969.

Mathé, G., Weiner, R.S.: Investigation and stimulation of immunity in cancer patients. Springer-Verlag, New York, 1974.

McKhann, C.F., Gunnarsson, A.: Approaches to immunotherapy. Cancer 34:1521, 1974.

Merigan, T.C., Regelson, W.: Interferon induction in man by a synthetic polyanion of defined composition. N. Engl. J. Med. 277:1283, 1967.

Miller, J.F.A.P., Basten, A., Sprent, J., Cheers, C.: Interaction between lymphocytes in immune response. Cell. Immunol. 2:469, 1971.

Morton, D.L.: BCG immunotherapy of malignant melanoma. Summary of seven years experience. Ann. Surg. 180:635–643, 1974.

Nauts, H.C., Swift, W.Z., Coley, B.L.: The treatment of tumor by bacterial toxins as developed by the late William B. Coley, M.D., reviewed in the light of modern research. Cancer Res. 6:2303, 1946.

Oettgen, H.F., Old, L.J., Farrow, J., Valentine, F., Lawrence, H., Thomas, L.: Effects of transfer factor in cancer patients. J. Clin. Invest. 50:71a, 1971.

Ohazaka, W., Purchase, H.G., Burmaster, B.R.: Protection against Marek's disease by vaccination with a herpes virus of turkeys. Avian Dis. 14:413, 1970.

Order, S.E., Donahue, V., Knapp, R.: Immunotherapy of ovarian carcinoma: An experimental model. Cancer 32:573, 1973.

Order, S.E., Kirkman, R., Knapp, R.: Serologic immunotherapy. Results and probable mechanism of action. Cancer 34:175, 1974.

Pilch, Y.H., Ramming, K.P.: Transfer of tumor immunity with ribonucleic acid. Cancer 26:630–637, 1970.

Pilch, Y.H., Ramming, K.P., Deckers, P.J.: Induction of anti-cancer immunity with RNA. Ann. N.Y. Acad. Sci. 207:409–429, 1973.

Plaque, R.E., Dray, S.: Monkey to human transfer for delayed hypersensitivity in vitro with RNA extracts. Cell Immunol. 5:30–41, 1972.

Rigby, P.G.: Prolongation of survival of tumor bearing animals by transfer of "immune" RNA with DEAE dextran. Nature 221:968, 1969.

Ruckdeschel, J.C., Codish, S.D., Stranahan, A., McKneally, M.F.: Postoperative empyema improves survival in lung cancer. Documentation and analysis of a natural experiment. N. Engl. J. Med. 287:1013–1017, 1972.

Scott, M.T.: Corynebacterium parvum as an immunotherapeutic anti-cancer agent. Semin. Oncol. 1:367–378, 1974.

Simmons, R.L.: Immunospecific regression of methylcholanthrene fibrosarcoma with the use of neuraminidase. Surgery 70:38–46, 1971.

Simmons, R.L., Rios, A.: Comparative and combined effect of BCG and neuraminidase in experimental immunotherapy. Nat'l. Cancer Inst. Monogr. 39:57–65, 1973.

Simmons, R.L., Rios, A., Ray, P.K., Lundgren, G.: Effect of neuraminidase on the growth of methylcholanthrene fibrosarcoma in normal and immunosuppressed syngeneic mice. J. Natl. Cancer Inst. 47:1087, 1971.

Sjögren, H.O. Hellstrom, I., Bansal, S.C., Hellstrom, K.E.: Suggestive evidence that "blocking antibodies" of tumor bearing individuals may be antigen-antibody complexes. Proc. Natl. Acad. Sci U.S.A. 68:1372, 1971.

Sokal, J.E., Aungst, C.W., Snyderman, M.: Delay in progression of malignant lymphoma after BCG vaccination. N. Engl. J. Med. 291:1226–1230, 1974.

Sparks, F.C.: Complications of BCG immunotherapy in patients with cancer. N. Engl. J. Med. 289:827–830, 1973.

Sparks, F.C., O'Connell, T.X., Lee, Y-T.N., et al.: BCG therapy given as an adjuvant to surgery: Prevention of death from metastases from mammary adenocarcinoma in rats. J. Natl. Cancer Inst. 53:1825–1826, 1971.

Stjeruswald, J., Levin, A.: Delayed hypersensitivity: Induced regression of human neoplasms. Cancer 28:628–640, 1971.

Thor, D.E., Dray, S.: Transfer of cell-mediated immunity by immune RNA assessed by migration inhibition. Ann. N.Y. Acad. Sci. 207:355, 1973.

Webb, H.E., Smith, G.C.E.: Viruses in the treatment of cancer. Lancet 1:1206–1209, 1970.

Zbar, B., Rapp, H.J.: Immunotherapy of guinea pig cancer with BCG. Cancer (Suppl.) 34:1532–1540, 1974.

26

Directions in the Design of Clinical Trials, Present and Future

Cancer has been with man since antiquity. It has been identified in fossil bones and recently in mummies. Tumors are currently identified according to their appearance, behavior, and location. A growing body of evidence indicates that although they look alike, they may not act alike. Within any group of tumors and indeed any stage of a given cancer, there are different degrees of malignancy. These differences must be understood if advances are to made in the field of anticancer drug therapy.

Tumors were finally identified and described according to their microscopic appearance. It became evident that cancer cells arise from normal cells and that there are at least as many cancers as there are normal cells. Carcinogenesis is the change from a new cell to one endowed with new growth (neoplastic) properties. The neoplastic cell transmits to its descendents components of the neoplastic cell as well as the original cell. Their function is often at a more primitive level than that of the normal cell. The cancer cell grows in an uninhibited manner and, unlike the normal cell, its growth is not controlled. This results in a nodule of neoplastic cells, resulting in a tumor. The only control on the growth of a cancer is the death of its hosts. It does not respond to normal growth controls, is not influenced by contact inhibition, and although its growth is inefficient, the cancer cell divides continuously. It possesses the characteristic properties of invasion and the ability to metastasize. Cartilage and dense fibrous tissues obstruct the easy spread of cancer, but bone is readily invaded. At the edge of most tumors there is a collection of lymphoid cells which represents an attempt at defense.

Cancer research has directed a great deal of energy, resources, and money toward finding specific and constant chemical, biologic, and immunologic differences between normal and cancer cells. It is important to identify the differences in the development and maintenance of the properties of cancer cells and, by understanding these differences, to control the cancer cell. It is hoped that the future reveals these differences and thus permits the selective destruction of cancer cells by the use of chemicals.

The long-term future belongs to the immunologist and the geneticist, and the intermediate future to the chemotherapist. But the present and the immediate future belong to the surgeon and the radiotherapist. To the extent that chemotherapy is developed first, surgery will be needed less, but in those fields in which early detection is developed first, it will be largely surgery which will convert these gains in information into cured patients by extirpation of the cancer before it has spread. Currently, progress in making an early diagnosis of malignancy is more advanced than is reported.

Surgery and radiation are effective only for localized disease. Chemotherapy (drugs and hormones) can be used effectively for disseminated as well as localized cancer. Chemotherapy has become a reality only in the past 30 years. It has been employed generally for palliation, but recently it has also proved its value as a primary therapeutic modality of therapy. Its prophylactic role after surgical removal or eradication of the cancer by radiation therapy has only recently been explored. A major goal of current chemotherapy is to achieve cures by prompt and vigorous treatment of cancer without producing an inordinate morbidity and some mortality.

Combinations of chemotherapeutic agents have been used with considerable success, particularly when each of the drugs used acts on the cancer cells in a different way. An improved knowledge of cell kinetics or cell divisions, as well as of the life cycle of the cancer cell, has provided the basis for a more rational approach to the use of anticancer drugs. Major improvements in treating certain types of cancer have been achieved by using several anticancer drugs simultaneously and by using different drugs in sequence.

Cell biology is complex and involves all of the metabolic, enzymatic, and hormone synthesis that is necessary for the cell to remain viable. The cells of the body have both internal and external functions. The individual functions in mature cells of parenchymatous tissues are concerned with the maintenance of metabolic cycles for energy and for the specialized synthesizing functions characteristic of differentiated tissues. These functions include the synthesis and maintenance of hemoglobin for gas transport; the synthesis of secretory products such as insulin, mucin, casein, and steroids; and the synthesis of constructive products such as cilia, keratin, and osteoid. The biochemical basis for these activities is the translation of genetic material contained in DNA into the specific RNA and proteins concerned in such specialized differentiated functions.

Certain tissues such as the intestinal tract, skin, and bone marrow require replacement of a great number of mature dying cells. There must be an internal function geared to rapid cell replication. This involves the cycle of DNA replication known as mitosis in mammalian cells. Since the neoplastic process involves the replication of unwanted cells, much chemotherapy is directed toward inhibiting the mitotic cycle of such cells, especially the steps in which new DNA molecules are produced.

The external function of tissue growth relative to the cancer problem concerns the process by which cell, tissue, and organ growth is restricted after a critical volume is reached and stimulated to resume after death or removal of part of an organ. Knowledge of how to measure this parameter is vital to the judicious use of immunotherapy. Cell growth is limited and organ size is controlled by a combination of local factors such as contact inhibition (allogeneic inhibition) in which normal cells become inhibited in replication and migration by contact with other normal cells, and distant factors such as humoral feedback mechanisms and controls. The latter is believed to result in the release of growth-inhibiting substances, chalones, from normal tissue. The accidental death of tissue cells by injury results in changes in this homeostatic mechanism, with the result that certain clonogenic cells, which have retained the capacity to divide, begin to do so in order to regenerate the lost normal tissue.

Cancer is a disease of the cell. An understanding of the life cycle of a cell, and in this instance the cancer cell, is important in planning therapy for a given malignancy. Cellular reproduction occurs by a series of different chemical steps known as the cell cycle (the cell cycle is measured from mitosis to mitosis). An understanding of the order of steps has allowed identification of the phase of cellular activity in which a specific anticancer drug acts. It is now evident that a drug for cancer must be defined not only by its chemical composition, but also by its specific dosage, specific route, and by schedule of administration, each of which significantly modifies its activity.

A study of tumor cell kinetics confirms that only some of the tumor cells are in an active growth cycle at any one time, and the synthesis of critical cellular constituents is known to occur during specific phases of that cycle. It is important and necessary to explore and understand the selective toxicity of anticancer drugs during different phases of the cell cycle. This is essential to a deeper understanding of a rational approach to chemotherapy. It is also important to elucidate the natural rate of death of cells within a tumor and to exploit this knowledge of tumor cell death. The fraction of cells in the tumor which has the ability to reproduce, as well as the selective killing of cancer cells, especially those that are not in the critical phases of synthesis is essential for carrying out options of therapy. These types of information are vital to an understanding of the cell kinetics of slow-growing tumors, particularly solid tumors such as ovarian carcinomas.

One important goal is to solve the problem of how to invade selectively the sanctuary of tumor cells. Malignant cells lodged at a distance from the closest capillaries or beyond the blood-brain barrier may enjoy a pharmacologic sanctuary where drug concentrations cannot reach them in concentrations that will have lethal effects. Experimental and clinical research must supply a method for eradicating the last cancer cell, no matter where it lodges or seeks sanctuary.

Structures with the cell are visible under the electron microscope. The description is taken from *Immunobiology for the Clinician*, pages 9–11 (Figure 2) and page 12.

Chemotherapy is no longer a modality reserved for palliation alone, it now constitutes a major and indispensable therapeutic approach, capable of producing cures in certain kinds of widespread cancer. The cancers that have been cured by drug therapy with a predictable rate are choriocarcinoma, metastatic hydatidiform mole, Burkitt's tumor, acute leukemia of children, Hodgkin's disease, embryonal carcinoma of the testis and ovary, adenocarcinoma of the uterine corpus, and cancers in the superficial layers of the skin.

Chemotherapy has been therapeutically beneficial in a significant number of cases, but it has not resulted in predictable cures as in the cancers listed above. These cancers are chronic myelocytic leukemia, chronic lymphatic leukemia, lymphosarcoma, reticulum cell sarcoma, multiple myeloma, polycythemia vera, mycosis fungoides, malignant melanoma, and neuroblastoma.

There are other types of cancer that have been significantly benefited by anticancer drug therapy. Clinical improvements occur and possibly the survival time is increased, but predictable long-term survival or long-term freedom from disease has not been observed. The cancers responding in this manner include cancer of the breast, large intestine, stomach, pancreas, prostate, head and neck, thyroid, ovary, and adrenal gland. Some cancers are notably unsusceptible to the anticancer drugs used to date. Major clinical benefit has not usually followed treatment of cancer of the lung, cervix, kidney, or bladder.

Anticancer drugs can occasionally produce cures in a broad spectrum of cancers. The cancers that can be cured by chemotherapy are not always those that grow most rapidly. Not all of the cancers are from the same primitive embryonic tissue; many organ classes and a variety of histologic types are represented. The chief block in the progress of anticancer chemotherapy is the lack of a predictable method for monitoring the volume of cancer and the inability to test the response of cancer cells in vitro to the action of the anticancer drugs.

Furthermore, curative chemotherapy is not usually a product of a single drug (except in choriocarcinoma) or of a single technique of drug use. Rather, many drugs in a variety of combinations are used. Surgery and radiation may be included in the therapy. It is obvious that no one drug, whether now in use or to be identified in the future, will serve as an overall cure. The number of combinations and regimens indicates that a drug that fails in the treatment of one kind of cancer may act against another.

There are many factors, not all of which are known, that play a role in the sensitivity of cancer cells to the action of anticancer drugs. It is logical to outline the path that an anticancer drug must take to effectively control a cancer cell (cancer cells divide continuously, although inefficiently). The anticancer drug must reach the surface of the cancer cell, enter the cell through its surface membrane, remain active or undergo activation by the necessary enzymes to accomplish this, reach a critical target site, and combine with it at a time when chemical processes on which the cell depends for its viability or reproduction are in progress. This complex process highlights the importance of a clear understanding of the life cycle of the cell or its kinetics.

Furthermore, competing and bypass pathways in the cell must not be able to compensate for the chemical injury which the drug inflicts. It is important to measure the number of mutations in a given volume of tumor cells to predict the development of resistance so that valuable time is not lost in pursuing a drug regimen that has lost its ability to control the cancer cell. Failure of the whole chain of events can result from the failure of any one step. Thus any drug given by the wrong regimen to a mass of cancer cells which are biologically insusceptible to its action at that time is a failure of chemotherapy. Better drug design and better understanding of the biologic characteristics of each cancer type, and indeed of each cancer, as well as a better understanding of the cell cycle, will advance the effectiveness of chemotherapy.

The dramatic and persistent change that accompanies the development of cancer has supported the somatic mutation theory of carcinogenesis. This theory bolsters the concept that the cancer is caused by a change in the cellular genetic material itself. It is important to know whether cancer is the result of a change in the genetics of the cell or of a change in the nongenetic material (epigenetic). If it affects the genetic material it is irreversible and can only be controlled by selective destruction, whereas if it affects the epigenetic material it may be reversible and controllable.

The last three decades have seen the development of more than 30 compounds that have shown their usefulness in the control of cancer. It is obvious that many more drugs are available, and the best are yet to be found. So far, most of the drugs identified with anticancer properties have followed from empirical screening. Most of the work is carried out by drug companies, governmental agencies, and cooperative groups. The National Cancer Institute has a division which revives and tests drugs from all kinds of sources throughout the world. The preparation and clinical use of these drugs are under the control of the FDA. The question should be raised whether this authority, as it relates to cancer, would not better be transferred to the National Cancer Advisory Board.

The use of active drugs for cancer may bring success even before there is a clear understanding of the malignant process. Indeed it may serve as a probe to explain the intricacies of neoplastic growth. Other medications, often derived from plants, gave predictable theraupetic results in many disease processes before the mechanism of the disease was clearly understood.

After the development or isolation of a new drug, several steps must be carried out under controlled conditions before the drug can be used in the treatment of cancer cases:

- The antitumor activity must be demonstrated in the same screening system.
- A broadscale study in other known biologic screening systems is necessary.
- After the activity of the drug has been confirmed, two general areas of study follow.
- It must be determined what the compound does and how it does it.
- The compound must be tested in animals.

PRECLINICAL TESTING

Careful preclinical pharmacology and toxicology are necessary to arrive at the optimum dose and route of administration for a new agent. Various rapidly growing systems are used to determine drug activity, e.g., bacteria, viruses, mammalian cells in culture, and transplantable and spontaneous tumors of small rodents. Specific organ toxicity is also determined in larger animals such as dogs and monkeys. General concepts of duration of action, blood levels achieved, tolerable routes of administration, usual routes of excretion, and possible modes of action are accumulated. At the end of each testing one should know, within 10%, the lethal dose to higher animals by single and repeated doses. This figure is often used as a basis for extrapolation to the first human trials, and hence every attempt should be made to gather high-quality data on the animal species closest to man. Commonly, the first human dosage level is one-fifth to one-tenth the LD_{10} in dogs.

Careful preclinical pharmacology and toxicity are necessary but the time required for these observations should be modified when the observations indicate that a stated time is not necessary for the completion of the study. For example, patients with advanced cancer have a finite life expectancy in the absence of effective treatment. One thousand cancer patients die in the United States every day. If a new compound shows appreciable activity against cancer, extensive pharmacologic studies can be made concomitantly with the subsequent clinical trials.

CLINICAL TRIALS

The study of a new compound in man requires skill in clinical pharmacology.

Stage I (Phase I)

In general, the primary aim of a phase I trial is to determine clinically the tolerated regimens of a drug that will later be used in trials to determine antitumor action in man. There should be no expectation that phase I patients will achieve remissions, although observations enabling a drug-induced remission to be recognized should be included as a matter of routine. Unfortunately, in most phase I trials the patients are normally those with far-advanced disease in whom chemotherapy has failed.

Stage I (phase I) testing consists of toxicity trials of host responses rather than trials in which the antitumor effects of the drug are even roughly assessed. The information that will hopefully be collected from stage I (phase I) trials are (1) an idea of useful routes of administration; (2) an idea of the doses which would be tolerable during the period of time necessary to observe remissons in the tumor types to be studied later, perhaps after 30 to 60 days; (3) early identification of intolerably toxic drugs and unfeasible routes of administration. Such drugs should be discarded as soon as possible. No drug should complete phase I trial if it has not been tacitly committed to be carried through phase II.

The time required to deliver a drug from its conception of first recognition in a testing system to clinical usefulness depends on the biologic factors and ability to produce the drug. A minimum of 2 to 3 years may be required, and in some instances it may take a decade to ascertain the optimal method of using the drug.

Stage II (Phase II)

Stage II (phase II) is a trial period in which an attempt is made to use the dose or doses of the drug determined in the stage I (phase I) trials to search for evidence of antitumor effect in man. A phase II trial requires about 20 patients with one type of tumor which can be evaluated for potential antitumor effect after treatment for a month or more at the maximum tolerated doses by the route administered. If several responses are observed among the 20 patients, further trials are in order, and if many responses are noted, a stage III (phase III) trial may be designed. In addition, a spectrum of tumors must be screened. Remissions must be carefully defined for each experimental approach. Frequency, duration, and extent of remission should also be recorded.

Stage II trials are mainly concerned with establishing optimum dosage schedules and combinations for chemotherapeutic agents. This type of clinical trial has produced such outstanding achievements as increasing the cure rate of metastatic choriocarcinoma from 0 to greater than 90%.

Stage III (Phase III)

The aim of this stage (phase) is to determine what should become standard therapy, usually by comparison of a standard form of therapy, with a new agent showing promise at the completion of phase II trials. In stage III (phase III) trials, careful definitions of subjective and objective remissions, and data on frequency, completeness, and duration of remission are mandatory.

It is a time for large-scale trials to compare the efficacy of different applications of the various therapeutic modalities. Each of these requires extensive evaluation in many patients, in different institutions, and with proper controls.

IMMUNOCHEMOTHERAPY

The property of specific recognition of the immune system is being evaluated in the field of antitumor chemotherapy. It is unnecessary to say that selective immunochemotherapy is of special therapeutic interest. However it would represent a major advance in anticancer therapy if it could be achieved with a predictable chance to selectively reach the cancer cell. Most of the drugs that are effective in controlling the growth of cancer cells are also toxic to normal cells. It is the small margin of safety between inhibiting the growth of a cancer cell and damaging normal cells that greatly limits the use of antitumor chemotherapeutic drugs. However, by exploiting the known principles of immunology, it is possible to attach antitumor drugs to antibodies prepared against specific or even tumor-associated antigens identified with that particular tumor. The antibodies directed against the antigen of the cancer cell would seek out the cancer cell or cells, attach to it or them, and thus deliver the drug selectively and in high concentrations where it is needed to carry out its lethal effect, but sparing completely the normal cell or cells. It is now technologically possible to experiment with this method. The concept of the "magic bullet" as a therapeutic method for control of cancer has been resurrected.

The concept of immunotherapy has expanded to include the use of BCG, given concomitantly with the antitumor drugs or immediately following their use. The concept also includes the use of allogeneic cells (genetically dissimilar but of the same species) that have been treated with 10,000 rads of radiation and then injected back into the patient. It is hoped that this method will destroy the malignant potential of cells while leaving the tumor-associated antigen intact. The patient is treated with a nonspecific immunopotentiator such as BCG, in the anticipation that the immune system will be excited and produce an antitumor effect. The potentials for combinations of immunochemotherapy treatment are great and offer the hope for another modality of administering anticancer chemotherapy.

NEW DRUGS

It is important to pursue a planned and empiric search for new drugs that have anticancer effect. With our present knowledge of pharmacology and new insights into cell kinetics, it is more logical to pursue a program of chemical synthesis of compounds or polymers designed to interfere with critical steps in cancer cell biosynthesis and metabolism. A coordinated program involving chemists, biologists, and clinicians must be directed to the specific targets and techniques of selecting the compounds for trial. This cooperative endeavor will insure immediate feedback and quick acceptance of drugs for clinical trial.

However empiric screening of natural products (particularly plant extracts), soil, and antibiotics continues to provide compounds that have major usefulness in clinical oncology. Approximately a dozen compounds derived from plants and bacteria are now in clinical use and have demonstrated significant therapeutic benefit. This type of program should be encouraged and can run parallel to a program of chemical synthesis of compounds without being competitive. The cooperative programs obviously should be expanded. The results of such studies are most urgently needed in the control and prevention of metastases.

Surgery and radiation therapy are already highly effective in controlling most primary cancer. The failure to prevent the dissemination of the cancer or to provide effective treatment after the disease has become widespread accounts for the greatest number of deaths. Certain drugs are now under clinical investigation which in animals are more effective in preventing metastases than in inhibiting growth of the primary tumor. The routine prevention of metastases would be a significant advance, if not a landmark in the control of cancer.

The search for botanical and antibiotic drugs against cancer should be extended, in close proximity with relevant biologic screening. To expedite the production, testing, and use of new drugs it would seem more appropriate to charge the National Cancer Advisory Board with the responsibility and control of the use of new anticancer drugs and to keep the control of all other drugs under the jurisdiction of the FDA.

AREAS IN WHICH RESEARCH IS NEEDED NOW

A great deal of research is needed to find the optimal use of the drugs that are available, and to search for new drugs and for methods of therapy with them. Although little has been achieved in delineating metabolic or enzymatic differences between normal and malignant cells, renewed efforts should be directed to this end with the new and advanced technology available. A recognition of even a small difference between the normal and cancer cell might lead to a new drug design. The advanced methods of testing drugs, particularly the many antibiotics identified, have revealed activity against many important biosynthetic enzymes. Drugs which may affect enzymes unique to oncogenic viruses hold particular promise for neoplasms found to be caused by viruses. Work with the reverse transcriptase enzyme may serve to unravel the mystery of the role of viruses in human cancer. Drugs that affect enzymes unique to oncogenic viruses could then be definitely applied to their control with a predictable response rate.

The pharmacology and metabolic disposition of known active compounds in human cancer patients must be explored in greater depth. Unfortunately, all of the anticancer drugs have an immunosuppressive effect. There is a small ratio between this effect and their cancer-controlling ability. The ratio must be explored or better drugs synthesized that have little or no immunosuppressive effect. The control of cancer would be advanced by the synthesis and understanding of the key structures in assembling the compound as well as by a knowledge of how and where to inhibit key enzymes and by discovery of species or tissues and/or cell differences in affinities for the anticancer drug.

Certain drugs now under clinical investigation in animals are much more effective in preventing metastases than in inhibiting the growth of the primary tumor. It is the tendency to spread that often makes cancer incurable. In fact metastases are the most important clinical feature of cancer because they usually determine whether the patient can be cured or not. An advance would be made by understanding the mechanism whereby certain drugs potentiate the destructive effects of heat on cancer cells. Research is needed to find new and effective drugs to produce radiosensitization of tumors that would kill cancer cells at a dose that would not destroy normal tissue.

Predictive testing of drugs before use in humans is mandatory, and better methods for such testing must be designed. The optimal dose, ideal route, schedule, and conditions of administration may be learned from experimental animals, as must the toxicities and side effects which may develop. Control of toxic effects is important. In addition, an in vitro test for the effectiveness of a drug on the patient's own cancer before its clinical use would help in selecting the proper drug for the cancer in that petient.

Current cooperative projects of clinical investigation in chemotherapy provide an essential link in cancer research, since it is directed to the ultimate goal of prevention and control of cancer in humans. The input of these cooperative group studies permits a comparatively quick evaluation of the results of treatment with greater precision and validity because of the variety and diversity of those investigators who have been screened for their material, program, and integrity. Accumulated data of this high quality with strict control provides a method of discarding the inferior plans of treatment and pursuing and expanding those that yield superior results.

SUMMARY

The finding that several disseminated human tumors can be cured by anticancer drugs alone demonstrates that selective toxicity does exist and that there is a potential cure. An effort must be made to understand the interaction of the drug, host, tumor, oncogenic agent, and host defense mechanisms. Research on which drugs to give for which tumors, in what combinations, and when in the course of the disease (before operation, after operation, with radiotherapy, after widespread metastases, etc.) are areas of great promise.

Only a portion of the tumor cells is in an active growth cycle at any one time, and the synthesis of critical cellular constituents is known to occur during specific phases of that cycle. The cell cycle is measured from mitosis to mitosis. It is important to accumulate knowledge on selective toxicity during different phases of the cell, and to know the time of the natural death of cells within the tumor and their regeneration time at the surface and the interior of the cancer, in order to discover the means to get cells into an active cycle or to kill them during the resting phase.

It has been shown that cells lodged at a distance from the closest capillary or beyond the blood-brain barrier enjoy a sanctuary from anticancer drugs. It is important to find means to deliver lethal doses of anticancer drugs to these areas.

A program to screen botanical and microbiological substances for anticancer activity must be expanded. Chemical syntheses of compounds or polymers designed to interfere with critical steps in cancer cell biosynthesis and metabolism are important. The specific targets and techniques of selecting the compounds for trial must be coordinated by chemists and biologists. The program must be streamlined and coordinated so that rapid feedback occurs from an area of the project that demonstrates anticancer activity.

Much research is needed (1) to study the metabolic or enzymatic differences between normal and malignant cells, in order to open programs for new drug designs; (2) to design new and sophisticated methods that test drugs, particularly those that affect enzymes unique to oncogenic viruses (this will be particularly important if viruses are ever identified as a causative agent in human cancers); (3) to study and fractionate pharmacologic products known to be active in controlling human cancer; (4) to study compounds that inhibit key enzymes, with the aim of discovering species or tissue differences in affinities for drugs; (5) to develop anticancer drugs that are not immunosuppressive; (6) to explore new classes of drugs that would inhibit invasion or act specifically on metastases; (7) to explore the mechanisms whereby certain drugs potentiate the lethal effects of heat on tumor cells; and (8) to search for new drugs that will be effective in producing radiosensitization of tumors.

New and better ways for predictive testing of anticancer drugs are needed. A method by which a drug can be tested in the laboratory before its clinical use would make a great contribution. Cooperative group studies (such as the gynecologic oncology group) bring earlier results of high precision and validity because of the positive intellectual input of several investigators in planning and reporting the research. It is hoped that clinical investigation in chemotherapy will provide an essential link in cancer research.

BIBLIOGRAPHY

Barber, H.R.K. (Ed.): Immunobiology for the Clinician. Wiley, New York, 1977, p. 9.

Bloomfield, R.D.: Current cancer chemotherapy in obstetrics and gynecology. Am. J. Obstet. Gynecol. 109:487, 1971.

Brule, G., Eckhardt, S.J., Hall, T.C., Winkler, A.: Drug Therapy of Cancer. World Health Organization, Geneva, 1973, p. 12.

De Vita, V.T.: Cell kinetics and chemotherapy of cancer. Cancer Chemother. Rep. 1:35, 1971.

Frei, E., III: Cytokinetics and clinical cancer, in Chemotherapy Oncology, Year Book Publishers, Chicago, 1970, p. 131.

Greenwald, E.S.: Cancer chemotherapy. NY State J. Med. 2:2641, 1972; 3:2757, 1972.

Greenwald, E.S.: Cancer chemotherapy. Medical Examination Publishing, Flushing, NY, 1973.

Hoffan, J., Post, J.: The effects of antitumor drugs on the cell cycle, in Drugs and the Cell Cycle. Edited by A.M. Zimmerman, G.M. Padilla, I.L. Cameron. Academic Press, New York, 1973, p. 219.

National Program for the Conquest of Cancer: Report of the National Panel of Consultants on the Conquest of Cancer. Report No. 91-1402. U.S. Government Printing Office, Washington, D.C., 1970.

Skipper, H.E., Schabel, F.M., Jr.: Quantitative and cytokinetic studies in experimental tumor models, in Cancer Medicine. Edited by J.R.Holland, E. Frei, III. Lea & Febiger, Philadelphia, 1973, p. 629.

Zimmerman, A.M., Padilla, G.M., Cameron, I.L.: Drugs and the Cell Cycle. Academic Press, New York, 1973.

Addendum

I t is difficult to devote an entire chapter to every topic related to the subject of ovarian cancer, even though these topics are important and should be understood by the clinician. And to incorporate such topics into other chapters, it would be necessary to sacrifice the individual attention which each deserves. Therefore it was decided to group these subjects into a separate chapter.

REVERSE TRANSCRIPTASE

Reverse transcriptase is a newly isolated RNA-dependent DNA polymerase which can transcribe the base sequence of a viral RNA onto a DNA strand, in vitro, so that now it is possible to synthesize relatively large quantities of such virus-specified DNA. If a virus is the cause of a particular cancer, its genetic material may be present in the cancer cells in the form of DNA, even though it may not reveal its presence. It is possible to extract cellular DNA from tumors, to purify it, and to separate its strands. This DNA can be mixed with synthetic single-stranded DNA, carrying the base sequence of the RNA virus. Should a complementary viral genome (i.e DNA specified by the same virus) exist in the tumor extract, the two should bind together, reconstituting double-stranded molecules. Such molecules can be recognized. Thus the identification of these double-stranded "hybrid" molecules would, in itself, prove the existence of the same viral genome in the tumor and, on the basis of present evidence would strongly indicate the tumor's viral etiology.

CYTOGENETICS OF OVARIAN CANCER

Reports describe definite patterns of numerical and structural chromosome changes in ovarian cancer. These reports support the current concepts that such changes in gynecologic tumors are not random and that patterns for invasiveness appear to be tissue-specific or organ-specific. Information available at this time suggests that many of the chromosome abnormalities in cancer are most likely secondary or coincidental, but that primary, significant chromosome changes exist as well. Identifying such changes is difficult because of the variability of cytogenetic changes among cancers of the same histopathologic type, because of their obliteration by coexisting coincidental changes, and, particularly in the case of solid tumors, because of technical problems.

Cytogenetics is the study of the chromosome complement of cells. It is now well known that the normal human chromosome number is 46. However neoplasms have been shown to have a wide variation in chromosome number and structure (aneuploidy), often differing from cell to cell within the same tumor. *Karyotype* refers to the chromosome characteristics of an individual or of a cell line. The cells are arrested in metaphase for study. Recently banding of the chromosomes has enabled a more accurate evaluation of the chromosomes being studied. Metaphase chromosomes, arrested by colchicine and recorded by microphotography of single-cell nuclei, are arranged in pairs in descending order of size and according to the position of the centromer. The Patau system, which is the most commonly used, arranges these pairs of chromosomes into seven groups, A to G. Karyotypes of neoplastic cells are examined for variation from normal, that is, the overall number of chromosomes falling into each of seven Patau groups is determined, and changes in individual chromosome structures are evaluated. Such structurally abnormal chromosomes are referred to as *marker chromosomes*, and they result from gaps, breaks, deletions, or rearrangements. Those marker chromosomes that are recurrent are of particular interest because they most likely represent specific rather than coincidental chromosome changes, changes that may be involved in the causation or progression of cancer.

Ovarian cancers seem to differ from other gynecologic tumors in their ploidy distribution and in the frequency of marker chromosomes. A variety of modes and consistent markers has been reported for primary ovarian cancers. In malignant ovarian tumors, the chromosome distribution varies with the degree of invasiveness.

Wakong-Vaartaja and Auersperg reported 59% of the differentiated and undifferentiated cancers of the ovary were in the hypodiploid (2n-x) group and 41% were in the triploid (3n $\pm$ x) group, whereas 100% of the undifferentiated were in the triploid group. Ovarian cancers that were localized had a high diploid mode, while those that had metastasized had a high triploid mode. The evidence suggests that a spread outside the ovary is associated with a change from the diploid to the triploid mode. The same authors report a higher incidence of larger marker chromosomes in ovarian cancer. Since benign, borderline, and invasive areas may be present in the same tumor, it is obvious that wide sampling must be carried out to determine accurately the chromosomal content of the cancer.

HIGH RISK PATIENTS

The most logical definiton of a high-risk patient would be any patient with an ovarian cancer or any patient with an adnexal mass that gets progressively larger or has any of the pelvic findings listed in chapter 7.

The first group of patients at high risk are those explored through an improper or inadequate incision. In dealing with ovarian cancer or a suspected malignancy of the ovary, it is important to operate through a vertical incision. The incision must not only be longer than the extent of the cancer but must allow easy access to the area between the liver and diaphragm. The initial operation often determines the success or failure of therapy. It is the height of professional integrity not to succumb to the wishes or demands of the patient, but rather to advise them of the importance of the contemplated incision. Inability to communicate this vital information to the patient is not a license for poor and inadequate treatment, and the surgeon is morally bound to withdraw from the case.

The other groups at high-risk for ovarian cancer are women with the following traits: nulliparity, involuntary infertility, group A blood type, positive family history, early menopause, severe dysmenorrhea, marked premenstrual swelling, spontaneous abortions, breast cancer, and residence in highly industrialized countries. These groups are discussed in chapter 3.

AREAS OF FUTURE PROMISE IN THE CONQUEST OF OVARIAN CANCER

The number two killer in the United States is cancer. Cancer kills one man, woman, or child every 2 minutes in the United States. Among women, cancer far exceeds any other disease as a cause of "working years lost."

There are approximately 670,000 new cases of cancer each year in the United States, and about 370,000 reported deaths. Estimates of cancer incidence show that gynecologic malignancies are the third most common cancer type in women, following breast and gastrointestinal cancer with approximately 67,000 to 68,000 cases each year. The gynecologic cancers are also the third leading cause of cancer deaths in women; they cause an estimated 22,000 to 23,000 deaths. In this group, cancer of the ovary accounted for about 17,000 new cases in 1976 and approximately 11,000 deaths, making it the fourth leading cause of death for women and yielding a crude death rate of 64%.

The Division of Cancer Treatment of the National Cancer Institute has been analyzing the gynecologic cancers from the standpoint of requirements for developing an overall strategy for combining systemic therapy, such as chemotherapy and/or immunotherapy, with the local modalities of surgery and/or radiotherapy in an attempt to increase their potential for long-term disease control. In an all out attack on a specific cancer (by site), it is imperative to know the overall incidence of disease; the frequency of presentation at diagnosis of local, regional, and metastatic stages; the patterns of failure; the prognostic variables; the therapy and survival by stage; and the potential for increased therapeutic efficacy with systematic therapy.

Ovarian cancer is difficult to diagnose early. It occurs in an organ that lies deep within the pelvis. In elderly, obese, tense women with an inelastic and conical vagina, it is difficult to feel pathology until the disease is advanced. A means for early diagnosis is receiving high priority. Preliminary reports indicate that an antigen is present on the surface of the ovarian cancer cell and that it is capable of stimulating an antibody response. There is fairly solid additional data that an antigen-antibody complex is present on the surface of the ovarian cancer cell as well as in the positive ascitic fluid. The challenge is to translate this knowledge into a serologic diagnosis for early ovarian cancer by employing immunologic techniques—techniques that take advantage of the extraordinary power of discrimination of the immune defense mechanism itself. If the tumor sheds malignant cells before it releases antigens, the test will have less value than if it releases antigens before it releases intact cancer cells. There is evidence that the antigen is released before intact cancer cells. Another question concerns the volume of tumor necessary before the release of tumor antigens. If the volume of cancer must reach a size of 1 cm^3 or more before shedding its antigen, the tumor at that time would contain a billion cells capable of originating a new focus of disease and would no longer be an early stage of cancer.

A serologic test may prove to be an all or nothing test—the patient either would have cancer or would not. Inability to detect precursors of cancer would reduce the significance of the serologic test as a method of early diagnosis, if it is assumed that ovarian cancer is a continuum of diseases progressing from atypia, to dysplasia, to cancer in situ, and on to invasive cancer. The serologic test would still serve to detect ovarian cancer in stages I or II instead of stages III and IV, where 70% of the cases of ovarian cancer are now diagnosed. This test may not provide the hoped for early diagnosis, but at least it would be an *earlier* diagnosis. In any event, it would provide a method of monitoring the cancer patient and could serve as the keystone in therapy.

OVARIAN CANCER AS AN AUTOIMMUNE DISORDER

Ovarian cancer not only acts like an immune suppressive agent, but produces a secondary type of autoimmune disorder or disease in a great number of patients with cancer. Nonspecific hemagglutinating antibodies have been identified in these patients. The presence of these antibodies make it difficult to cross-match these patients. They often respond in a relatively short time to cortisone therapy and are then cleared of these antibodies after successful treatment with surgery, radiation, or chemotherapy. The polyglandular imbalances seen in certain endocrine syndromes may have a counterpart in the cancer patient, i.e., the multiimmunologic syndrome that accounts for the variety of problems that arise in the cancer patient. Stage III and IV ovarian cancer have characteristics similar to those found in autoimmune disorders and indeed in autoimmune disease. Whether there is a clearcut relationship between ovarian cancer and immunodeficiency diseases remains to be seen.

AUGMENTING THE IMMUNITY OF
PATIENTS WITH OVARIAN CANCER

Ovarian cancer is associated with an immunosuppressive state and methods to reverse this state would make a significant contribution to its control. As a corollary, selective immunosuppression and strengthening of the immune responses would be an ideal modality of treatment. A method that would selectively suppress the enhancing and blocking antibodies while stimulating the production of a strong cell-mediated response would be an advance in the control of the cancer.

A possible mechanism of action is the arming of nonsensitized cells. Certain sera taken from either animals or human patients during the period of tumor remission have been found to increase the cytotoxic effect of immune lymphocytes. This process has been referred to as *potentiation.* One may speculate that potentiation is related to the unblocking phenomenon and operates by removing (or neutralizing the action of) blocking serum factors present in the lymphocyte suspensions tested, but other mechanisms, including arming of nonsensitized cells, are equally possible.

The origin, nature, function, chemical composition, and role of complement must be explored. Although the cell-mediated response is the primary path to tissue rejection and tumor control, additional work remains to be done with cytotoxic antibodies and complement. Even a sufficient supply of cytotoxic antibodies is not able to kill tumor cells unless an ample supply of complement is present. Perhaps an understanding of the nature and function of complement could expand its role in tumor control.

Theoretically, immunotherapy is potentially the perfect therapeutic modality for the treatment of cancer. An important distinction must be made between immunotherapy, which is the treatment of established tumors and/or their metastases, and immunoprophylaxis, which is the induction of transplantation resistance by immunization prior to tumor cell grafting. The development of more precise techniques for measuring the presence of small numbers of cancer cells would be useful in detecting cancer and also in quantitating the response to various types of therapy. It has been shown that immunotherapy can eradicate a small volume of tumor, but even a strong and maximally magnified tumor rejection mechanism cannot eradicate large established tumors.

Because the immune mechanism is depressed in the very young and the very old and parallels the level of hormone production, the relationship between these two mechanisms should be explored. Most of the antigenic determinants are on the cell surface membrane, and the hormone receptors are found in the same place. The role and interaction of immunology and endocrinology remain to be explored.

NEW ANTIOVARIAN CANCER DRUGS

New anticancer drugs must be found and those available must be explored in greater detail. Attack on the DNA of a tumor cell stands at the forefront of tumor therapeutic models: the use of antimetabolites introduces the wrong building blocks, or prevents synthesis of the correct ones, and alkylating agents simply hammer away at the completed DNA. Perhaps methods may be evolved to starve the cancer cell in the same way that asparaginase starves the leukemia cell. The role of combination therapy should be expanded with prospective protocols. The basic principle of multistep therapy is to set off cytolytic mechanisms that are strictly localized in cancer tissue. This approach should be explored.

The knowledge that may be contributed by applying the reverse transcriptase enzyme to the identification of viruses in human cancer is accumulating. If a virus is identified, antiviral remedies may work preventatively, but probably will have no effect on gross tumor.

Cellular engineering has been employed by Robert Good for the treatment of leukemias. In patients with primary immunodeficiency diseases, he is able to completely reconstitute the immunity system by transplanting bone marrow cells from matched donors. It is conceivable that this approach, coupled with very aggressive chemotherapy, can provide powerful new approaches to the management of solid tissue cancers.

Woodruff has reported that the ovary and the peritoneum of the abdominal cavity are mesothelial tissues. The question of whether the millet seed implants represent metastatic disease or multiple primaries has not yet been answered. Since the latter theory suggests a common stimulus to produce the multiple primaries, it is important to explore this suggestion. The common stimulus may enter the peritoneal cavity by way of the cervix, endometrial cavity, and tubes, or perhaps there is another common etiologic explanation. Epidemiologic evidence suggests that environmental factors are major etiologic factors in ovarian cancer. Because the highest rates for ovarian cancer are recorded in highly industrialized countries, it has been suggested that physical or chemical products of industry are major causes of these neoplasms. A major exception is highly industrialized Japan, which has one of the lowest rates of ovarian cancer in the world. A possible explanation is that the causative factors are present in higher concentrations in the environment in the United States than in Japan. This possibility is supported by the higher rates of cancer of the ovary in Japanese migrants and their offspring in the United States. The search for causative carcinogens is being focused on the immediate environment: food, personal customs, and the chemical carcinogens used in industry are being investigated. Of the main industrial products known or suspected of human carcinogenic activity, only asbestos and talc have been seriously considered. There is no hard data at this time to implicate them in ovarian cancer.

BIBLIOGRAPHY

Barber, H.R.K. (Ed.): Immunobiology for the Clinician. Wiley, New York, 1977.

De Vita, V.T., Todd, H., Wasserman, H.R. Young, R.C., Carter, S.K.: Prospectives on research in gynecologic oncology. Cancer (supplement) 38:509, 1976.

Fraccaro, M., Mannini, A., Tiepolo, L.: Karyotypic clonal evolution in a cystic adenoma of the ovary. Lancet 1:613, 1968.

Gelender, A.B., Cohen, J.A.: A review of cytogenetic studies of gynecologic neoplasms. Chicago Med. School Q. 32:59, 1973.

Greene, W.H., Marsh, J.C.: Infection in malignant disease: Diagnosis and treatment. Forum on infection. Clinical Views from Research and Practice 3:3, 1977.

Kayayama, K.P., Toews, H.A.: Chromosomes of metastatic ovarian carcinoma treated with a progestogen and alkylating agents. Am. J. Obstet. Gynecol. 104:997, 1969.

The National Health Education Committee: The Killers and Cripplers—Facts on Major Diseases in the United States Today. David McKay Company, New York, 1976, p.51.

Patau, K.: Identification of individual chromosomes, especially in man. Am. J. Genet. 12:250, 1960.

Rapp. F.: Herpes viruses and cancer. Adv. Cancer Res. 19:265, 1974.

Rashad, M.N., Fathalla, M.F., Kerr, M.G.: Sex chromatin and chromosome analysis in ovarian teratomas. Am. J. Obstet. Gynecol. 96:461, 1966.

Slot, E.: Karyologic study of the cancer of the ovary and the cancer cells in the ascitic effusion. Neoplasma 14:3, 1967.

Spiegelman, S., Axel, R., Baxt, W., Kufe, D., Schlom, J.: Human cancer and animal viral oncology. Cancer 34:1406, 1974.

Süss, R., Kinzel, V., Scribner, J.D.: Cancer Experiments and Concepts. Springer-Verlag, New York, 1973.

Wakonig-Vaartaja, T., Auersperg, N.: Cytogenetics of gynecologic neoplasms. Clin. Obstet. Gynecol. 13:813, 1970.

Wakonig-Vaartaja, R., Hughes, D.T.: Chromosome studies in 36 gynecological tumors of the cervix, corpus uteri, ovary, vagina and vulva. Eur. J. Cancer 3:263, 1967.

Weiss, R.R., Richart, R.M., Okagaki, T.: DNA content of mucinous tumors of the ovary. Am. J. Obstet. Gynecol. 103:409, 1969.

Glossary

Accessible antigens. Antigens of self that are in contact with antibody-forming tissues and with the host, which is normally tolerant.

Active immunization. Direct immunization of the intact individual or immunocompetent cells derived from the individual and returned to him.

Active immunotherapy. May be divided into two groups: specific immunogens and nonspecific adjuvants. Active specific immunotherapy is attempted by the immunization of a tumor-bearing patient with autologous tumor cells that have been altered chemically or by radiation. Nonspecific immunotherapy attempts to augment antitumor immunologic activity with nonspecific stimulants such as BCG or phytohemagglutinin.

Adaptation. The process whereby protection accorded to a foreign graft from the immune reaction of the recipient renders the graft less vulnerable to immunologic attack by the host.

Adoptive immunization. The transfer of immunity from one individual to another by means of specifically immune lymphoid cells or materials derived from such cells which are capable of transferring specific immunologic information to the recipients' lymphocytes.

Adjuvant. A substance which, when mixed with an antigen, enhances its antigenicity.

Agglutinin. An antibody that produces aggregation or agglutination of a particulate or insoluble antigen.

Allergy. The specifically altered state of reactivity of a host following exposure to an allergen. The term applies to either hypersensitivity or immunity.

Allogeneic. Pertaining to genetically dissimilar individuals of the same species or referring to tissues originating in different individuals of the same species or in members of a different inbred strain.

Allogeneic inhibition. In vitro damage to cells caused by contact with genetically dissimilar cells. When two antigenetically different lymphocytes are cultured in the presence of phytohemagglutinin (a substance which activates lymphocytes), there is a mutually damaging effect—the opposite of syngeneic preference.

Alpha fetoprotein (AFP). A serum protein synthesized in the fetus by perivascular hepatic parenchymal cells and found in a high percentage of patients with hepatomas and malignant teratomas, especially of the endodermal sinus type. It is present in concentrations up to 400 mg/100 ml in early fetal life, falling to less than

3 μg/100 ml in adults. Increased levels may be detected in the serum of adults with hepatoma (80% positive) and teratoma (40% positive) and may be used to follow the progress of the disease.

Alpha ray. A stream of alpha particles, which are helium nuclei.

Anamnestic response. A recall mechanism; the accelerated response of antibody production to an antigen which occurs in an animal that has previously responded to the antigen; synonymous with secondary immune response.

Anergy. A deficiency in the response to agents which normally induce an immune response, especially delayed hypersensitivity.

Aneuploid. Having a chromosome number that is not an exact multiple of the haploid number.

Antibody. A specific globulin (immunoglobulin) produced in response to stimulation by an antigen and capable of reacting specifically with that antigen. A paratope is the site or area on an antibody molecule complementary to the epitope on the antigen molecule. The number of paratopes per molecule is the valency of the antibody.

Antigen. A substance that is capable of inducing the production of specific immunity. The antigens may be extrinsic (an antigen that is not a constituent of the cell), intrinsic (an antigen that is a constituent of the cell), or occult (a self-antigen that does not reach antibody-forming tissues).

Antigen determinant (epitope). The small three-dimensional configuration of the everted surface of the antigen molecule which combines with a specific antibody. The total number of antigen determinants per antigen molecule is the valence of that antigen.

Antiserum. A serum containing antibodies and obtained from animals exposed to antigen(s) of a certain nature.

Atopy. An hereditary predisposition to develop immediate-type hypersensitivity on contact with certain antigens (atopens or reagins).

Autoantigen. A substance in a person's tissue to which he or she is immunologically sensitive.

Autochthonous. Tissues of any sort originating in the same host or tumor borne by the host of origin.

Autologous. Derived from the subject itself.

Axiom. An established principle, for example, that a neoplasm is named from its most differentiated portion and graded from its least differentiated parts.

B cell or B lymphocyte. A bone marrow cell. These cells mediate humoral immunity and are thymus-independent cells. In the avian species, B cells are derived from the bursa of Fabricius. In man, no discrete bursa has been identified.

Bergonie and Tribondeau 1906. The radiosensitivity of cells and tissues in proportion to their reproductive capacity and in inverse proportion to their degree of differentiation.

Binding site. Antibody-combining sites and other sites of specific attachment of macromolecules to one another.

Blast transformation. The transformation of small lymphocytes with minimal cytoplasm, condensed nuclei, and few cytoplasmic organelles into a lymphoblast characterized by abundant cytoplasm, numerous organelles, and a large nucleus with multiple nucleoli. Blast transformation may be induced by a number of mitogens.

Blocking factor (enhancement antibody). A humoral antibody or an antigen-antibody complex that acts as a noncytotoxic antibody. Instead of damaging the cell, it coats it with a protective covering so that neither complement nor killer lymphocytes can attack the cell.

Brachytherapy. (from the Greek *brachy*—short, and *therapy*—treatment). A term used to distinguish the therapeutic use of encapsulated radionuclides *close to* the tumor from their use *at a distance from* the tumor. For the latter, the term *teletherapy* (from the Greek *tele*—far) has been used.

Cancer. (From the Latin *cancri*—crab). An inclusive term used to describe a variety of malignant neoplasms.

Cancerous growth. A cancerous growth measuring 1 cubic centimeter (approximately 1/16 cubic inch) and weighing about 1 gram (approximately 1/30 ounce) is about the smallest that can be detected by palpation or by x-rays, yet it contains about one billion cancer cells, each perhaps capable of originating a new focus of disease.

Carcinoembryonic antigen (CEA). An antigen found originally in fetal tissues of endodermal origin as well as in malignant tumors of adult tissues of endodermal origin. It probably results when a gene is derepressed by some stimulus. Since other tissues have been found to contain CEA, it is possible that the CEA molecule has more than one antigenic surface determinant.

Carcinoma: In modern medicine, all malignant tumors.

Cell-mediated immunity (CMI). Specific immunity that is mediated by small lymphocytes. They are thymus-dependent cells and are referred to as T cells, as opposed to the thymus-independent cells which are called B cells. The T cells are probably the most important cells in cancer immunity and organ rejection.

Central venous pressure. The following data have been helpful in interpreting central venous pressure (measured in centimeters of water), assuming there is no significant abnormality of cardiac output:
0—5 cm H_2O pressure=hypovolemia
6—12 cm H_2O pressure=normovolemia
over 12 cm H_2O pressure=hypervolemia

Chalones. A group of naturally occurring substances which are sensitized by cells and appear to be importantly involved in the regulation of the cell division as well as in differentiation of such normal cell types as epidermal cells, liver and kidney cells, granulocytes, and certain other cell types. Since the antimitotic effect of these substances is tissue-specific and since they are essentially nontoxic, they would appear to represent an almost ideal group of substances for use in the suppression of growth of those tumors that have lost the ability to synthesize their own chalones but remain sensitive to their inhibitory effects.

Chimerism. A state in which two or more genetically different populations of cells coexist.

Chromosome. Carriers of genetic information composed of DNA on a framework of protein. They are in the cell nucleus and are visible in a dividing cell as deeply staining rod-shaped or J-shaped structures.

Citrate intoxication. Intoxication characterized by hypotension, a narrow pulse pressure, and elevated left ventricular end diastolic and central venous pressures.

Clonal selection theory of acquired immunity of Burnet. A theory which suggests that immunity and antibody production are functions of clones of mesenchymal cells. Each clone is able to react immunologically with a small number of antigens, and each cell is immunologically competent because it carries on its surface a receptor that is able to react with a given antigen.

Clone. A population of cells derived from a single cell by asexual division.

Cobalt 60. A radioactive isotope with a half-life of 5.3 years which emits beta and gamma radiations (1.17 and 1.33 Mev) and is used as teletherapy.

Common epithelial ovarian cancers. These cancers are composed of one or more of several types of epithelium and stroma in a variety of combinations. They are generally considered to be derived from the surface epithelium (mesothelium) covering the ovary and from the underlying ovarian stroma. The word *common* has been applied because most ovarian tumors belong in this general category.

A. *Serous tumors* are composed of epithelium resembling that of the Fallopian tube or the surface epithelium of the ovary. Ciliated epithelium is found on the benign tumors but rarely in the presence of cancer. Psammoma bodies may be present and any mucus produced is extracellular.

B. *Mucinous tumors* are composed of tumors whose epithelial element includes a prominent component of mucin-filled cells. The epithelial may resemble endocervical or enteric epithelium, occasionally containing argentaffin cells and rarely Paneth cells. From time to time the question is raised whether these tumors should be included among the germ cell tumors as teratomas. The differential diagnosis should include metastatic adenocarcinoma from the large bowel.

C. *Endometrioid tumors* have the microscopic features of one or more of the typical forms of endometrial neoplasia. A small number of endometrioid tumors can be shown to arise in endometriosis, but the demonstration of such an origin is not required for the diagnosis. Endometrioid carcinomas may have a markedly papillary pattern, which is unusual in carcinomas of the endometrium.

D. *Clear cell (mesonephroid) tumors* are composed of cells containing glycogen and resemble those of the renal cell carcinoma and/or the hobnail or pig-shaped cells lining small cysts and tubules. Hobnail cells are characterized by scant cytoplasm and large nuclei that project into the lumen. The clear cell tumor must be distinguished from the endodermal sinus tumor, the dysgerminoma, and the lipid cell tumor.

Complement. A system of serologically nonspecific proteins present in fresh normal serum which are necessary for the lysis or death of cellular antigens in the presence of antibody.

Concomitant tumor immunity. The ability to reject a second tumor graft while the first tumor graft continues to grow. A piece of a tumor removed and implanted close to the original tumor will usually continue to grow, while the same piece of tumor transplanted at a distance from the original tumor may be rejected.

Curie. The quantity of any radioisotope which disintegrates at the rate of 3.7×10^{10} disintegrations per second. Subunits of the curie (C) unit are the millicurie (μCi) = 1/1000 of a C; microcurie (μCi) = 1/1000 of a mCi; and millimicrocurie (μCi) = 1/1000 of a μCi.

Cytophilic antibody. A globulin component of immune serum which becomes attached in vitro to certain normal cells in such a way that these cells are subsequently capable of specifically absorbing antigens.

Deblocking antibody. An antibody capable of overcoming the inhibitory effect of blocking factor, thereby permitting immunologic destruction of malignant cells.

Delayed hypersensitivity. See *Cell-mediated immunity.*

Dinitrochlorobenzene (DNCB). A drug used to test for cell-mediated immunity. When applied to the skin it acts as a hapten attaching to a protein in the skin, producing an antigen that has the potential to sensitize lymphocytes. In 2 weeks the challenge produces a marked local response in patients with good cell-mediated immunity.

Disseminated intravascular coagulation (DIC). Characterized by a triad of thrombocytopenia, hypofibrinogenemia, and lysis of a blood clot within 2 hours.

Electrophilic atom. An electron-deficient atom, for example, a carcinogen. See *Nucleophilic atom.*

Enhancement antibody. See *Blocking factor.*

Epidemiology. Cancer epidemiology seeks to correlate differences in the incidence of different types of cancer with already established differences in the external or internal environments of the persons developing these cancers; for example, the relationship identified between cigarette smoking and lung cancer.

Epigenetic change. A change due to an alteration of a nongenetic biochemical process which sometimes affects the hereditary material. It is theoretically a reversible process.

Epithelial ovarian cancers. See *Common epithelial ovarian cancers.*

Epitope. See *Antigen determinant.*

Established tumor. In tests of substances for antigrowth activity against transplantable tumors in animals, the test substance is sometimes given before there is any visible growth of the tumor. If, on the other hand, the tumor implant is allowed to grow before the test substance is administered, it is referred to as *established.*

Etiology. Cancer etiology is the study of the causes of cancer. Its ultimate goal is cancer prevention. Three types of agents have now been shown to cause cancers: chemicals, radiation, and viruses. Of these, two (chemicals and radiation) clearly cause cancer in man, and the third (viruses) are highly suspect on the basis of present knowledge.

Ewing's histologic grading. Ewing influenced many pathologists when he presented his material using only three grades. In the Ewing-inspired grades, Broders' grades III and IV are combined and called grade III. The histologic classification is based on the uniformity or lack of uniformity of the cells, whether the nucleus is regular or not, the ratio between the nucleus and cytoplasm, the number and size of the nucleoli, and the number of mitoses per highpower field.

Favored or privileged site. The anatomic region where foreign tissues tend to survive because of the diminished ability of an immunologic reaction to be incited there.

Forbidden clone. A hypothetical clone of immunologically competent cells with specificity for self-antigens which, according to the clonal selection theory, has been suppressed in fetal life and which may regain activity in adult life and cause autoimmune disease.

Freund's adjuvant. *Complete:* Freund's water-in-oil emulsion of mineral oil, plant waxes, and killed tubercle bacilli used to incorporate with antigen to stimulate antibody production. *Incomplete:* Freund's mixture without tubercle bacilli.

Gene. An elementary germinal unit, situated in chromosomes, which carries an hereditary transmissible character. It is composed of distinctly arranged deoxyribonucleic acid chains. Histocompatibility genes are special entities, the nature of which determines the fate of grafts.

Genotype. The sum of the genes of an organism.

Germ cell tumors. Undifferentiated tumors; in some, extraembryonic structures predominate; in others the predominant structures are immature and/or mature structures which may be derived from any or all of the three embryonic layers— ectoderm, mesoderm, and endoderm.

A. *Dysgerminoma* is composed of germ cells that have not differentiated to form embryonic or extraembryonic structures. The tumor has a uniform appearance and is composed of large, rounded, clear cells which resemble primordial germ cells, both morphologically and histochemically. Its stroma is almost always infiltrated with lymphocytes and often contains granulomas similar to those of sarcoid.

B. *Teratomas*

1. *Extraembryonal forms:* The endodermal sinus tumor is composed of embryonal cells lining a network of spaces. The most specific feature is the presence within some of the spaces of isolated papillary projections containing single blood vessels and having a peripheral lining of neoplastic cells. The tumor resembles the endodermal sinuses of the rat placenta. It contains intracellular and extracellular hyaline bodies resembling Russell bodies. When, on rare occasions, these vesicles form a major portion of the neoplasm, it is called a polyvesicular vitelline tumor.

2. *Choriocarcinoma* is a rare tumor composed of both cytotrophoblast and syncytiotrophoblast. It may be associated with precocious puberty.

3. *Adult teratoma* is composed exclusively of mature (adult) structures. It may be solid or cystic. The cystic is commonly called a dermoid. It is made up mainly of ectodermal elements but may contain endodermal and mesodermal tissue.

4. *Embryonal teratoma* is one that contains immature (embryonal) structures. Mature tissue may be present as well. The tumor is highly malignant and usually radioresistant. *Polyembryonic embryoma* is a very unusual and poorly differentiated form of embryonal teratoma. Myriads of early embryos make up a large portion of the tumor.

5. *Struma ovarii* is a teratoma in which thyroid tissue is exclusively present or constitutes a grossly recognizable component of a more complex teratoma.

6. *Carcinoids* arise most often from respiratory or gastrointestinal epithelium in a dermoid cyst, but may develop within a solid teratoma or a mucinous cystic tumor.

C. *Gonadal stromal tumors*

1. *Female type:* The granulosal cell tumor is the most common. It may contain not only granulosa cells but also varying numbers of spindle-shaped, collagen- producing cells, elements resembling theca cells, and lutein cells. A variety of microscopic patterns may be encountered: microfollicular, macrofollicular, trabecular, cyclindromatous, insular, gyriform, solid-tubular, and sarcomatoid or diffuse.

2. *Male type:* The Sertoli-Leydig cell tumor contains Sertoli and Leydig cells of varying degrees of maturity; indifferent gonadal cells of embryonal appearance are present in certain cases. The designation *arrhenoblastoma* has been abandoned because not all of these tumors produce masculinization.

D. *Gynandroblastoma* is a very rare tumor in which collections of granulosa cells with typical Call-Exner bodies coexist with hollow tubules lined by Sertoli cells.

E. *Gonadoblastoma,* a rare ovarian cancer, is composed of germ cells (dysgerminoma) and gonadal stromal cells (granulosa-Sertoli). Sex chromatin studies usually show a negative nuclear pattern (46 XY) or a sex chromosome mosaicism (XO/XY). Most patients are intersexual with phenotype female habitus, amenorrheic, and possibly virilized. The malignancy rate is very low.

Gold, radioactive (^{198}Au). A radioactive isotope with a half-life of 2.7 days which emits beta (960 Kev) and gamma (412 Kev) radiation; used in small sources in a colloidal form to suppress malignant serous effusions and to control free-floating cancer cells in the peritoneal cavity.

Graft-versus-host reaction. In the presence of an immune-deficient host, the graft may produce lymphocytes that react to the host antigen, producing hepato-splenomegaly, lymphopenia, diarrhea, and skin rash. In the very young a disease called *runt disease* (allogeneic disease), which develops after injection of allogeneic lymphocytes into immunologically immature experimental animals, produces a picture similar to the one outlined above plus the failure to thrive and often death.

Half value layer (HVL). The thickness of a specific material which reduces the flux of radiation by one-half;. a function of voltage, filtration, and target material, it is used as a rough gauge of radiation quality.

Haploid. Having a single set of unpaired chromosomes in each nucleus, a characteristic of gametes.

Hapten. A partial antigen which contains at least one of the determinant groups of an antigen. It can react specifically with antibodies, but in itself it does not induce the formation of antibodies unless it is complexed with a carrier molecule such as a protein.

Helper factor. Sensitized T-lymphocyte subpopulations release a helper factor which enables immunocompetent B cells to respond to antigens which they would otherwise be unable to recognize. The stimulated B lymphocytes differentiate into plasma cells, which are the main producers of antibody. The helper factor also stimulates the B lymphocyte to produce a variant of the B cell, the *killer (K) cell,* which is able to attack tumor cells only after the tumor cells have been exposed to specific antibody. Complement is not required for this action. See *Killer cell.*

Hepatitis-associated antigen (Australian antigen). This antigen (Au antigen), first detected in the serum of an Australian aborigine, has been detected in the sera of patients during the incubation period and early clinical course of serum or transfusion hepatitis, but not in the sera of patients with a short incubation form of infectious hepatitis. The serum of patients carrying the antigen has been shown, under the electron microscope, to contain aggregates of pleomorphic particles and tubules. The aggregates have been interpreted to be antigen-antibody complexes, and the particles are thought to be antigen derived from the virus causing the infection.

Heterophil. Pertaining to antigenic specificity shared between species.

Heterozygosity. The occupancy of dissimilar genes in the same chromosome.

Histocompatibility. The ability to accept transplants of tissue from another animal of the same species. Such ability depends on the identical genetic constitution of donor and recipient.

Histologic grading. The Broders classification consisted of four numerical grades (I, II, III and IV) for both epidermoid and adenocarcinoma of the cervix. The basis for this classification is the well-known observation that the degree of malignancy keeps pace with the degree of cell differentiation, grade I being the most highly differentiated and grade IV the most immature. The original Broders grading method is cumbersome to apply, because as many as 13 different cytologic characteristics have to be observed and evaluated. The following factors are recorded for each grade: epithelial pearls, individual keratinized cells, intercellular bridges, tumor giant cells, and mitosis per high-power field. Most pathologists now use a simplified version. See *Ewing's histologic grading.*

Histologic type and grading. The parameters which classify the microscopic characteristics of the tumor.

HL-A antigen (human leukocyte antigen). A genetic locus containing two closely linked groups of several alleles, i.e. subloci. It is present on the cell membranes of all nucleated cells and plays a major role in determining graft rejection.

Horizontal transmission of viruses. Transmission of viruses between individual hosts of the same generation. See *Vertical transmission of viruses.*

Host. An organism whose body serves to sustain a graft; loosely interchangeable with *recipient.*

Humoral immunity. Pertaining to the body fluids, in contrast to cellular fluids. It is initiated by the thymus-independent B cells. These B lymphocytes proliferate and differentiate into plasma cells that secrete immunoglobulins (IgG, IgM, IgA, IgD, and IgE).

Hybrid. An animal whose parents belong to different species. Ordinarily procreation is dependent on a fixed sexual role of one or the other species partners. When it occurs, regardless of the sexual identity of the mated species, the offspring is a reciprocal hybrid (mutual hybrid).

Immunogen. An antigen that induces a specific immunologic response.

Immunologic surveillance. Described by Sir F. MacFarlane Burnet, effective immunological surveillance depends on the presence of tumor-specific antigenic determinants on the surfaces of neoplastic cells, which enable these altered cells to be recognized as nonself and to be destroyed by immunologic reactions.

Immunoreaction. Reaction between antigen and its antibody.

Interferon. A protein released by cells in response to virus infection. It represents nonspecific immunity.

Killer cell (K cell). Sensitized T lymphocytes produce a helper factor that acts on the immunocompetent cell to produce a population of cells, possibly variants of the B cell, termed killer cells (K cells), which are able to attack tumor cells that have been exposed to a specific antibody. Unlike the usual humoral antibody (immunoglobulin) response, complement is not needed to destroy the cell.

Krukenberg tumor. A metastasis of distinctive appearance characterized by the presence of mucus-filled signet-ring cells accompanied by a sarcoma-like proliferation of the ovarian stroma. This tumor is usually secondary to gastric cancer, but may originate in any organ in which mucinous carcinomas arise, including the breast and intestine. On rare occasions a tumor with the pattern of a Krukenberg tumor appears to be primary in the ovary.

Linear energy transfer (LET). A measure of the average rate of energy loss along the track of an ionizing particle, expressed as energy units per unit track length. It is the energy released (usually in kev) per micron of medium (tissue) along the track of any ionizing particle.

Locus. The precise location of a gene on a chromosome. Different forms of the gene (alleles) are always found at the same position on the chromosome. A complex locus is a locus within which mutation and recombination can occur at more than one site.

Lymphokine. Substances released bysensitized lymphocytes when they come in contact with the antigen to which they are sensitized. There are at least four mediators of cellular immunity, including transfer factor (TF), lymphocyte-transforming activity (LTA), migration inhibition factor (MIF), and lymphotoxins.

Lysogeny. A virus joins up with the DNA of the cell and is carried along through many generations. It is inactive unless some noxious agent stimulates it to become active. In *lysogeny*, the virius is part of the DNA of the cell, and, in *transduction*, some of the DNA is carried along as part of the virus.

Macrophage. A large mononuclear phagocyte; in the tissues this cell may be designated a histiocyte and in the blood a monocyte. Macrophages in the spleen, lymph nodes and thymus are known as the sinus-lining macrophages (sometimes called reticulum cells). An antigen must contact or pass through a macrophage before it can become a processed antigen with the ability to encounter and then sensitize a small lymphocyte.

Macrophage activating factor (MAF). The sensitized T lymphocytes release a nonspecific macrophage activating factor which creates a cytotoxic population of macrophages that appears to distinguish malignant from normal cells, killing only malignant ones.

Migration inhibition factor (MIF). A lymphokine produced when a sensitized lymphocyte is cultured in the presence of an antigen to which it is sensitized. It inhibits the migration of these lymphocytes.

Mitogen. A substance that induces lymphocytes to undergo blast transformation, mitosis, and cell division (causing mitosis or cell division).

Mixed lymphocyte (leukocyte) culture (MLC). The transformation of small lymphocytes to blast cells, with synthesis of DNA, in mixed cultures of blood leukocytes from normal allogeneic individuals. The magnitude of the reaction reflects the degree of disparity between histocompatibility antigens of the two donors. In identical twins, neither set stimulates the other, whereas in unrelated pairs there is almost always stimulation of each cell by the other. The degree of stimulation is analyzed either morphologically by blast transformation or biochemically by measuring tritiated thymidine incorporation into newly synthesized DNA.

Mosaic. An individual composed of two or more cell lines but from the same species. This can come about either through somatic mutation or by grafting cells between individuals of a very close genetic constitution, such as dizygotic twins.

Nuclear grade. The nuclei of the tumor cells are graded from 1 to 3 according to the classification of Black and Speer; grade 1: markedly enlarged, irregular in outline with chromatin clumping and prominent nucleoli; grade 2: intermediate degree of differentiation; grade 3: similar in size and appearance to each other and to normal ovarian tissue when present. Grade 1 is the most anaplastic and grade 3 the least anaplastic.

Nucleophilic atom. An atom with excess electrons. The information-containing macromolecules of the cell (DNA, RNA, and protein) are relatively rich in nucleophilic sites and, in those cases that have been adequately studied, derivatives of chemical carcinogens have been found to be firmly bound to the

DNA, RNA, and protein of target tissues. Furthermore, in some cases, susceptibility to cancer formation by chemical carcinogens has been correlated with the kinds and amounts of these macromolecule-bound carcinogens.See *Electrophilic atom.*

Nude mice (nu nu mice). Mice born with a congenital absence of the thymus. The blood and thymus-dependent areas of the lymph nodes and spleen are depleted of lymphocytes. These mice are homozygous for the gene "nude"—which is abbreviated *Nu,* hence *nu nu*—and they have no hair. They should be distinguished from mice carrying other genes that cause a lack of hair, e.g. shaven, *sha;* hairless, *hr;* bare, *br;* hair loss, *hl;* etc. All of these latter strains have normal thymuses.

Ovary. A *supernumerary ovary* is one which is independent of and equal in size to the normal ovary. It is extremely rare.
Accessory ovaries are usually attached to the normal gland by peritoneal bands in the mesovarium or adjacent part of the broad ligament, near the hilum of the ovary. They have clinical significance if they undergo pathologic changes or when bilateral oophorectomy is carried out; their presence may result in continued ovarian activity. Accessory ovaries *occur in about 3% of women.*
Ectopic ovaries may be congenital or acquired, but the aquired type is much more common. Congenital displacement may be due to nondescent, a phenomenon by which the ovary remains above the pelvic brim, or it may be due to the ovary having been pulled into the inguinal canal or large labia by the gubernaculum. The acquired type is common and may follow pregancy with prolapse of the ovary into the cul-de-sac.

Overgrowth stimulating factor (OSF). This factor can cause normal cells in culture to adopt the appearance and growth habit of the transformed cell. Stimulated cells revert to normal when the overgrowth stimulating factor is removed.

Oxygen enhancement ratio (OER). The ratio of the radiation dose under anoxic conditions to the dose under fully oxygenated conditions required to produce an equivalent effect. The oxygen enhancement ratio (OER)for most mammalian cells is about 3.

Paratope. See *Antibody.*

Passive transfer of immunity. The transfer of specific antibody from one individual to another.

Penumbra. The radiation just outside and adjacent to the full beam arising from the finite size of the source; its usage usually includes components from scatter in tissue or from incomplete beam collimation.

Phosphorus (^{32}P). A beta emitter with a maximum energy of 1.7 Mev and a half-life of 14.2 days, which may be given orally,intravenously, or intraperitoneally. It is maximally incorporated into cells with short turnover times, and is used to suppress malignant serous effusions and to control free-floating cancer cells in the peritoneal cavity.

Phytohemagglutinins. Lectins extracted from the red kidney bean, *Phaseolus vulgaris* or *P. communis.* They can be purified to yield a glycoprotein mitogen, which stimulates lymphocyte transformation and causes agglutination of certain red cells. Phytohemagglutinins provide a method for estimating the pool of thymus-dependent lymphocytes (T cells).

PMPO syndrome (postmenopausal ovary syndrome). Palpation of what is interpreted as a normal-sized ovary in the premenopausal woman represents an ovarian tumor in the postmenopausal woman.

Pneumocystitis carinii. An example of a parasite of low-grade virulence which presents a clinical problem only in the *immunologically compromised* host. The organism induces a pneumonitis with characteristic clinical and pathologic findings. Three groups of susceptible hosts have been defined: (1) premature or debilitated infants, (2) individuals with primary immunologic deficiency disorders, and (3) individuals with a malignancy or who are receiving immunosuppressive therapy and who demonstrate an immunologic deficit. There is an increasing state of dyspnea, progressive cyanosis, and a dry, nonproductive cough. Most remarkable is the lack of systemic reaction to this infection, and many patients are usually dyspneic and cyanotic, even in the absence of fever, malaise, or anorexia. The laboratory findings include the demonstration of a ventilation perfusion deficit, with a relatively normal pH and pCO_2 and a low pCO_2. Serologic techniques for the diagnosis of the diseases are hindered in humans, because most affected individuals have immunologic deficiency states and are therefore incapable of an antibody response.

Pokeweed mitogen (PWM). A mitogen extracted from the pokeweed plant which can be purified to yield a glycoprotein. The pokeweed mitogen stimulates blast formation of both B and T cells.

Prophylactic immunization. Immunization of an individual against a causative agent (e.g., a virus) or tumor-specific antigen,before any natural encounter with the agent or tumor.

Rad. A unit of absorbed dose of ionizing radiation equivalent to the absorption of 100 ergs per gram of irradiated material.

Radioactivity, artificial. Emission of radiant energy arising from the breakdown of nuclei which have been energetically unstable, for example, ^{60}Co and $^{137}C_5$.

Radioactivity, natural. Emission of radiant energy arising from the breakdown of nuclei which are unstable in their natural states, for example, radium.

Reverse transcriptase (RNA-dependent DNA polymerase). This recently isolated factor can transcribe the base sequence of a viral RNA onto a DNA strand, in vitro. It is now possible to test human cancers for association with any one of a number of RNA viruses.

Second look operation. The reoperation of a patient at a stated time without evidence of any clinical disease.

Selective IgG deficiency. A deficiency associated with a variety of disorders, but most frequently with diseases of an autoimmune nature. The immunoelectrophoretic pattern shows absence of IgA. Cellular immunity is intact, and all other immunoglobulins are present, e.g. IgG, IgM. IgD, and IgE. Selective IgG deficiency affects 1 in 700 individuals.

Sequestered antigen. Any antigen or antigenic determinant that is hidden from contact with immunologically competent cells or antibody and thus cannot stimulate an immune response. They may be intracellular antigens or hidden determinants on cell surfaces or on soluble molecules.

Serology. The study of antigen-antibody reactions in vitro.

Serum sickness reaction. A systemic allergy to the administration of a large amount of serum or purified foreign protein. Its appearance coincides with, and is caused by, the interaction of newly formed antibody with excess antigen circulating in the blood and tissue fluids.

Shock lung. An entity which has long been confused with such pathologic diagnoses as bronchopneumonia, patchy atelectasis, and agonal changes. Pulmonary edema can be the result of sepsis, fat embolism, cardiac failure, lung contusion, or oxygen toxicity. The resulting pulmonary insufficiency is a major cause of death in injured patients and patients receiving intensive care. A single cause for shock lung has not been described, and any or all of the above may be implicated.

Specific stimulation. The utilization of tumor cells or their antigenic products for immunization directed specifically towards that tumor or other tumors sharing the same antigens.

Staging of ovarian cancer. A clinically determined estimate of the extent of the disease and the size of the tumor, whereas histologic type and grading classify the cancer's microscopic character.

Stem (primitive) cell. A cell which is capable of proliferation and may give rise to differentiated cells.

Stromal reactions. Chabon, Takenchi, and Sommers have employed a stromal evaluation in a breast study. The stroma of each epithelial ovarian cancer was graded according to the number of lymphocytes, plasma cells, and polymorphonuclear leukocytes present. Lymphocytes, plasma cells, and polymorphonuclear infiltration in the stroma and around small veins were graded 0 to 3: 0 = none, 1 = 2 = moderate, and 3 = marked.

Supervoltage radiation. High-energy radiation with ill-defined limits usually extending beyond energies which no longer are preferentially absorbed in bone (i.e. 500 Kev) to peak energies of several Mev.

Suppressor T cells. An important set of feedback controls, centered around sensitized T lymphocytes, through which inhibitory populations of these cells suppress the production of sensitized lymphocytes and antibody-forming cells.

Syngeneic. Pertaining to genetically identical or nearly identical animals such as identical twins or highly inbred animals.

Syngeneic preference. Unlike allogeneic inhibition, syngeneic preference represents improved growth in syngeneic recipients.

Teletherapy. Treatment with the radiation source at a distance from the body. See *Brachytherapy.*

Template theory. An instructive theory of antibody production in which it was supposed that an antigen was taken into a cell and acted directly as a template that determined the shape of the combining site of the antibody which is produced by that cell. The theory was originally proposed by Haurowitz, Mudd, and Alexander.

Tests for evaluating a clotting disorder. *Bleeding time* can be unreliable because of variations in puncture technique; it may also be abnormal because of platelets deficient in number or function or because of von Willebrand's disease. Normal= *less than 4 minutes..*
Clotting time (glass) is an insensitive test. It does, however, test for all intrinsic coagulation factors except VII, XIII, and platelets. Normal = less than 15 and usually less than 10 minutes.
Prothrombin time (one-stage) is a reliable and sensitive test for the extrinsic system coagulation factors (V, VII, and X) as well as for fibrinogen (I) and prothrombin (II). Normal = less than 20 seconds (check control value).
Prothrombin consumption tests are reliable in testing platelet function (unlike bleeding time) and have acceptable sensitivity for the intrinsic system coagulation factors (unlike the clotting time). This test checks V, VIII, IX, X, XI, and XII. Normal = less than 20% (alternatively expressed as greater than 80%).

Partial thromboplastin time (PTT) (activated partial thromboplastin time) is a sensitive screening test for detection of alterations in coagulation mechanisms such as previously undiagnosed hemophilia, various coagulation deficiencies, and circulating anticoagulants, Normal = 20 to 45 seconds.
Thrombin time, when prolonged, indicates over-heparinization, defibrination, or fibrinolysis.
The quantity of platelets can be rapidly estimated from a smear. Platelet counts considerably below 100,000 may implicate massive bank blood transfusions as a cause of bleeding. Normal = over 100,000.

Tetraploid. Having four times the haploid number of chromosomes.

Therapeutic immunization. Any therapy initiated after the patient shows clinical manifestations of malignancy.

T lymphocyte (T cell). Lymphocytes that have matured and differentiated under thymic influence are termed thymic-dependent lymphocytes. These cells are primarily involved in the mediation of cellular immunity, as well as in tissue and organ rejection.

Tolerance. Failure of the antibody response to a potential antigen following exposure to the antigen. Tolerance commonly results from prior exposure to antigens.

Transcription stage. The transcribing of genetic information from nucleus to cytoplasm, i.e., from DNA to RNA by messenger RNA.

Transduction. This form of recombination depends upon bacteriophage for its completion. A phage particle can carry some DNA from the lysed cell in which it was formed to the new cell it infects. There, instead of multiplying, it remains inactive, and the transferred bacterial DNA may become incorporated into the DNA of the new host. Apparently only a small portion of the genetic material undergoes transduction at any one time. In *Salmonella,* a genus of bacteria to which many pathogenic intestinal bacteria belong, the ability to resist certain drugs can be transferred by transduction. See *Lysogeny.*

Transfer factor. A heat-labile, dialyzable extract of human lymphocytes that is capable of conferring specific antigen reactivity to the donor. See *Lymphokine.*

Transformation. The process that occurs when a bacteria absorbs the DNA of a dead bacterium and incorporates some of it into its own genetic constitution. The incorporated DNA is then transmitted to later generations. Usually only a small part of the genetic material is involved in transformation, and usually the process occurs only between members of the same species; however streptomycin resistance has been transferred in this way from pneumococci to streptococci.

Translation stage. The translation of the base sequence code in RNA into an amino acid sequence in proteins.

Tumor angiogenesis factor (TAF). The tumor angiogenesis factor represents the induction of the growth of blood vessels by a stimulant released by tumor cells. The growth of the tumor parallels the development of new blood vessels.

Vertical transmission of viruses. Transmission of viruses from one generation to the next, i.e., from mother to offspring. See *Horizontal transmission of viruses.*

Xenogeneic (heterologous). Pertaining to individuals of different species.

Index

314